The Children of Santa María Cauqué

International Nutrition Policy Series

General Editors
Nevin S. Scrimshaw, Massachusetts Institute of Technology International
Nutrition Planning and Policy Program, and Michael C. Latham, Cornell
University Program on International Nutrition and Development Policy.

Editorial Board
Lance Taylor, Massachusetts Institute of Technology; Eugene B. Skolnikoff,
Massachusetts Institute of Technology; Milton J. Esman, Cornell University;
and David L. Call, Cornell University.

1. *Morinda: An Economic Analysis of Malnutrition Among Young Children
in Rural India*, F. James Levinson, 1974

2. *The Children of Santa María Cauqué: A Prospective Field Study of Health
and Growth*, Leonardo J. Mata, 1978

All correspondence about submission of manuscripts and allied matters should be sent to
International Nutrition Policy Series, Mass. Inst. of Tech., 20A-222, 18 Vassar Street,
Cambridge, MA 02139. Correspondence about ordering books or subscribing to the
series should be sent to The MIT Press, 28 Carleton Street, Cambridge, MA 02142.

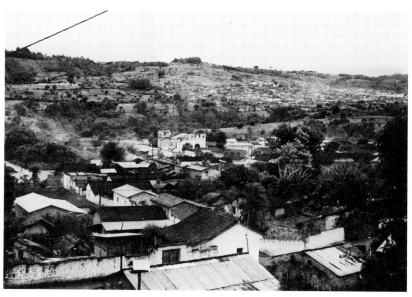

Santa María Cauqué, nestled in a little valley in the Guatemalan highlands. In the background the village of Santiago Sacatepéquez.

The Children of Santa María Cauqué:
A Prospective Field Study of Health and Growth

Leonardo J. Mata

The MIT Press
Cambridge, Massachusetts, and London, England

This book was set in IBM Composer Press Roman by The Blue Ridge Group, printed and bound by Halliday Lithograph Corporation in the United States of America.

Library of Congress Cataloging in Publication Data

Mata, Leonardo J
    The children of Santa María Cauqué.

    (International nutrition policy series ; 2)
    Bibliography: p. 363
    Includes index.
    1. Children—Care and hygiene—Guatemala—Santa María Cauqué—Longitudinal studies. 2. Children in Santa María Cauqué, Guatemala—Growth—Longitudinal studies. 3. Malnutrition in children—Guatemala—Santa María Cauqué—Longitudinal studies. 4. Communicable diseases in children—Guatemala—Santa María Cauqué—Longitudinal studies. I. Title. II. Series. [DNLM: 1. Child welfare—Guatemala. 2. Health surveys—Guatemala. 3. Indians, Central American. W1 IN827B v. 2 / WA320 M425c]
RJ103.G8M37   618.9'23'90097281   78–70
ISBN 0-262-13135-8

To John Everett Gordon
and to María Gabriela, Juan Luis, Adriana, and Eugenia Isabel

Contents

Series Foreword   x
Preface   xii
Acknowledgments   xv

PART I
FOUNDATIONS OF THE STUDY
Chapter 1
Foundations of the Study   3
Chapter 2
The Village and Its People   6

PART II
STUDY PLAN AND PROCEDURES
Chapter 3
Operational Procedures and Approach   43
Chapter 4
Operational Procedures and Analysis of Data   54

PART III
RESULTS
Chapter 5
Maternal Environment   95

Chapter 6
The Newborn Infant   121
Chapter 7
Maternal Factors and Fetal Growth   137
Chapter 8
Survival   152
Chapter 9
Growth and Development in Infancy and Early Childhood   167
Chapter 10
Feeding Practices   202
Chapter 11
Infection and Colonization of the Intestine   228
Chapter 12
Diseases and Disabilities   254
Chapter 13
Malnutrition   293
Chapter 14
Multivariate Analysis of Physical Growth   304

PART IV
**SYNOPSIS, INTERVENTIONS, PRIORITIES, AND FUTURE
ALTERNATIVES**
Chapter 15
Synopsis, Interventions, Priorities, and Future Alternatives   321

Appendix A
Staff   333
Appendix B
Advisors and Consultants   335
Appendix C
Code for Signs, Symptoms, Illnesses, Diseases, and Injuries, 1964-1972   337
Appendix D
Variables of the Cauqué Study   342
Appendix E
Anthropometric Data   345

References   363
Index   385

Series Foreword

The magnitude and complexity of the malnutrition problem and its relationship to national development have been increasingly recognized by governments in low-income and industrialized countries, bilateral and international assistance agencies, foundations, and the academic community. Although large-scale program success to date has been limited, a capacity, backed up by field experience, is being developed to address the problem and to carry out effective nutrition planning.

Unfortunately there has been no means of systematically making available to concerned persons information on alternative approaches to nutrition planning and programming and on actual nutrition intervention programs that have been attempted.

To meet this need, the MIT International Nutrition Planning and Policy Program and the Cornell University Program on International Nutrition and Development Policy jointly initiated the *International Nutrition Policy Series*. This continuing series will focus on two main categories of monographs: (1) national or regional planning studies, utilizing tools of the natural and social sciences to identify and refine appropriate nutrition policy instruments; and (2) reports and reviews of specific nutrition intervention programs, providing accounts of actual projects, information on projected costs and effectiveness, and evaluation of the impact and significance of such programs.

The editors and editorial board bring to the task both considerable professional competence in the natural and social sciences and a great deal of international experience. The board has set for itself the highest standards of excellence to assure a series that will be of professional quality and of value in the application and teaching of international nutrition policy.

Preface

This study of the natural history of health and growth of children was conceived in Boston, was born and grew in Guatemala, and matured in Seattle.
In Boston the concept of a study in a developing rural region and the plans
to carry it out were developed and fertilized by discussions with teachers and
friends. The choice of Guatemala for the field work was logical in view of my
own origin in Central America and a personal familiarity with the area. Later,
as the task got under way in Seattle of putting together the results from nine
years of observation in a little mountain village several thousand miles away,
my thoughts turned inevitably to the Mayan Indian villagers with whom I had
worked and to the circumstances that dictated the change in locale.

The move to Seattle was decided in large measure by the friendship and
technical help offered by John P. Fox and other colleagues at the School of
Public Health and Community Medicine of the University of Washington. A
main determinant, however, was the need to get away from administrative
and other obligations of my home base at the Institute of Nutrition of
Central America and Panama (INCAP) in Guatemala, and especially to avoid
the fascination of continued data gathering and the generation of new
research projects.

In a well-appointed office in Seattle, instead of in the field and laboratory,
with the comparative cold of a northern temperature climate substituting for
the sunny days of the "Land of Eternal Spring," I came to appreciate fully
my good fortune in having directed the studies in Santa María Cauqué and
being accepted as a friend by the people of that Indian village. My regular
visits to the community, close collaboration with a variety of field workers,

and personal participation in so many affairs of the village were the genuinely rewarding parts of that endeavor.

By standards of more advanced societies, the villagers of Santa María Cauqué would be characterized as primitive, in some respects barely emerging from the Middle Ages. Working with them, however, brought realization of a distinctive civilization that functions most humanely, of a community that conducts itself peacefully according to firm values, and with a sense of purpose that stems from the necessity to live, to create, to share with each other, and to suffer and die together—enviable qualities so frequently absent in many western societies.

Continued interaction with the villagers in their daily activities brought appreciation of a sobriety and maturity of behavior, yet an overriding graciousness never wholly marred by a necessarily stoic and austere life of hard work, much suffering, and death that so often comes so early. How wonderfully they accept, understand, and help not only their fellows but also the strangers who come to their community from another culture. They talk readily and easily, and greet friend, acquaintance, or traveler with a smile, offering hospitality and such food as they have amidst a dominant poverty.

Nine years of study and a growing familiarity with Santa María Cauqué changed earlier ideas of field workers in the village about society, man, and his environment, and particularly about what can best be done to remedy some of the health and social problems of this village and others like it.

Life in the village centers around an incredibly complex framework of traditional attitudes that permeate all spheres of existence, challenging the stand of those observers who conceive of the spiritual world of the Indian as simple, monotonous, and dull. The highly constructive attitudes of the Indian toward birth, mother-child interaction, and childrearing, the ceremonial cultivation of maize, and the deeply felt respect for authority all challenge that viewpoint. Life in the village is full of occupational and social activities in which practical life and routine are closely interwoven with spiritual, religious, and even superstitious elements. The complete pattern of life in villages such as Santa María Cauqué causes one to meditate on whether man is really better off in the supposedly more enlightened western industrial world. How much harm might be inflicted by recommending or implementing social or other interventions becomes a worry, once one gains insight into the ways of village life.

The outsider from another culture or another way of life is inevitably impressed with how well the Indian society is equipped for survival—past any extent one would anticipate. Through millennia, the Mayans and their descendents have survived natural and man-made disasters, once rising to a cultural eminence yet to be matched by many societies presently resident on the American continent. Now in cultural decline, the Indian tries to find his own destiny.

During their reproductive years Indian women have a succession of babies of whom all too many begin life with low birth weight. Somewhat more than a half of their children survive unbelievably adverse environmental conditions to become fit and hardworking young adults. They are of low stature yet capable of maintaining themselves with little more to eat than a dozen tortillas per day.

At an early age the men learn how to find water, whether from high in the mountains or deep in the ground. With soil and water they make adobe to build houses that protect them from heat and cold. They learn the traditions involved in the cultivation of maize, beans, and other plants. Above all, they grow up to respect and maintain the principles of village authority and of private property, and those that decide the important issues within a home. Boys are educated in these traditions with no shouting or beating. Physical punishment of children is rare.

The housewife is hardworking and devoted to her home, yet kind and gracious. Through a daily part in household chores a girl learns from her mother to be a companion and an eventual wife and mother. She gains specific knowledge in the traditional preparation of maize. She visits the fields carrying food to the men and often helps in the harvest.

In this way life in the village proceeds under an almost complete self-dependence. World economic crises, wars, and major catastrophes have little effect on established patterns of existence; indeed, these events often pass unrecorded in the village. In more recent times this satisfying picture has been changing. The economic system of the world industrial powers is increasingly reflected in the simple penny economy of the villages. In the course of its survival the village suffers from malnutrition and infectious diseases and many children die. For ill-defined reasons, infant mortality began to decline forty to sixty years ago. Birth rates continued high. The result has been an accelerated population growth, a serious shortage of land, overcrowding of households, and ultimately a beginning migration from villages to the larger urban centers. Excessive population growth is the most important deterrent to the continuation of a village life so much to be admired. The more tangible problems of malnutrition and infectious disease are interrelated and contributory. The study summarized in this book had its primary concern with these elements; the findings are directed toward an improved understanding and a solution of the underlying health problems. In that endeavor many of the unique aspects of this culture inevitably will be neutralized or destroyed. The hope remains that we will be sufficiently astute to encourage preservation of its positive values.

Leonardo J. Mata
Guatemala, December 1974

Acknowledgments

This study was conducted at the Institute of Nutrition of Central America and Panama (INCAP), the established regional nutrition center of the Pan American Health Organization with headquarters in Guatemala City, Guatemala. Other organizations and institutes made important contributions. A major part of data handling and analysis was done at the Department of Biostatistics, School of Public Health and Community Medicine, and the John L. Locke, Jr., Computing Facility, University of Washington in Seattle, an arrangement favored by my appointment as Visiting Professor in the Department of Epidemiology and International Health during the academic year 1973–1974. Much technical assistance was also provided in producing the book.

The Pan American Health Organization gave administrative and partial financial support. The National Institutes of Health of the US Department of Health, Education, and Welfare (National Institute of Allergy and Infectious Disease and National Institute of Child Health and Human Development) provided most of the funds to conduct the study and to prepare this report. Additional financial support came from the US-Japan Cooperative Medical Science Program of the National Institutes of Health, the US Army Research and Development Command, the World Health Organization, the Guatemalan Ministry of Health, and American Cyanamid International.

Many scientists contributed significantly in the development of the study. While I was in Boston (from 1959 to 1962) Nevin S. Scrimshaw of the Massachusetts Institute of Technology and the first Director of INCAP urged me to undertake a study of the interaction of nutrition and infection upon my return to Guatemala. Many discussions with John E. Gordon, Thomas H.

Weller, Franklin A. Neva, and George Hutchison of the Harvard School of
Public Health were fundamental in conceptualizing the ideas and design of
the study. The then new course in Epidemiology by Brian MacMahon and
colleagues influenced my choice of a cohort approach for the study. The
advice and support of many teachers and friends, among whom John Gordon
was outstanding, constituted a key force in the development of the project.
In Guatemala just before the project began Joaquín Cravioto and Ian
McGregor gave crucial advice on making the study interdisciplinary, without
which the present data would not have resulted.

Significant and invaluable participation in the analysis of data was derived
from my colleagues Richard A. Kronmal, John Gordon, John P. Fox, and
Claire Joplin. The philosophic and scientific contributions of John Gordon,
Nevin Scrimshaw, John Fox, René Dubos, Joaquín Cravioto, Edgar Mohs,
Abraham Horwitz, and many others, and the warm memories and example of
my teachers, Thomas H. Weller, Alfonso Trejos, Rodrigo R. Brenes, and
Renato Soto have instilled modesty in moments of success and brought
consolation in times of frustration.

I am profoundly grateful to the residents of Santa María Cauqué who for
so many years were friendly, patient, and cooperative. Their cordial attitude
assured that staff members were always welcome; it relieved much of the
distress so reasonably associated with continued work in a prevailing atmosphere of poverty. I thank the leaders and authorities of the village for their
help in official and public matters, and extend special gratitude to the Indian
midwives and school teachers for unconditioned commitment in aid of the
field staff.

A final and almost sentimental word is reserved for the skillful, persever-
ing, loyal, and truly dedicated workers in the project, the staff of the field
and laboratory. They believed and worked in the project, some of them for
the entire study, through cold and heat, mud and dust, political upheaval and
economic crisis. To all, my enduring gratitude.

Analyses hardly are the work of any one person. During twelve months
devoted to interpretation of data and the writing of the book I received
invaluable assistance from professors and friends John Gordon, John Fox,
Richard Kronmal, Nevin Scrimshaw, Merrill S. Read, John H. Kennell,
Gerald T. Keusch, and Richard Stark who read most chapters, gave support,
and advanced sound criticism. Numerous faculty members of the University
of Washington gave significant advice: Peter Kunstadter, Gerald La Veck,
David J. Erickson, Irvin Emanuel, Russell E. Alexander, Lowell E. Sever,
Cyril Enwonwu, Samuel Preston, David W. Smith, Ronal C. Scott, Bonnie
Worthington, Marion K. Cooney, Carrie Hall, Ricardo Marroquín, and Mary
Coyle. I am indebted to many of my colleagues who reviewed parts of the
manuscript—Juan José Urrutia, Bertha García, Jean-Pierre Habicht, Guillermo

Arroyave, Charles Teller, and Robert Stickney—and to Jessie R. Janjigian who helped with the final editing of the book.

With patience and endurance, efficient secretaries typed and proofread repeated drafts of rather imposing lots of material: Nellie Neumayer from the University of Washington, Claire Butler from Harvard University, and my personal secretaries Yomila Lürssen, Magda Medrano, and Miriam Molina.

Che ré ri jun ishoc utz qui bech,
Che ré ri ishoc natural Santa María Cauqué

To her, who deserves all,
To the Indian woman of Santa María Cauqué

PART I
FOUNDATIONS OF THE STUDY

Chapter 1
Foundations of the Study

That poverty, disease, and malnutrition still prevail among more than half of the world's population is a challenging paradox in the face of man's achievements in science and technology. Part of the failure of less developed societies to attain better standards of living and health rests in their inability to perceive the nature and magnitude of the existing problems. This failure is abetted by inadequate or nonexistent knowledge about feasible measures for prevention or control. Of themselves, these two reasons justify long-term epidemiological field studies with an emphasis on human values, especially among the large rural populations that dominate so much of the world.

This study of the village of Santa María Cauqué is an example of that kind of approach. Throughout nine years of investigation the driving force, the justification for this particular kind of research, was the conviction that a thorough understanding of the nature, causation, and magnitude of disease processes would provide the scientific foundation for the design, implementation, and evaluation of immediate and long-term action programs directed toward a specific attack on identified problems. Development planners would thus have information which they could use to convince and convert local and foreign intellectuals and political leaders to the desirability and advantage of action in accordance with observed facts.

Many factors entered into the genesis of the conceptual idea from which the Cauqué study followed. For two reasons the health and growth of infants and young children in a rural and economically disadvantaged area was the natural choice. The first was a demonstrated need for such study. Attention centered on malnutrition and infectious disease because in combination they constituted the main health problem of Central America. The second reason, tempered perhaps by sentiment, was exposure of the principal investigator to new ideas and approaches to health investigation during graduate training at the Harvard School of Public Health (1959–1962), and especially to the philosophical considerations on interactions between nutrition and infection as advanced by Nevin S. Scrimshaw, C. E. Taylor, and John E. Gordon (1959). To launch a study design and introduce a methodological approach that at the time (1962) was rather unorthodox and, in the opinion of many, too ambitious and unrealistic, also required a degree of independence and aggressiveness.

The particular concept was to recruit a small cohort of infants at birth but observed from gestation, to be studied in depth, systematically, and intensively in prospective fashion; this was in contrast to the more usual dependence on large numbers for significance, and with observations sufficiently long to obtain full data on the critical stages of growth during infancy and preschool years. Furthermore, observations of one kind or another were to be made on practically every person of the village in order to permit a clear idea of the community health situation.

To satisfy specifications implicit in its concept, the study was to be conducted in a small rural population judged representative of larger rural populations of the country. Population migration in such locality should be practically negligible, and malnutrition and infectious disease had to be sufficiently prevalent to ensure collection of meaningful data. Many Guatemalan Indian villages, Santa María Cauqué among them, met these three requirements. Living conditions within Santa María Cauqué were relatively traditional, yet the village was so located as to be readily accessible to the established and well-equipped headquarters, a necessity in view of methodologies to be used in the study, specifically, isolation of viruses, cultivation of anaerobic bacteria, and a systematic evaluation of field and laboratory procedures and findings.

A distinctive feature of the Cauqué study was the incorporation of a multidisciplinary approach in study design and collection of data, along with interdisciplinary analysis and interpretation. Furthermore, the study design specified that staff members and methods were not to be altered to any extent that would significantly affect the nature and quality of observations made. To this end the disciplines of infectious disease, nutrition, microbiology, pediatrics, and public health became integral parts of the study. This book is not, however, directed specifically to specialists in pediatrics, growth and development, nutrition, microbiology, infectious disease, or the sciences of man, although it touches on each of these disciplines. It represents the attempt of a biologist to describe the health of a typical Guatemalan Mayan village in the 1960s, to assess the human values and attitudes of its inhabitants, and to appraise their situation and the prospects for future development.

Part I discusses the foundations of the study and describes the village and its people. Part II gives a detailed account of experimental design and of the study plan, with emphasis on field, laboratory, and statistical techniques and methods used to collect and interpret observations. Part III presents the results of the study, beginning with a biological and clinical characterization of the pregnant woman and newborn infant. This leads to an analysis of maternal factors and fetal growth and how they relate to survival and to growth and development of the child. Other sections discuss feeding practices and growth and development in infancy and early childhood. The impact of infection and infectious disease on the infant and young child is examined next. These chapters extend into an appraisal of the problem of protein-calorie malnutrition in the village.

The last section contains a brief summary of the main findings of the Cauqué study and a discussion of the health implications in this and similar societies, with considerations of underlying socioeconomic factors.

Chapter 2
The Village and Its People

Although no written history of Santa María Cauqué has ever been found, elderly residents, those more than eighty-five years old, say that their great-great-grandparents lived in the village. That the community must be more than three hundred years old, probably dating from pre-Columbian times, is a reasonable assumption. Like many Indian villages, the name of Santa María Cauqué is of two parts: one Spanish, Santa María, the name of the Virgin Mary, and the other Indian, Cauqué, its meaning unknown. The closest native word is *cashuque*, "to kneel down." An old folk tale tells of the founders of the village who, having tired after walking many miles, decided to settle where their women had stopped temporarily to kneel on the ground.

The village was relatively isolated until the Inter-American Highway, which cuts across the outskirts of the locality, was opened around 1950. The years 1944–1955 marked an era of social reform in which the Central Government of Guatemala made a strong effort to raise the standard of living of its rural population, and particularly of the Guatemalan Indians. Several important events of distinct relevance to the quality of village life occurred during this period. A village public health nurse was appointed by the government in 1944; an elementary school for boys and girls was built and a communal system for water supply installed in 1949; a Health Center was constructed in 1955; and in 1956 a public shower bath, the first latrines, and two slaughter-houses were built. All these things tended to improve the nutrition, hygiene, and health care of the village, as did the various medical services and health measures instituted by the Institute of Nutrition of Central America and

This chapter was written jointly with Bertha García.

Panama (INCAP), which had chosen Santa María as one of the first locations for a dietary survey in 1950 (Flores and Reh, 1955). The Health Center acquired great prominence in the life of the village during the INCAP Nutrition-Infection Study carried out from 1958 to 1963 (Scrimshaw et al., 1967a, 1967b), which was followed by the present investigation (1963 to 1972).

Like most Guatemalan villages, despite a relatively uneventful historical background, this little community has a long record of suffering, as evidenced by the records of births and deaths, epidemics of disease, and population growth that constitute the substance of this book. This chapter summarizes the considerable amount of information on the village and people of Santa María Cauqué obtained in 1963, the first year of the study, a year devoted entirely to the establishment and testing of field methods and logistic preparation. This information was augmented throughout the study until its termination in 1972. (The methods used are in chapters 3 and 4.)

THE VILLAGE

Location and Climate

Santa María Cauqué is a village of the Municipality of Santiago, Department of Sacatepéquez, in the Republic of Guatemala (figure 2.1). It is 22 miles (35 kilometers) from Guatemala City on the Inter-American Highway, 6,200 feet (1,900 meters) above sea level, and rests off the slopes of secondary hills of the Sierra Madre along with many other similar highland communities. The setting of the village is relatively flat. A small creek runs just beyond the village limits, and peripheral forests line the hilly side.

Although Santa María Cauqué is geographically in the tropics, its specific location in the highlands accounts for a varying spring-summer climate without severe extremes. The lowest temperature recorded during the study period was 41°F (5°C) and the highest 84°F (29°C); in a single day, however, variations of as much as 59°F (15°C) can be observed. The dry season extends from mid-November to mid-May. The heaviest rains are in September and October. The combination of altitude and tropical location, rain and sunshine, results in some chilly nights but warm days.

The soil is fertile and enriched by volcanic deposits of the remote past and, in recent years, by ashes from the nearby Fuego volcano. Characteristics of terrain and climate account for the existence of pine, cypress, and oak forests.

As in most Guatemalan highland villages, dwellings are closely clustered along well-defined streets, forming blocks of varying sizes and shapes (figure 2.2). The central square is bordered by the municipal building, Catholic and Protestant churches, and the Health Center (INCAP village headquarters). The streets are unpaved, and according to the season they become either muddy or extremely dusty.

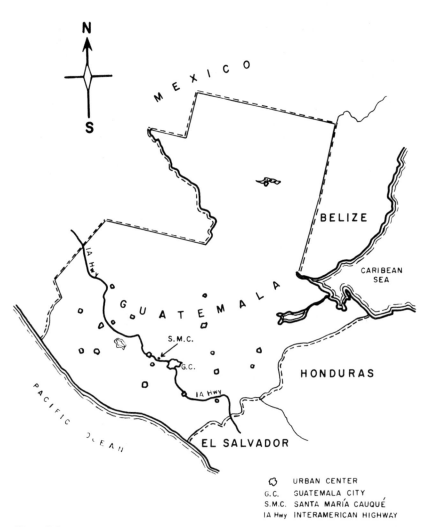

Figure 2.1
Location of Santa María Cauqué

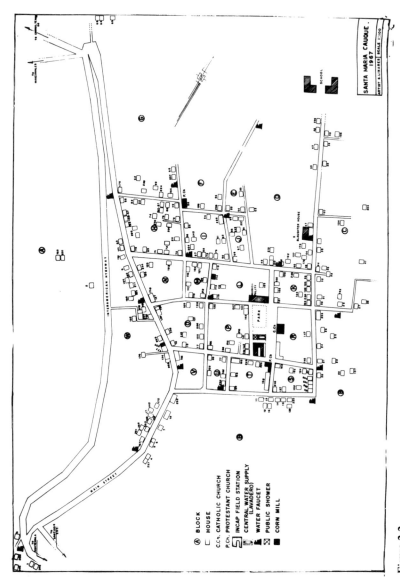

Figure 2.2
Map of Santa María Cauqué

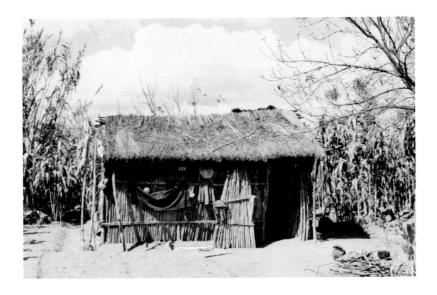

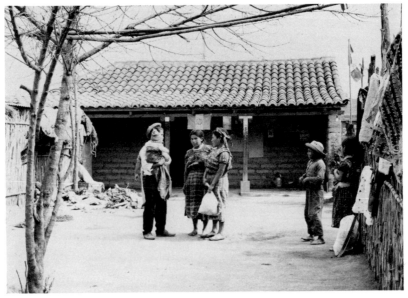

Figure 2.3
Various types of housing

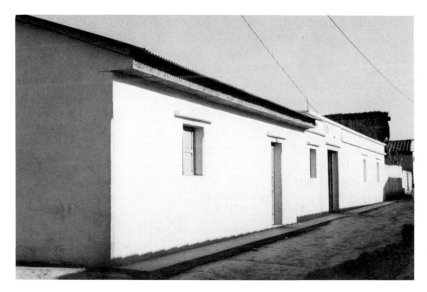

Table 2.1
Building Material of Houses, by Survey Year and Number and Percentage of Families

	Number of families (percentage)		
	1963	1967	1971
Floors			
Earthen	185 (91.1)	199 (86.5)	227 (88.3)
Tile	3 (1.5)	9 (3.9)	8 (3.1)
Cement	5 (2.5)	20 (8.7)	18 (7.0)
Combination	10 (4.9)	0	1 (0.4)
Unknown	0	2 (0.9)	3 (1.2)
Walls			
Adobe or brick	112 (55.2)	198 (86.1)	236 (91.8)
Corn stalk	31 (15.3)	30 (13.0)	18 (7.0)
Adobe and stalk	60 (29.6)	0	0
Unknown	0	2 (0.9)	3 (1.2)
Roofs			
Tile	66 (32.5)	124 (53.9)	133 (51.8)
Palm or straw	65 (32.0)	43 (18.7)	23 (8.9)
Metal	15 (7.4)	61 (26.5)	98 (38.1)
Tile and other	26 (12.8)	0	0
Metal and other	31 (15.3)	0	0
Unknown	0	2 (0.9)	3 (1.2)
Number of families	203	230	257

Housing

A typical family has a one- or two-room house, as well as primitive granary or *troje*, and a place for worship, the *oratorio*. Although some families may have separate sleeping and cooking quarters under one roof, or two independent buildings that serve these purposes, most families still use the same room for sleeping and cooking. Several kinship families may group together in a compound, although this is not the rule.

The walls of the village houses are variously constructed of cornstalk, adobe, brick, or combinations of these materials; floors are earthen or tiled. Roofs are made of thatch, tiles, or corrugated iron, or again of various combinations (figure 2.3). In recent years, the quality of walls and roofs has improved appreciably, with an increased tendency to use materials such as bricks, corrugated iron, tiles, and cement (table 2.1), in contrast to earlier descriptions (Otzoy, 1949).

The oratorio is a place for keeping images or statues of one or more saints. Whether located within the living quarters as is usual, or in an independent structure, the oratorio has a special distinction; if separate, it is likely to be better built than the house itself. The family prays or gathers socially in the oratorio and works there occasionally preparing vegetables or flowers for market.

The *tuj* or *temascal*, an oven-like structure of adobe used for steam baths, is a common feature of adjacent household premises present in about half of the homes (figure 2.4). Steam is generated by pouring water over stones previously heated by a fire of burning cornstalks fed through a smaller door of the bath. A latrine and a corral for domestic animals are other usual features of a compound, usually located near the temascal or similar facilities (figures 2.4a, b, c, and d). If a latrine does not exist, a special area of the premises is designated for defecation.

A slight decrease in home ownership was noted between 1967 and 1971, a situation that, together with land ownership, reflects the increased crowding the village is experiencing. The size and distribution of homes remained wholly constant, as evidenced by the number of rooms and their use (table 2.2).

Electricity was introduced into the village in November 1966. Of 200 homes surveyed in 1968–1969, sixty-three (30.3 percent) had electricity. Of this number, twenty-one (33 percent) had two bulbs, thirty (48 percent) had three to four bulbs, and twelve (9 percent) had five or more. Some families purchase electrical service for light bulbs only. No electrical applicances were found in any home with less than five bulbs, not so much because of lack of familiarity with electric current but more because of its high cost and the prohibitive price of appliances.

Sanitation

Household and environmental hygiene is markedly deficient. Few houses have

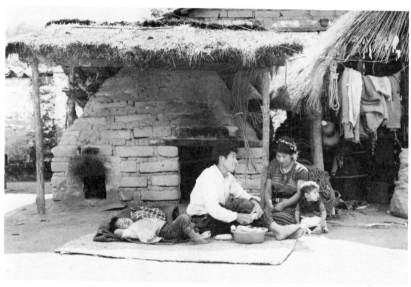

Figure 2.4a
Temascal (steam bath)

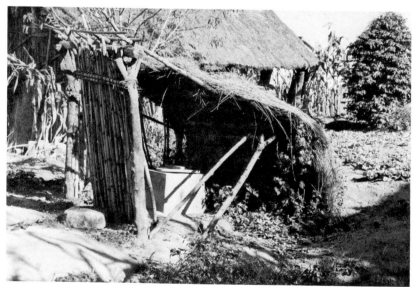

Figure 2.4b
Latrine

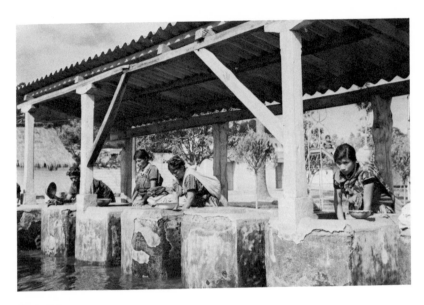

Figure 2.4c
Public reservoir and laundry

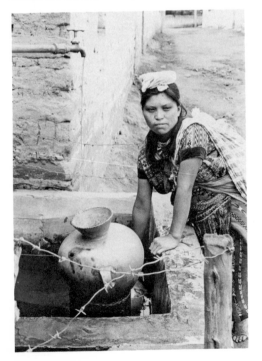

Figure 2.4d
Public faucet

Table 2.2
Housing, by Survey Year and Number and Percentage of Families

	Number of families (percentage)			
	1959	1963	1967	1971
Tenure				
Owned	159 (85.5)	171 (84.2)	199 (86.5)	204 (79.4)
Rented[a]	27 (14.5)	32 (15.8)	30 (13.0)	50 (19.5)
Unknown	0	0	1 (0.4)	3 (1.2)
Number of rooms				
One		166 (81.8)	188 (81.7)	200 (77.8)
Two		33 (16.3)	37 (16.1)	47 (18.3)
Three		3 (1.5)	3 (1.3)	6 (2.3)
Unknown		1 (0.5)	2 (0.9)	4 (1.6)
Oratorio[b]				
None		186 (91.6)	217 (94.3)	245 (95.3)
One		17 (8.4)	11 (4.8)	9 (3.5)
Unknown		0	2 (0.9)	3 (1.2)
Number of families	186	203	230	257

[a]Usually land outside the village limits.
[b]A room of the house or a separate installation devoted to worship.

Table 2.3
Household Sanitary Facilities, by Survey Year and Number and Percentage of Families

	Number of families (percentage)			
	1959	1963	1967	1971
Temascal[a]				
None		96 (47.3)	95 (41.3)	131 (51.0)
Present		107 (52.7)	129 (56.1)	123 (47.9)
Unknown		0	6 (2.6)	3 (1.2)
Water				
Carried from public fountain	171 (91.9)	183 (90.2)	213 (92.6)	67 (26.1)
Private (piped or well)	15 (8.1)	18 (8.9)	17 (7.4)	157 (61.1)
Combined	0	1 (1.0)	0	29 (11.3)
Unknown	0	0	0	4 (1.6)
Cooking				
Fogón[b] on floor	178 (95.7)	189 (93.1)	204 (88.7)	236 (91.8)
Fogón, elevated	8 (4.3)	3 (3.9)	13 (5.6)	9 (3.5)
Unknown	0	6 (3.0)	13 (5.6)	12 (4.7)
Number of families	186	203	230	257

[a]An oven-like structure for steam baths.
[b]A hearth fed by wood.

Table 2.4
Number and Use of Latrines, by Survey Year and Number and Percentage of Families

| | Number of families (percentage) | | | |
	1960	1963	1967	1971
Families				
With latrine[a]	115 (62)	208 (90)	157 (68)	181 (68)
Without latrine	72 (38)	6 (3)	73 (32)	85 (32)
Total	187	214	230	266
Usage				
All family members	45 (39)	177 (85)	51 (32)	99 (54)
Certain family members	59 (51)	25 (12)	88 (56)	71 (39)
No one	11 (10)	6 (3)	18 (12)	11 (7)
Total	115	208	157	181

[a]Includes a few flush toilets.

running water in the house although more have a water faucet now than when the study started, as a result of government installation of a central water supply in 1968. Most people still carry water from the main public reservoir which also serves as the laundry or from public faucets (figure 2.4). By necessity bathing facilities continue to be the temascales. Food is prepared on a hearth fed by wood at the level of the floor (table 2.3).

Environmental sanitation is a serious problem. No effort has been made to build sewers or to provide adequate disposal of feces or other wastes. Waste water from cooking or washing of dishes is discarded in the yard or in the street. Garbage and animal fecal waste is common around the outside of the house. Only about a third of the population actually uses latrines, which almost invariably are in poor condition. An INCAP program to install latrines, accompanied by an educational effort in sanitation, began in 1959 as a feature of a field experiment (Scrimshaw et al., 1967b). The effort ended when the study terminated in 1961. An evaluation of this intervention was made at various stages of the Cauqué study by visual appraisal of latrine maintenance and by an assessment of frequency of use. Availability of latrines increased from a base level of 60 percent to 97 percent as a result of promotion and distribution of materials (table 2.4). A few years after the experiment had ended, however, the proportion of homes without a latrine had returned to its original level. The number of indiscriminate squatters, who had become few by 1963, rose again to numbers comparable to those before the program began, a situation that has remained essentially fixed for eight years. Furthermore, at the end of the study, fewer families were disposing of garbage by soil fertilization and more were discarding it.

Flies prevail throughout the year; during the colder months of December and January they are scarce but they become abundant as the rainy season

Table 2.5
Seasonal Harvest of Food Crops

	Crops per Year[a]	Planting Season	Harvest Season
Maize	1	May–July	January–March
String beans	4	All year[c]	All year
Black beans[b]	1	April–May	July–August
Peas	1	April–May	September–October
Hot peppers[d]	1	February	July
Cabbage	4	All year[c]	All year
Peaches, pears, plums	1		July

[a]Excluding foods produced in the village not regularly consumed.
[b]Approximately 10 families grow black beans, others buy them in markets or local stores.
[c]Planting is more intense in the rainy season (May through October).
[d]Not given to children under three years of age.

begins and reach a peak in April and May. Mice and rats, together with insects and fungi, contribute to significant destruction of stored grain.

Economy
The soil in the highlands is generally fertile and yields are relatively good. The small land parcels, called *minifundios*, are devoted almost exclusively to a traditional agriculture of food crops, predominantly maize and string beans but also peas and other legumes, and to cash crops of vegetables, flowers, and fruits. These cash crops include cabbage, chard, carrots, radishes, root beets, lettuce, coriander, celery, pears, peaches, plums, apples, carnations, roses, chrysanthemums, and dahlias. Wild leaves and bushes are also gathered for food, for instance, chipilín, macuy, berro, bledo, and mushrooms.

Leveled land is preferred for cultivation, but crowding and scarcity often force the Indians to work hilly or mountainous land, sometimes at an angle of 45°. Times of cultivation and harvest are well defined by the seasons. The first step is clearing the forest and is often done by fire. The land is then turned over using the *azadón*, a simple hand tool. Terracing is done on the slopes. From March through May the land is carefully prepared to receive the maize seeds. Children and women help in the preparation of the land and often other Indians are hired as laborers. Maize is well adapted to the region; it grows two to three meters tall without the aid of chemical fertilizers, each stalk producing one to three ears at the annual harvest. In recent years people have begun to use chemical fertilizers in moderate amounts. This practice became more popular after 1970, but was halted by the energy crisis in 1974. The usual crop requires only two weedings. The seasonal harvest of food crops is indicated in table 2.5.

Table 2.6
Land Owned and Rented per Family and Use by Principal Crops, by Survey Year

	Total cuerdas (cuerdas per family)		
	1963	1967	1971
Amount of land			
Owned	1,904 (9.7)	2,174 (9.5)	1,883 (7.7)
Rented	219 (1.1)	57 (0.2)	28 (0.1)
Total	2,123 (10.8)	2,231 (9.7)	1,911 (7.8)
Land use			
Maize	1,255 (6.4)	1,416 (6.2)	1,193 (4.8)
Beans	414 (2.1)	199 (0.9)	184 (0.7)
Wheat	0	0	0
Potatoes	2 (0.01)	9 (0.04)	1
Vegetables	341 (1.7)	338 (1.5)	219 (0.9)
Fruit	6 (0.03)	4 (0.02)	3 (0.01)
Flowers & other	90 (0.5)	151 (0.7)	36 (0.1)
Not used	15 (0.1)	114 (0.5)	275 (1.1)
Total	2,123 (10.8)	2,231 (9.7)	1,911 (7.8)
Number of families	197	229	249

Note: One cuerda = 0.3 acres. Figures show total amounts with land per family in parentheses. To do the computations, the land rented by one person to another, within the
community, was generally subtracted from the total land owned. In this way each cuerda
was counted only once.

Land cultivated by the villagers may be privately owned or rented. Originally most Indians received titles to such land as was available after large
plots had been taken or claimed by Europeans. Land titles are passed from
parents to children, both sons and daughters. Most families possess only small
plots, ranging from one to twenty-five *cuerdas**, a circumstance that restricts
the practice of modern agriculture. In recent years, as noted by observation
in the Cauqué study, the amount of land under cultivation showed a slight
decline; fewer families owned land than when the study started, and the
proportion of landless families had increased significantly (tables 2.6 and
2.7). Land continued to be devoted to the same crops, although cultivation of
maize declined somewhat and cultivation of beans declined significantly as
did that of vegetable crops, though to a lesser extent.

Most families raise chickens and occasionally other fowl, about half own
dogs and cats, but few possess cattle, hogs, or horses (table 2.8). At best,
the total number of cattle, hogs, and fowl per family remained small.

Most families grow enough maize to meet their own needs. Any surplus

* One cuerda = 0.3 acres; one acre = 3.3 cuerdas. A cuerda in the lowlands is of different size from one in the highlands, and the equivalence in acres should be brought out if
data from different regions are compared.

Table 2.7
Land Owned or Rented per Family and Used for Principal Crops, by Survey Year and Percentage of Families

	Percentage of families		
	1963	1967	1971
Amount of land per family (cuerdas)			
Owned			
0	15	16	24
1–3	14	6	9
4–9	34	34	28
10–24	33	44	35
Unknown	4	0	4
Rented			
0	75	94	94
1–3	8	2	1
4–9	13	4	1
10–24	2	0	0
Unknown	2	0	4
Land use by crop			
Maize			
0	5	15	28
1–3	20	6	4
4–9	50	56	49
10–24	20	23	16
Unknown	5	0	3
Beans			
0	21	55	60
1–3	48	34	34
4–9	24	11	4
10–24	4	0	0
Unknown	3	0	2
Vegetables			
0	32	29	40
1–3	49	60	54
4–9	15	10	3
10–24	1	1	0
Unknown	3	0	3
Number of families	203	230	257

Table 2.8
Domestic Animals per Family, by Survey Year and Percentage of Families

	Percentage of families		
	1963	1967	1971
Cattle			
0	77	62	67
1	14	28	23
2	7	8	8
3	2	2	2
Hogs			
0	80	64	90
1	15	23	6
2–4	5	13	4
Fowl			
0	28	30	30
1–3	14	12	9
4–9	30	26	23
10+	28	32	38
Goats			
0	99	99.6	99.2
1–9	0.5	0	0.4
10–20	0.5	0.4	0.4
Horses			
0	90	88	94
1	7	11	4
2	3	1	2
Number of families	203	230	257

of maize or of the particular cash crops constitutes the main source of income, negotiated either individually in the locality or in the large markets of Guatemala City. The average annual per capita income in the village is difficult to determine; the mean gross domestic product (MGDP) per capita for the Department of Sacatepéquez, where Santa María Cauqué is located, has, however, been declining. This reflects the general impoverishment of the rural Guatemalan population, judged by the 26 percent decline in per capita MGDP from U.S. $142 to U.S. $105 between 1951 and 1966 (table 2.9). The Department of Sacatepéquez showed a marked reduction of 38 percent in MGDP during this period. The increase of 26 percent for the country as a whole is accounted for almost wholly by the Department of Guatemala, and within it, by the economic growth of Guatemala City (Smith, 1973). In summary, the rich are getting richer while the poor are getting poorer. Under such circumstances the future of the villages is difficult to forecast. The indicators discussed in this chapter, however, are of interest. The country as a

Table 2.9
Mean Gross Domestic Product per Capita, Selected Regions of Guatemala

	Product (U.S. dollars)		Percentage change in 15 years
	1951–1952	1965–1966	
Department of Guatemala[a]	847	1,071	+26
Department of Sacatepéquez[b]	197	123	-38
All Guatemala, except 3 Departments[c]	144	104	-28
Rural Guatemala	142	105	-26
Total	265	329	+24

Note: After Smith (1973).
[a]Includes Guatemala City with about 15 percent of the total population of the country.
[b]Santa María Cauqué is a village of this Department. The area borders on the Department of Guatemala.
[c]The Departments of Guatemala, Escuintla, and El Petén stand alone in showing an increase in the gross domestic product.

whole shows a tendency toward a reduction in the output of maize and important complementary foods such as beans. Meat is being exported and in progressively larger amounts, mainly to the United States. Even village agriculture has changed since the Cauqué study ended, from a basically subsistence agriculture to a mixed one including cash crops (vegetables, fruits, flowers) that are sold in the Guatemala City market. The mean gross domestic product is decreasing and per capita availability of the basic foods—maize and beans—has also decreased in recent years.

The changes in land ownership and crop pattern would not be so important had they been counterbalanced by improvement in agricultural practices through development of local craftmanship or industrialization, or by other activities leading to extra income. Such collateral events did not occur, however. This resulted in a progressive decrease in the purchasing value of the quetzal,* while other factors, including wages, remained constant (table 2.10). The increase in cost of living was alarming, particularly when items such as transistor radios, plastic utensils, and carbonated beverages appeared in the markets at reasonable prices, presenting an opportunity for deviation of money that otherwise could have been destined for food and shelter. Such developments have been compounded by the present energy crisis and by worldwide inflation.

THE PEOPLE

Ethnicity
The villagers of Santa María Cauqué readily identify themselves as belonging to one or another of two ethnic groups, Indian or ladino, categories that are

* 1 Quetzal = US $1 = Central American $1.

Table 2.10
Prices of Land, Animals, Groceries, and Other Items

	Prices (quetzales)			Percentage increase		
	Feb. 1963	Feb. 1972	Feb. 1974	1963–1972	1972–1974	1963–1974
Work						
Farm labor, 8–10 hrs[a]	0.50	0.50	0.80	0	60	60
Mason, 8–10 hrs	1.50	1.50	2.00	0	33	33
Salaried farmer, monthly	20.00	20.00	30.00	0	50	50
Midwife services	3.00	3.00	5.00	0	67	67
Harp ensemble, 24 hrs[b]	6.00	6.00	6.00	0	0	0
Land (cuerdas)						
In town	150.00	250.00	300.00	67	20	100
Outside town	60.00	80.00	100.00	33	25	67
Pig						
Medium size	6.00	6.00	12.00	0	100	100
Piglet	2.50	3.00	6.00	20	100	140
Groceries						
Maize, 100 lbs						
Harvest time	2.50	3.00	5.00	20	67	100
Off-season	4.00	4.50	8.00	13	78	100
Black beans, lb	0.08	0.12	0.20	50	67	150
Stewing beef with bone, lb	0.20	0.35	0.45	75	29	125
Beef, round, lb	0.40	0.60	0.75	50	25	88
Eggs, dozen	0.48	0.50	0.72	4	44	50

Clothing

Güipil,c traditional	12.00	18.00	35.00	50	94	192
Morga,d traditional	12.00	18.00	40.00	50	122	233

Note: 1 Quetzal = US $1 = Central American $1.
aIncludes midday meal.
bThree people, fed and provided with alcoholic beverages.
cBlouse.
dSkirt cloth.

Table 2.11
Population by Ethnic Group and Sex, by Survey Year and Number and Percentage of
Total Population

	Number (percentage of total population)[a]							
	1959		1963		1967		1971	
Indian[b]								
Male			531	(49.6)	613	(48.9)	665	(48.5)
Female			493	(46.0)	585	(46.7)	667	(48.7)
Total	887	(96.1)	1,024	(95.6)	1,198	(96.6)	1,332	(97.2)
Ladino[c]								
Male			21	(2.0)	25	(2.0)	20	(1.5)
Female			26	(2.4)	31	(2.4)	18	(1.3)
Total	36	(3.9)	47	(4.4)	56	(4.4)	38	(2.8)
Total population	923 (100.0)		1,071 (100.0)		1,254 (100.0)		1,370 (100.0)	
Number of families	186		203		230		257	
Persons per family	5.0		5.3		5.5		5.3	

[a]Children under 15 were grouped with their parents.
[b]An Indian (natural) is a person who follows Indian traditions and speaks primarily the
Indian dialect. Women wear traditional Indian costumes.
[c]A ladino is a person who does not follow Indian traditions, speaks primarily or only
Spanish, has a varying degree of non-Indian blood, and is maybe of direct European
descent. Women do not wear Indian costumes.

based on ethnic background rather than genetic endowment. An Indian, or
better a *natural* as they prefer to designate themselves, is a person who speaks
the dialect as a principal language and follows many of the traditions and beliefs of the Indian culture; Indian women wear the traditional colorful cos-
tume, and generally go barefoot. A ladino speaks Spanish as the primary
language and has customs and traditions more in accord with the accepted
western pattern; ladino women do not wear Indian clothing. According to
this classification the village population is almost wholly of naturales (table
2.11). The relatively greater proportion of Indians in the population at the
end of the study was due to the migration of a few ladino families and to a
higher fertility rate among the Indians.

About one half of the five million people of Guatemala are classed as
Indian. They live predominantly in the highlands at altitudes ranging from
3,000 to 10,000 feet. As in Mexico and Peru, Indian cultures survived in the
highlands of Guatemala where fertile soils favored domestication and perpetuation of food crops and where there was relative protection from heat,
drought, and the typical fevers and ailments of the lowlands.

Most naturales are descended directly from the pre-Columbian peoples of
the region; in Santa María Cauqué they are of Mayan origin and of the
Cakchiquel linguistic group. The ladino group generally is of mixed European
and Indian descent. Many individuals of the Indian group appear to have an

admixture of caucasian genes, and among the ladinos an Indian component is often evident. As would be expected, some Indians eventually take on a ladino way of life; occasionally an Indian marries a ladino woman, and more than one young Indian girl dresses in non-Indian clothes.

The distribution of blood groups demonstrates the great homogeneity of the population; among 300 villagers examined, 98 percent were O(IV) Rh positive. The mongolian spot is a general occurrence; a high prevalence of bilateral rotation of the middle deciduous incisor teeth has been demonstrated; and a few surnames occur at high frequency. All these considerations attest to the high rate of endogamy.

Social and Cultural Characteristics

Tradition strongly determines the way of life in this little community. Village authority is centralized in local municipal officials and Indian leaders, usually middle-aged and elderly working males (figure 2.5). In the home women have most of the authority for decisions on child rearing, health, food, and shelter; they also have a say in land transactions.

The municipal government consists of the mayor, three assistant mayors, one pipe layer, and three rotating groups of eight *ministriles* (policemen), each group subordinate to an assistant mayor and all appointed *ad honorem* by a committee of honorable elderly men who have served the community previously as mayors or assistant mayors. Service in all lower levels is a prerequisite to becoming mayor. Mayors have been appointed from each of the political parties and from the two religions. Appointment is for one year only, with no second term.

In carrying out important duties, the ministriles carry a black rod as a symbol of authority. If a person is arrested because of drunkenness or scandalous behavior (and these cases are rare), the rods are sufficient symbols of power. Except for a few shotguns for hunting, there are no firearms or other weapons in the village. Machetes with three-foot steel blades are owned by almost every male, but are fundamentally tools for work.

All clerical work relating to civic, legal, and political affairs is handled by the secretary of the neighboring larger village of Santiago Sacatepéquez to which Santa María is politically subordinate. This secretary, who is almost always a ladino, receives a salary, is literate, and can type.

The village government has relative freedom for independent action, yet is also the channel through which the Central Government implements its actions. Customarily, the party in office exerts an appreciable influence on local village governments. Political individuality and independence, however, are on the rise; for example, in recent years the ruling party has lost the popular elections in many villages, including Santa María Cauqué. Village people are developing political awareness, yet involvement in national politics is relatively minor when judged by standards of western industrial societies.

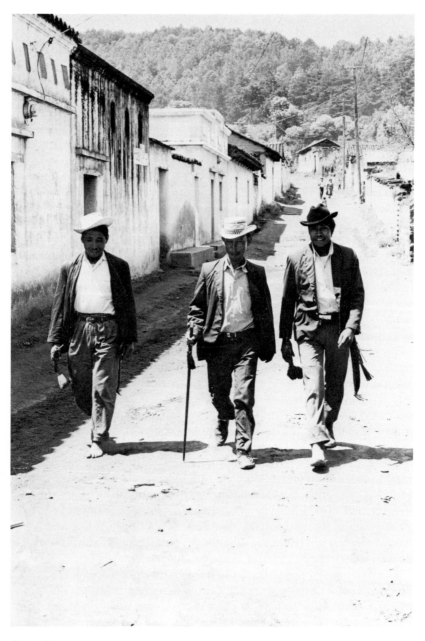

Figure 2.5
Three municipal officials

A respect for authority and a sense of cohesiveness derive from religious activities. The village has three churches, one Catholic and two Protestant Christian, with respective enrollments of 210 and 35 families. A visiting priest comes for one to two hours to hear confessions and to celebrate Sunday mass, baptisms, weddings, and Patroness's Day, August 15, the Feast of the Assumption of the Virgin Mary. Occasionally the priest may visit the village on a weekday to hold a private mass or to give the last sacrament. Women and men visit the church often and are responsible for its care and maintenance. More nonclerical activity is evident in the Protestant churches because some Indians have learned to read the Bible and give sermons. No conflicts relating to religion were observed during the study period.

More importance is attached to the *cofradías* or religious organizations than to formal religious activities. The three main cofradías in Santa María Cauqué are those of the Virgin of the Assumption, of Saint Michael, and of the Virgin of the Rosary. A cofradía is an aggregation of several families under the guidance of two men and two women drawn from different family groups. Each cofradía celebrates at least one great fiesta annually with music, food, and alcoholic drinks, usually for three days and two nights. As many as 300 persons may attend the more important cofradías. The meetings are both social and religious. The people pray and burn incense, eat and drink heavily, and dance in an open and happy way. Candles are lighted to the Saint and gifts of food, money, and alcohol are brought by guests. In these activities women tend to pray more and appear more devoted than the men. The men, however, invariably perform the key rituals, direct the preparation of the fiesta, supervise the ceremonies and processions, handle the distribution of liquor, and control the finances.

Traditional belief and instinct still play a part in the village imagery of disease (Rosales et al., 1964) and are very evident in many superstitions and concepts of cause and recovery. Early records reveal the existence of indigenous medicine men who treated and cured diseases. More recently the *curandero*, usually a professional of ladino ancestry, is sought out by villagers for the alleviation of their problems (Solien-González, 1957). In the more traditional and isolated villages the Indian witch-doctor continues to care for the more serious diseases and health problems so often assumed to be of supernatural origin, through curses, magical influences, the use of herbs, and other ancient practices. Western medicine, nevertheless, had been accepted rather thoroughly when the Cauqué study began in 1963, and many villagers had a firm appreciation of the decline in mortality and often attributed it to the introduction of Western medicine.

No medicine man or curandero practiced in the village during the Cauqué study, although some villagers sought consultation and treatment from curanderos and pharmacists in the larger neighboring communities of Sumpango, Chimaltenango, and Santiago, or in the cities of Antigua or

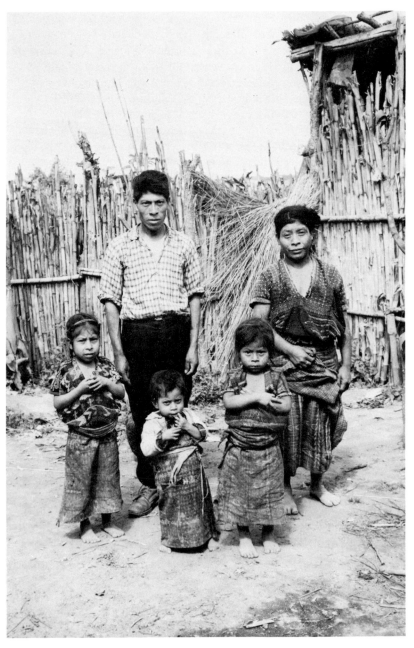

Figure 2.6
Typical village family

Table 2.12
Population by Family Components, by Survey Year and Number and Percentage of
Total Population

	Number (percentage of total population)		
	1963	1967	1971
Fathers or heads[a] of families	208 (19.4)	229 (18.3)	260 (19.0)
Mothers	169 (15.8)	200 (15.9)	229 (16.7)
Children (including relatives and adopted)	602 (56.2)	736 (58.7)	774 (56.5)
Parents of father or mother	17 (1.6)	11 (0.9)	6 (0.4)
Other adult relatives	70 (6.5)	71 (5.7)	92 (6.7)
Brothers and sisters of father or mother	2 (0.2)	5 (0.4)	7 (0.5)
Others without family relationship	2 (0.2)	1 (0.1)	1 (0.1)
Servants	1 (0.1)	1 (0.1)	1 (0.1)
Village population	1,071	1,254	1,370
Households	203	230	257

[a]The mother could become head of family when father dies or is away for a long period.

Guatemala. Occasionally villagers went to the clinic of a qualified missionary physician in Chimaltenango. The great majority of the sick and afflicted were attended by the staff of the Cauqué clinic, who kept records of the disabilities they treated and, when possible, of those people who were known to have sought services elsewhere.

Except for the occasional elderly childless woman or couple, all villagers live as family units of parents and children, often including grandparents and other relatives (figure 2.6). The 1963 census by family components is shown in table 2.12. The family is generally ruled by the father, but the mother may become the head at his death or because of his prolonged absence. Husband and wife constitute a stable union, although marriage is not a societal requirement. When a religious marriage ceremony is performed, it is a status symbol that provides an opportunity for a great fiesta for relatives and friends. More commonly, a ritual marriage is performed months or years after the union, often after enough money has accumulated for the proper celebrations.

Youngsters generally start courtship when the girls are fourteen to seventeen years old and the boys seventeen to twenty years old. Unmarried girls who become pregnant are almost always engaged; the usual occurrence is for the couple to elope, with the girl moving to the in-laws' house where she generally is welcome. Rarely does the boy move to the home of the girl, an act implying loss of prestige. Common-law and formal marriages are mostly between village residents; occasionally a woman marries a man from another community. Boys from neighboring villages initially are not altogether welcome in the village and may suffer some physical punishment. Should persistence in his suit lead to acceptance, the man takes up residence in the village of the woman if he has no land of his own and she does.

The custom in marriages among residents is for the parents of the bridegroom to request the bride from her parents. By protocol, the suit is invariably rejected and repeated two or three times. Normally at the third request the boy's parents bring food, liquor, and approximately ten quetzales in cash; approval follows and plans for the wedding begin. If the parents of the girl continue to reject the proposal because of the boy's limited economic capacity or because of a difference in religion, elopement is still possible in which case the girl must leave her personal possessions.

The civil marriage contract is simple, inexpensive, and ordinarily performed on a weekday. The religious wedding takes place on a Saturday or Sunday, traditionally at six in the morning in a well-decorated church. After the ceremony the couple departs to the bridegroom's house for the three-day fiesta. The house is decorated with pine garlands, flower and paper decorations, and pine needles on the floor. Traditional Indian music is played on the marimba and other indigenous instruments, such as the harp, *chirimía* (flutes) and *tamborón* (drum). Dancing starts in the afternoon, usually by the first person to become excited by the alcohol, commonly an older woman, while the other guests form circles and hold hands. The newlyweds do not drink, or, if they do, they do not overindulge; they spend most of the fiesta entertaining guests and listening to the advice of parents, ushers, and other prominent people. As in all celebrations, food plays an important role. Hot chocolate and bread are served for breakfast; soup, *pulique* (a dish made with beef), tortillas, coffee, and bread are served for lunch and dinner. Tripe, beans, and tamales are other favored foods.

Women's occupations are largely those concerned with the care of children, cooking and housekeeping, agricultural activities, and the selling and buying of produce in the markets. In former days women spent as much as half a day in the laborious preparation of maize. During the past three decades the introduction of community mechanical mills, usually of European import, has allowed more time for other activities. The same can be said about hand weaving, which, in this village, has become rare in recent times due to greater availability of low-cost machine-woven fabrics.

A woman's typical day starts at 5:30 A.M. and ends at 8:30 P.M. It includes such activities as lighting the fire, going to the mill to grind the *nixtamal* (corn that has been boiled for one hour with lime water), preparing the meals, washing the dishes, helping with the crops, washing clothes and mending, gathering wood, and visiting neighbors and friends. Older girls and school children aid their mothers in household chores.

The day allotted to attending the great market in a nearby city or town is commonly a family event. It begins at 1 A.M. when members of the family

Table 2.13
Occupations, by Survey Year and Number and Percentage of Male and Female
Population

	Percentage of men and women[a]		
	1963	1967	1971
Men			
Farmers	81	67	49
Day Laborers	4	15	35
Soldiers or unoccupied	6	11	6
Masons	2	2	1
Other[b]	6	5	8
Total number of men	292	343	388
Women			
Housewives	96	97	98
Other[c]	4	3	2
Total number of women	261	301	349

[a]Includes only persons aged 15 years or more.
[b]School teacher, storekeeper, mason, fixer, butcher.
[c]School teacher, merchant, farmer, weaver.

depart by bus, carrying legumes, fruits, or flowers to be sold. These products
have been carefully selected, cleaned, and bundled the preceding day, a most
laborious occupation. The return home is at noon, after the produce has been
sold and needed supplies purchased. Profits are often low, sometimes no more
than enough to cover the bus fare, but sales may reach as much as 50
quetzales when the produce represents the harvest of a whole season.

Men have less complicated schedules, but their work is physically harder.
The day's work extends from 6 A.M. to 6 P.M., although at harvest time they
occasionally sleep during the night in improvised huts in the fields. As with
women, their activities are extremely varied. Changes in the weather and variations in moons and rains are watched carefully, and propitious times are
noted for clearing land, cultivating, weeding, and harvesting. These operations
are surrounded by a degree of mystery and hope for the Indian, since he de-
pends on the land to live. A few men have subsidiary occupations other than
farming; there are several masons in the village, a butcher, two barbers, and
two carpenters, but craftmanship, in general, is not developed.

While there were significantly fewer farmers at the end of the study
period than at the beginning, the proportion of day laborers had increased
(table 2.13). A farmer is a man who cultivates his own land; a day laborer
does the same work but for wages and on someone else's property. The overall proportion of men engaged in agriculture, however, remained rather fixed
over the study period. The observed shift relates to the increase in landless
men as a result of population growth and land shortage, a grave problem in

Table 2.14
Languages, Literacy, and Educational Attainment, by Survey Year and Percentage of
Total Population

	Percentage of total population[a]		
	1963	1967	1971
Languages			
Spanish only	2.4	4.0	3.3
Cakchiquel only	6.8	2.0	1.1
Cakchiquel and Spanish	90.1	93.0	95.3
Unknown	0.6	1.0	0.4
Literacy			
Read and write	51.1	55.9	62.8
Read, only	1.5	0.4	0
Illiterate	47.1	43.4	36.8
Unknown	0.3	0.3	0.4
Educational attainment			
No schooling	32.8	29.3	29.4
Elementary school			
1st year	14.7	23.1	17.8
2nd or 3rd year	27.4	29.3	32.4
4th to 6th year	14.7	16.8	19.5
High school			
1st to 3rd year	0.4	0.3	0.1
4th to 6th year	0	0.6	0.6
Technical school	0	0	0.1
University	0	0	0
Unknown[b]	10.0	0.5	0.1
Population	789	931	1,045

[a]Includes only persons aged seven years or more.
[b]Information could not be obtained for a large number of people in 1963.

Guatemalan villages, which eventually will affect urban areas even more. A
greater proportion of men employed as soldiers in 1967 appears to reflect
increased recruitment because of larger military operations during the study
period. No change was recorded in women's occupations.

In Santa María Cauqué men and women find time to chat and smile while
working. No direct provision is made for sports or leisure activities, but a
general feeling of contentment and security is evident in the village. Fences
do not exist, doors are not locked, there is no haste or violence, and most
residents are willing to give attention, to listen, and to smile when approached
in their work or on the street.

Education

A public primary school for boys and girls was built in 1954. It is an outstanding structure in the village and currently has six grades. For almost thirty years village children, who enter the school when they are seven to nine years old, have been taught Spanish there. Before that age most children speak only Cakchiquel, but school instruction is almost wholly in Spanish. Because the national Guatemalan educational system is of the European pattern, transferred from the urban capital city to the rural areas without significant alteration, the school program has little relation to the Indian culture or to village life and its problems. Despite such shortcomings, some progress has been made over the years in literacy and educational attainment (table 2.14). Over half of the population over seven years old is literate, which, however, does not imply that all of these can read, write, and handle numbers effectively. The increased proportion of Indians speaking Spanish, as well as the increased proportion of literate persons, reflects the influence of schooling and radio broadcasts in Spanish. No technical training is available in the school system, and opportunities to pursue a technical or college education remain minimal.

Hygiene and Sanitary Practices

Tradition, illiteracy, and poverty at the village and individual levels are reflected in hygienic practices. Water supply is limited. The temascal is the traditional method of bathing used by women and, to a lesser extent, young men. While not all homes have a temascal, most women use the facility about twice a week, if necessary through a neighbor's unit. Women bathe after the menstrual period, postpartum, and in case of illness. Men bathe less frequently. They use creeks, public showers, and temascals. No care of teeth, nails, or ears is customary. Clothing is washed once a week, and most people sleep with their clothes on. Water in the house is stored in large earthen jars, from which it is taken by any handy receptacle. The family sleeps in one room, on a simple pallet, a *tapesco* (slightly elevated bed), or, less often, a *petate* (mat) on the floor. Ordinarily, the sick are not isolated.

Defecation on the ground is frequent; at the time of the first village survey more than two-thirds of the population were recorded as indiscriminate squatters. The rest used latrines, although even in houses with latrines older people and children often made no use of them. Garbage and animal waste ordinarily is thrown away indiscriminately or, more rarely, buried or used for fertilizer. Living quarters ordinarily are unkempt; beds are not made and a disarray of objects and articles characterizes most households. Floors and yards of houses, however, are neatly swept and maintained free of garbage. Considering economic resources and education, the Indians evidently appreciate cleanliness and manage to accomplish a great deal under difficult conditions.

Diet

The present dietary pattern of families indicates a slow change toward a greater diversity of foods than was present in the diets of Santa María Cauqué in 1950 (Flores and Reh, 1955). Maize, however, continues to contribute 60 percent of total calories and protein to pregnant women and 47 percent to preschool children, with no observed changes in overall protein and caloric intake except for a few novel items that contribute little or nothing to the diet, such as flours, edible starches, potato chips, and carbonated beverages. The last item is a significant drain on the village economy since it is purchased at an equivalent cost of one bottle of beverage for every two pounds of maize or half pound of black beans.

An average family of five—parents and three children under ten years of age—consumes approximately 1,600 pounds of maize and 180 pounds of black beans per year. This intake has been estimated from dietary surveys of the Cauqué study; it is nutritionally deficient in beans. To grow this amount of produce without fertilizer a family needs about ten cuerdas of land, an amount that agrees with land status as recorded in the 1963 census (table 2.6). Significantly more land would be required to grow the larger amount of beans necessary to balance the diet.

Births, Deaths, and Population Growth

In general, Santa María Cauqué has a young population; approximately 50 percent of the inhabitants are less than fifteen years old. Relative stability in age composition, reflected in the shape of the pyramids in figure 2.7, is evident at all ages throughout the twelve years of the present study. The population pyramids are characteristic of underdeveloped societies. How such composition came about becomes evident in examining the birth and death rates over the years.

Santa María Cauqué has exceptionally high birth and death rates, which early biomedical surveys recognized as characteristic of much of Guatemala (Shattuck et al., 1938). Birth rates per 1,000 population for the years 1936 through 1972 are shown in figure 2.8.* Birth rates for the period, by five-year intervals, are shown in table 2.15. Both displays reveal a decline from 1936 to 1949 and from 1960 to 1971.

The profile of mortality, expressed as the crude death rate per 1,000 population, is also shown in figure 2.8 and table 2.15. Greater variability was noted in annual crude death rates because of severe epidemics of whooping cough, measles, diarrhea including dysentery, and acute respiratory

---

* In general, births tended to be slightly more numerous in the rainy months from August to November. Conception was most frequent in the dry season from December to March. Whether this is related to an increased caloric intake in that period, to the fact that men spend more time at home, or to the influences of weather, the agricultural calendar, or social variables is little more than speculation.

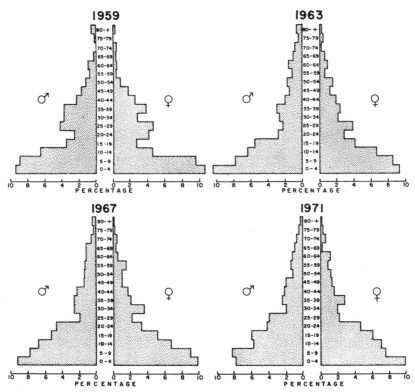

Figure 2.7
Population distribution, by age and sex, 1959, 1963, 1967, 1971

disease. The average annual rate was 51 per 1,000 in 1940 to 1944 through the influence of a combination of measles, whooping cough, and diarrheal disease epidemics in 1940 to 1942. Notably high mortality rates were 54 per 1,000 population in 1943; 72 in 1942; and 43 in 1950. In those years more than one of every twenty persons in the village died, with excess fatalities among adolescents and adults as well as among children. Epidemics are vividly remembered by older people of the village. Several deaths commonly occurred within a single day, a traumatic experience sometimes prolonged for weeks at a time, disrupting social equilibrium and decimating the cohorts not only of children but of adolescents and persons in the reproductive ages. The latter group had, perhaps, the most serious impact, because it is the main support of the village economy. Since 1952 no more epidemics of large proportion have been recorded. At the conclusion of the writing of this book, however, an earthquake destroyed the whole village, except for six buildings, on 4 February 1976. All of the adobe houses were destroyed, resulting in 78 deaths and 357 injured among 1,500 people. This natural disaster affected preschool children primarily and was reminiscent of past tragedies.

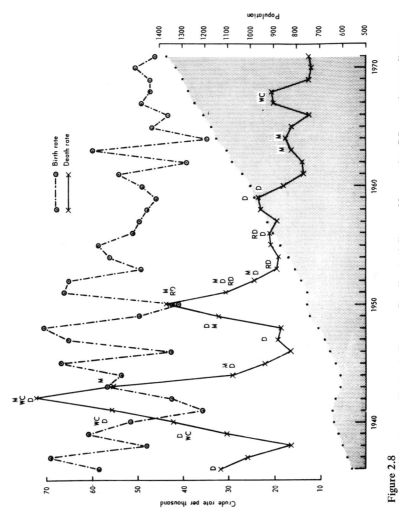

Figure 2.8
Birth and death rates. Epidemic diseases: D = diarrheal disease; M = measles; RD = respiratory disease; WC = whooping cough. Key words at the top of epidemic peaks indicate that the base of the epidemic was formed by those diseases.

Decrease in childhood and crude death rates during the years from 1946 to
1960 (table 2.15) coincided with a greater availability of health services and
particularly with the beginning of INCAP activities in the village (Flores and
Reh, 1955; Scrimshaw et al., 1967a; Mata et al., 1967a). Excessively high
death rates were not observed after 1954. The reduction became even more
pronounced—the crude death rate had declined by 1960 to 16 per 1,000 per
year—with the establishment of a treatment center as part of the Nutrition-
Infection Study (Scrimshaw et al., 1967b). The rate continued to drop
throughout the Cauqué observations, reaching a low of 9 per 1,000 population at the end of the study.

Age-specific death rates by quinquennium from 1940 to 1972 are presented in table 2.16. Reductions in postneonatal and preschool mortality
were evident after the period from 1940 to 1944 despite the occurrence of
serious epidemics. (The factors that led to the remarkable decline in severity
of epidemics and associated fatality in the period from 1945 to 1954 are not
wholly understood.) After 1954 the decline in rates occurred more slowly,
although in the later years of the Cauqué study postneonatal mortality and
schoolchild mortality were markedly reduced. Consequently, there was an
overall effect on infant mortality. The markedly increased neonatal and preschool mortality from 1965 to 1969 relates to an epidemic of whooping
cough in 1968; these rates then declined during the period from 1970 to
1972.

The relative distribution of deaths among the various age groups expectedly has changed over the years (table 2.17). While the relative proportion of deaths among infants and persons aged fifteen years or more has
remained fairly fixed, dramatic decreases have occurred among children two
to fourteen years old. In the period from 1960 to 1969 not a single death was
recorded among children ten to fourteen years old. Furthermore, toward the
end of the Cauqué study (1970 to 1972) there was a further decrease in
deaths of children one to four years old.

Estimates of population growth in table 2.15 demonstrate a slow decline
in both the birth and death rates and a well-marked and steady rate of population growth dating from the oldest village records, except for the years
1940 to 1944 when deaths exceeded births, giving an overall estimated population decrease. Rates of population growth in Santa María Cauqué during
recent years have increased from 2.8 percent per year in the period 1950 to
1954 to 3.6 percent in the period from 1970 to 1972. Figure 2.8 demonstrates that the population has doubled in twenty-five years. Although this
increase was due in part to the availability of a health center and better health
services, it was not wholly based on these factors; measurable increments
were recorded before these interventions occurred. That the village situation
is not exceptional is revealed by similar growth in the nation as a whole;

Table 2.15
Population Growth, 1936–1972

Period	Average annual birth rates per 1,000	Average annual death rates per 1,000	Average annual percentage growth per year	Remarks
1936–1939	59.1	26.2	3.29	
1940–1944	47.8	51.0	-0.32	
1945–1949	58.7	21.9	3.68	Social reform began in 1944
1950–1954	55.4	27.1	2.83	Health Center established in 1955
1955–1959	50.4	21.5	2.89	Nutrition-Infection study began in 1958
1960–1964	47.1	15.8	3.13	Cauqué study began in 1963
1965–1969	46.7	16.3	3.04	
1970–1972	47.4	10.9	3.65	

Note: Data for the years 1936 to 1949 are of low reliability (see Part II).

Table 2.16
Age-Specific Death Rates by Five-Year Periods: Infancy, Early Childhood, Late Childhood, Adolescence, and Adulthood, 1940–1972

	Number of deaths						
	1940–1944	1945–1949	1950–1954	1955–1959	1960–1964	1965–1969	1970–1972
Early neonatal (0–7 d)	20	30	37	26	20	17	15
Late neonatal (8–28 d)	40	15	27	26	12	24	21
Neonatal (0–28 d)	60	45	64	51	32	42	36
Postneonatal (29 d–11 mo)	99	90	82	56	63	52	26
Infant (0–11 mo)	159	134	146	107	95	93	62
Preschool (1–4 yr)	115	65	43	46	32	39	13
5–9 yr	37.6	12.8	4.7	8.1	3.5	4.0	0
10–14 yr	22.6	0	3.9	1.7	0	0	1.9
15–24 yr	10.0	1.5	1.3	4.5	1.0	2.6	1.2
25+ yr	28.9	13.8	11.2	19.0	12.0	13.8	11.2
Crude death rate	51.0	21.9	27.1	21.5	15.8	16.3	9.0

Note: Infant mortality, deaths per 1,000 live births; preschool mortality, deaths per 1,000 population aged one to four years; thereafter, deaths per 1,000 population of the specified age. Information on stillbirths was not tabulated because records of this variable in the Official Register are unreliable.

Table 2.17
Deaths and Percentage of Distribution by Age, 1940–1972

| | Number of deaths (percentage) | | | |
	1940–1949	1950–1959	1960–1969	1970–1972
< 1 yr	51 (22.9)	67 (36.6)	51 (29.8)	12 (32.4)
1 yr	35 (15.7)	27 (14.8)	38 (22.2)	3 (8.1)
2–4 yr	47 (21.1)	27 (14.8)	20 (11.7)	4 (10.8)
5–9 yr	26 (11.7)	9 (4.9)	7 (4.1)	0
10–14 yr	10 (4.5)	3 (1.6)	0	1 (2.7)
15–24 yr	7 (3.1)	5 (2.7)	4 (2.3)	2 (5.4)
25+ yr	47 (21.1)	45 (24.6)	51 (29.8)	15 (40.5)
Total	223	183	171	37 (99.9)

indeed, Guatemala's population increase is one of the largest in the world. Improvement of health services and nutrition as isolated measures, however, will only lead to greater demographic pressure, unless a multidisciplinary approach effects concomitant changes such as a reduction of births and improvements in the standard of living.

PART II
STUDY PLAN AND PROCEDURES

Chapter 3
Operational Procedures and Approach

No manual is known to the author on general procedures for the successful conduct of field work similar to those designed to guide the house staffs of modern hospitals. While principles of field epidemiology have been outlined (Gordon, 1963), the methods and techniques needed to initiate field work and conduct operations have not been detailed. In fact, the orientation and goals of the Cauqué study required that many available procedures had to be modified or adapted and others had to be developed specifically to meet the intended purpose.

Experience gained with the Cauqué study distinguished at least six fundamentals of this kind of field work. The first three relate primarily to human relations, and in order of importance they are: (a) recruitment of a hard-working, capable, and loyal field staff; (b) establishment of good relations with the subject population, together with continuing efforts to maintain or improve that rapport; and (c) provision of compensating services to the community in a systematic and reassuring fashion. The remaining three conditions are technical: (d) adequate physical and administrative support facilities; (e) full coverage of the designated population, whether a sample or the whole, in order to guarantee an adequate interpretation of results; and (f) systematic supervision of field operations to ensure good quality information. If a study plan calls for prospective observations over a long period, the need for the first three conditions is unequivocal. Failure in any or all will result in a loss of study subjects, perhaps enough to affect the results significantly or even to bring the research to a premature end. At best, deficiencies in the first three conditions will require a more exacting analytic effort in testing hypotheses.

On the other hand, deficiencies in the last three conditions may be compensated for by such means as the introduction of technical procedures for data quality control.

These six conditions are best addressed in the planning stage of a field study. They warrant special attention at the time data collection begins. They require continued effort throughout a long-term investigation if handicaps to eventual success are to be avoided. Some difficulties are bound to occur; the aim is to minimize them. The operational procedures of the Cauqué study were designed with this in mind.

Physical and Administrative Support Facilities

The headquarters of the Cauqué study were located in the Division of Microbiology of INCAP in Guatemala City, Guatemala. The study benefited throughout from its close association with INCAP. The elaborate procedures in research and field operations and the extensive experience and efficiency of INCAP administrators in helping scientists conduct their investigations was an important advantage. INCAP's link with the Pan American Health Organization also brought stability and ensured independence from local political intervention.

The study's headquarters at INCAP included a well-equipped assembly of laboratories and offices, capable of handling techniques and procedures of field epidemiology, clinical microbiology and nutrition, and the processing of large volumes of data.

The laboratories include units for tissue culture, virology, immunology and serology, enteric bacteriology, anaerobic bacteriology, and parasitology, all equipped with the necessary apparatus and instruments. Facilities for dish washing, media preparation, and sterilization jointly serve the various units. Offices house the professional staff with independent provision for data analysis and for conferences. Other units of INCAP, particularly the Computer Center, supported the work of the study through technical aid and consultation on special problems.

The facilities for data handling deserve special mention. During the first three years most study records were kept in the office of the Division Chief or of the Field Director. Eventually a data flow office was organized; it grew to house a staff of three assistants, one with a knowledge of Fortran programming.

INCAP's Computer Center had one IBM 1620 computer with disk drives. Most of the terminal analyses were done at the John L. Locke, Jr., Computing Facility of the Health Sciences Division, University of Washington, where a General Automation SPC-16/65 computer with 32K words, two 12.5 million word disk drives, two 9-track tape drives, and associated equipment was available. For the analyses the Conversational Computer Statistical System (CCSS), Biomedical Computer Programs (BMD), and Statistical

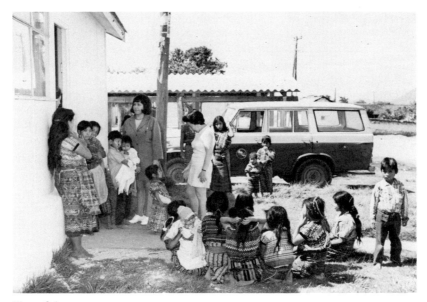

Figure 3.1
Dietician and nurse meeting children and adults in front of health center

Package for the Social Sciences (SPSS) were employed, the latter two available at the CDC-6400 computer of the University of Washington.

The field station used during the study also included the village Health Center (figure 3.1). Built in 1956, the station had been under INCAP administration since the start of INCAP's Nutrition-Infection Study in 1958. The building had areas for an outpatient waiting room, a nurses' clinic, physician's office, dietician's office, a prenatal clinic, storeroom, field laboratory, kitchen, dining room, and nurses' dormitory.

Since electric current was not available in the village at the beginning of the study, propane gas was used for the burners and stove, a kerosene-operated egg incubator was employed for the bacterial cultures, and daylight served for the single microscope. Electricity was installed at the end of 1966, and by May 1967 the laboratory and clinic were operating with it.

Living conditions in the field were modest yet adequate for the staff, particularly for the nurses who lived at the clinic. Material comforts included electricity, a shower, a flush toilet, a clean and spacious dining room, a refrigerator, and a modestly equipped kitchen for preparing meals.

The outpatient clinic ensured delivery of adequate medical assistance within the framework and limitations of a field station. Facilities of the prenatal and pediatric clinics were fully adequate to develop reliable information. The nurses' clinic and the dietician's office also served as general field headquarters for data collection through home visits.

Equipment at the field station included scales and balances, an infant-meter, calipers, otoscope, sphygmomanometer, pelvimeter, and equipment for minor surgery. The field station also had a portable X-ray machine for studies of bone maturation, refrigerators, a stove, a mechanical calculator, and a clinical laboratory.

Once electric current was available, modern incubators, refrigerators, a high-speed refrigerated centrifuge, and full equipment for processing samples for microbiological study were installed. At this point the field laboratory was as well-equipped as the base laboratories at headquarters in Guatemala City, with full capability for isolation of the labile *Shigella* organisms or growth of the fastidious anaerobic bacteria in the logarithmic concentrations found in biological specimens. These technical advantages, combined with ready access to patients, permitted an unusually prompt processing of specimens under optimal conditions for incubation, isolation, and identification of microorganisms. A technical laboratory staff in the field added still another dimension of importance, the identification of the laboratory worker with field activities and with the human problems under study.

Supervision

Daily supervision of research and service operations by professional workers was done through field visits by the physician or project director throughout the study, including weekends and holidays. Visits to the field station by persons unconnected with the study were also supervised. At irregular intervals of two to four times a year, parties of visiting scientists were escorted to the village, either singly or in groups rarely exceeding five persons. The scientists were usually from other lands, North America in particular. Their visits included a meeting with villagers and authorities, who usually were interested in the visitors' country of origin and occupation. These visits made the study more widely known in scientific circles and in turn enhanced funding and scientific interchange.

Coverage

An outstanding feature of the study was the continuous complete coverage and thorough surveillance of the village population. In addition to the efforts made in initial acquaintance and the cultivation of cooperation, a functioning staff was maintained in the village at all times. One auxiliary public health nurse was in residence at the Health Center and on call day and night, including weekends, under a rotating system that required added compensation. That service became an established tradition in the first year of the study. It was useful in medical and surgical emergencies and was of paramount importance in collecting information on births and deaths and in permitting thorough observation of childbirths as well as in maintaining good relations with villagers.

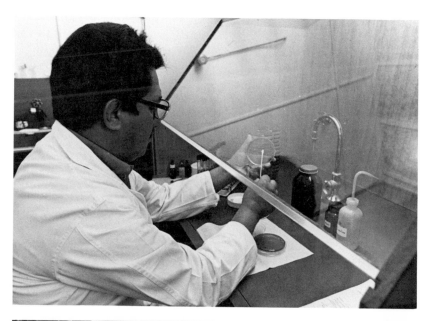

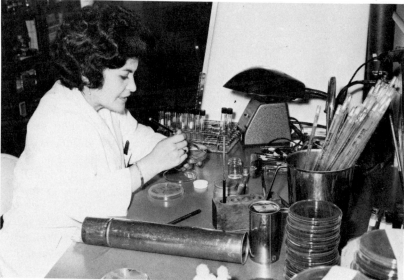

Figure 3.2
Processing fecal specimens, taking bacteria counts at the field laboratory

Field Staff

Three native Guatemalans, reliable and qualified women field workers, two of whom were from similar rural areas, were recruited to collect data through home visits. Two had previous experience in health work with Indian communities. By the end of the study this field staff had grown to ten, three men and seven women, all with similar characteristics and qualifications. One spoke Cakchiquel fluently; the others had a limited vocabulary in the dialect but acquired facility in the course of field operations.

Field work developed steadily and smoothly throughout the study. Even though the staff received no wages beyond accepted local levels, they made the work their primary concern and rendered unnecessary any use of the administrative regulations and prescribed disciplinary action developed in anticipation of difficulties. The staff, moreover, remained in the project largely through personal motivation and appreciation of the significance of the study, the quality of the methods employed, and the mystique that develops from group action in a village like Santa María Cauqué.

Rapport

The first contact in the village was between two groups, the local authorities—primarily the mayor and ministriles—and the project director, the field physician, and nurses. A message of good will was delivered to the authorities by the project director. Explanations in simple words then followed on the nature, scope, and general procedures of the study. Main emphasis was on reinforcement of the facilities of the Health Center and the provision of medical services without charge. More direct discussions with the authorities of the community and with elderly residents and established leaders, who soon were identified, followed this initial formal meeting. The two midwives who delivered all babies in the village were interviewed to explain the staff's need for surveillance of pregnant women, the recruitment of newborn infants for observation, and the collection of umbilical cord blood (figures 3.3 and 3.4). Midwives were assured that the field staff would not enter into competition for patients and that they were present in the village solely to promote health affairs.

These informal meetings almost invariably resulted in general acceptance of the study proposal for long-term observation of mothers and newborns and in an expression of willingness to participate. Occasionally, a villager or a group of villagers reacted negatively, and additional efforts were made to gain their cooperation. Almost all noncooperating families eventually joined in study activities. In a few instances collaboration was only partial with little information obtained but even these families used the services of the Health Center.

The early contacts were repeated many times in informal and subtle fashion during home visits or in the course of other field work as opportunity

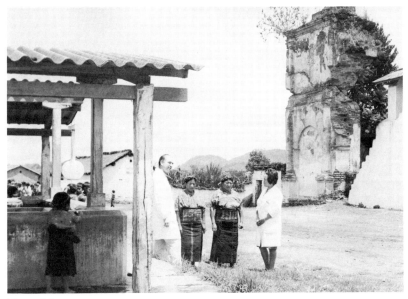

Figure 3.3
Physician and nurse chatting with the two midwives who attend most of the deliveries in the village

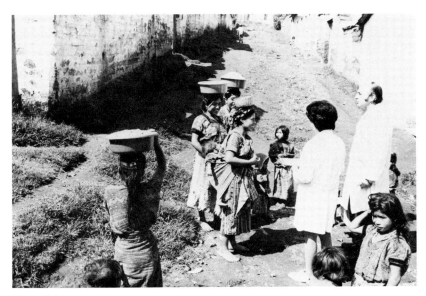

Figure 3.4
Physician and nurse meeting women carrying *nixtamal* (cooked maize kernels) to the mill, an everyday occurrence throughout the study

grew for more extended acquaintance and understanding. In most instances the obvious cultural barrier was overcome successfully but not wholly, and then mainly because the field workers, although native to Guatemala, were not Indian. This proved to be of some advantage, however, in that it precluded any deep involvement by observers in the private sphere of a family. In carrying out their tasks the field staff avoided personal involvement in problems inimical to the study.

Whenever difficult situations arose or new phases of the study were to begin, formal meetings were held with village authorities and leaders to dispel any doubt about proposed activities and to seek their cooperation. Formal meetings of this nature were scheduled each year, if for no other reason than to keep the community informed. Never in the history of the study was there an instance of hostility, or aggressive rejection of an examination or an interview.

Efforts to maintain good rapport were furthered at the village level as staff from the field, and on occasion from headquarters, participated in a number of village social activities—a baptism, a marriage, or the celebration of the cofradía. Social activities in which the entire INCAP staff participated were celebration of the village Patroness's Day (the Assumption of the Virgin Mary, August 15) and the Birth of Christ (December 24). For the August 15 celebration INCAP contributed to the limited funds of the municipality. Members of the staff visited officials to express their appreciation of village collaboration. This inevitably was followed by a formal exchange of *guaro* (the indigenous rum) after which the staff returned to the Health Center. There a social hour for field and headquarters staff brought the two groups together and reinforced the field members' assurance that they were the solid foundation of the project. Such meetings had a highly desirable effect on morale; they also provided a means for the laboratory staff, including secretaries and data clerks, to visit the field and see the study in perspective.

Over the years INCAP participation in this celebration became an established custom, accepted and welcomed by the villagers who in turn honored the staff by performing their traditional masked *Bailes de la Conquista* (Dances of the Conquest), a ceremony that dates from the time of the Spanish colonizers.

The social activity that outdistanced all others was the celebration of Christmas, an occasion for distributing gifts to young children and for breaking *piñatas* (decorated earthen jugs filled with candies) in the area fronting the Health Center. Attendance at the afternoon party was villagewide, with mothers and older children expressing much anticipation. Gifts were simple— a doll, a ball, candy—and care was taken that all shared equally. The combined field and laboratory staff joined in a Christmas social hour similar to the Patroness's Day celebration.

At certain intervals the field personnel were consulted on matters dealing with petitions to regional or central government or in other related matters, and advice was given to the extent that knowledge permitted.

From the beginning of the study, field workers were convinced of the respect they enjoyed from the village people. Perhaps the crucial factor was that all staff members had the conviction that the Indian deserves the same treatment as the non-Indian. Indian dignity, pride, problems, and way of life were respected and understood. The villagers knew this. Without doubt, it was the key to much of the success of field operations.

Services

Before INCAP came to the village in 1950 (Flores and Reh, 1955), no health, nutritional, or medical assistance was available other than the traditional advice and medicines given by curanderos, grandmothers, or the native medicine men. In 1956 a Health Center was opened by the Central Government and staffed by an auxiliary health nurse with three years of training in nursing school, after six years of primary school. When INCAP began its first studies on nutrition and infection in 1958 (Scrimshaw et al., 1967a), the staff was augmented by a part-time physician, an additional health nurse, and two field workers. Medical care included antimicrobial drugs in treatment of infectious disease, limited use of smallpox and diphtheria-pertussis-tetanus vaccines, but no nutritional education or food distribution. The study ended in 1963. The Health Center then was reorganized in accord with the design and plans of the Cauqué study, a key feature of which was to cultivate the collaboration of the villagers. Care of patients was the main aspect of that effort, regardless of their interest or willingness to participate in study observations.

Staffed by a full-time pediatrician, two auxiliary public health nurses, and two field workers for dietary surveys and other activities, the center provided far more medicine and attention than the program of the Guatemalan Health Services in comparable villages. Not only was medical care free and on demand but facilities for treatment were more elaborate than usual. The physician in charge was available full-time instead of through periodic visits at weekly or biweekly intervals for two hours or often less, as was the practice in neighboring villages. The competence of the field staff was above average; patients with medical or surgical emergencies were provided transportation to central hospitals, and dietetic treatment was available for patients with severe protein-calorie malnutrition.

Activities in preventive medicine were more limited. This situation was virtually forced upon the study by a combination of circumstances ranging from the cultural pattern of the village to the kind of health program provided by the Ministry of Health. The intent was to maintain and comply with national plans and government norms for rural regions.

No programs of general health education, nutrition, use of latrines, mass treatment for intestinal parasites, treatment of water supplies, or vaccination were prescribed or effected by the central government during most of the study. Vaccination with DPT was offered by the Health Center but distributed only on a small scale, mainly because the villagers had little sympathy with immunization procedures. After a serious epidemic of whooping cough in 1968 the community developed more interest with the result that in recent years the proportion of children immunized against this and other diseases has increased. A safe, inexpensive, and well-tested vaccine against measles was not available in Guatemala before 1968. Early vaccines caused numerous clinical manifestations resembling the natural and much feared disease. An adverse reaction by a single village child would have been damaging to the staff and the study as well. The decision therefore was to await a nationally sponsored governmental program which did not materialize until June of the year the Cauqué study ended (Mata et al., 1974c).

Focusing their attention on health care in addition to their research obligations, the physician and nurses of the field staff provided services through the outpatient clinic and through home visits, in the case of emergencies. At the start the field staff included only one native of the village. Other nurses stayed overnight in quarters specially provided. One nurse promptly decided to rent a house in the village, evidence that she liked the village and the work. A common activity of the project director or physician was to visit the field on nonwork days for social visits that rather routinely came to include their families.

The daily routine of field work began on Sunday, around 7 A.M., when the nurse on call started home visits, mainly to take rectal temperatures of ill children and to distribute cardboard boxes for fecal specimens. From Monday through Friday the physician, the dietician, and the laboratory technicians traveled by car from Ciudad de Guatemala to Santa María Cauqué, leaving the city about 8 A.M. and returning around 6 P.M. On Saturdays and Sundays a nurse was always at the field station; a professional visit to the field on weekends by the physician or director was routine throughout the study.

An outpatient clinic administered by the field physician and one of the nurses operated three afternoons a week (figure 3.5). The nurse recorded temperatures, and the physician examined all children and seriously ill adults after screening. The nurse attended patients visiting the clinic on days that alternated with the scheduled outpatient clinic days and screened them for a later examination by the physician. He was available on any day, however, in case of emergencies and through calls by village authorities, school teachers, or other prominent persons.

Home visits were commonly made to sick children on the assumption that this limited the spread of infectious agents to other attendants at the clinic. Home visits also gave special attention to a search for the origins of disease.

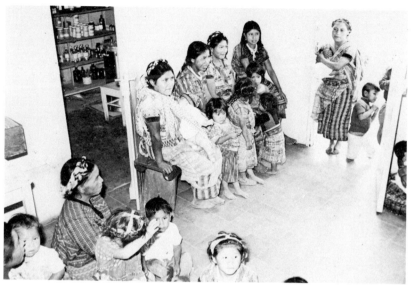

Figure 3.5
Waiting room of the clinic

Along with the continued surveillance, this practice contributed to early recognition and treatment of disease. During outbreaks of measles and whooping cough frequent home visits were made to most households in order to find new cases. Also, acutely ill patients and emergency needs were treated in the home. As much as half of the time devoted to medical care by the physician and his staff was outside the clinic.

The impact of these activities on the kind and quality of information derived became evident in the recorded results of the study.

Chapter 4
Operational Procedures and Analysis of Data

The preceding chapter described the concept, objectives, logistics, and overall accomplishments of field operations in Santa María Cauqué; this one details the methods, variables, and techniques employed in the collection and analysis of information. Field and laboratory data were recorded on special, individual forms, most of them precoded to facilitate card punching and computer processing. Appendix C lists the codes for the symptoms and illnesses studied, and appendix D lists all the variables tabulated.

During the formative stages of the Cauqué study and prior to the selection of subjects, ethical aspects of the research were assessed carefully by qualified scientists. A committee of active investigators in pediatrics, public health, biochemistry, anthropology, nutrition, and infectious disease was appointed for that specific purpose, primarily in relation to funding of the study by the National Institutes of Health, US Department of Health, Education, and Welfare. The study design, as eventually formulated, complied with the Institutional Guide to HEW Policy on Protection of Human Subjects (1971) in that no damage or injury was imposed upon the individuals concerned and the project, as conceived, reacted to their benefit. The descriptive nature of the Cauqué study settled most questions of ethics; the strict and severe position of the World Medical Association was fully met.

The study was instituted after visits and meetings with community principals and leaders over the course of a year; the study was explained and discussed in words that could be grasped by them, since more than half of the village adults did not read or write. Emphasis was placed on the benefits of free medical services and the potential gains—to the local community, to the country, and to nations with similar problems—from information the study would produce.

FIELD PROCEDURES

Births, Deaths, and Population Estimates
The data used for births, deaths, and population estimates for the years 1936 through 1963 were gathered from the village Municipal Registers. Items for the years 1964 to 1972 were obtained directly from the field staff of the Cauqué study. The census of 1967, carried out at midstudy, was judged the best estimate of the total population at that time. This population was the starting point from which annual populations of study years were estimated by adding deaths and subtracting births of the immediately preceding year. Populations for the years 1936 to 1962 were estimated by the same procedure. The post-1967 numbers represent people resident in the village as of January 1 each year. In view of the negligible migration documented for 1967 to 1971 and the completeness of birth and death registrations, our population estimates presumably do not contain significant errors.

The existence of relatively accurate and complete birth and death registers in a Guatemalan Indian village is a rare circumstance; its occurrence in Santa María Cauqué permitted an appraisal of the pattern of population growth through retrospective analysis (Luna-Jaspe et al., 1965) and provided the background for reasonable speculation as to the course of future changes.

The records of births and deaths for Santa María Cauqué have been kept in large books housed in the Municipal Building of the neighboring village of Santiago Sacatepéquez, the county seat. Complete records were available for all years since 1936. Books containing older data were too damaged to be used. For study purposes data for the years 1936 through 1963 were transferred from the registers to a prepared form indicating month and year of birth; month, year, and cause of death; and age at death.

While the recorded dates for both births and deaths were fairly accurate, two problems arose in using data from the registers. First, diagnoses of indigenous medicine men, relatives, friends of the family or, in some cases, the community secretary or other official had been entered as causes of death. In order to interpret these causes of death in conformity with modern medical criteria, ten of the leading village men were consulted on the meaning of the folk terms used in the registers. These meanings were then "translated" into most likely causes by qualified physicians. Over nine years of clinic work these equivalences have proved fairly accurate. Deaths from diarrhea, measles, and whooping cough are so dramatic and well known in the community that normally they are correctly recorded. Thus dysentery is readily characterized if blood and mucus are seen in the stools. Malnutrition, however, is a common cause that goes unrecognized. Worms are frequently the recorded cause of death among children dying of malnutrition and other diseases because of the frequency with which round worms (*Ascaris*) are expelled as death ensues or shortly thereafter (Béhar et al., 1958). Severe protein-calorie malnutrition may be designated as hydropexia, but usually a death is not recorded as being from kwashiorkor because an intercurrent acute infection is more obvious and outranks all other evidence in the judgment of the relative who reports the death. For purposes of analysis, therefore, only the number of deaths caused by measles, diarrhea, whooping cough, or pneumonia were considered.

The second problem in using the register data concerns an almost certain underreporting of females in the records for 1936 to 1948. Table 4.1 gives the number of recorded births by sex and the corresponding sex ratios in three arbitrarily determined periods: 1936 to 1948, the period from the first available data until the establishment of a health service in the village; 1949 to 1963, the period from that date until the start of the Cauqué investigation; and 1964 to 1972, the duration of the Cauqué study. Apparently, female births were underreported during the period from 1936 to 1948 to the extent of 25 to 30 percent. Improved health services and a better attitude toward registration in rural areas, perhaps, account for the subsequent differences. Infant morality rates before 1948 were probably underestimated as well, not only in the village but in other similar regions. Since infanticide is unknown among these people the figures for 1936 to 1948 were corrected arbitrarily by adding 25 percent to the female births in that period, on the assumption that the reporting of male births had been accurate. Since the annual populations were estimated retrospectively by adding deaths and subtracting births, the adjustment for underreporting of female births was incorporated into the population estimates.

Data for the years 1964 to 1972 presented fewer problems since three complete enumerations of the village population were made by the Cauqué field staff during the course of the study, the first in 1963 when the study began, the second at midpoint (1967), and the third near the end (1971). A similar although less complete census of 1959 was available and used for comparison. The four censuses were taken by the same field worker ac-

Table 4.1
Recorded Births by Sex, 1936–1972

| | Number of births | | | Ratio male/female |
	Male	Female	Total	
1936–1948	233	160	393	1.46
1949–1963	364	339	703	1.08
1964–1972	249	275	524	0.91

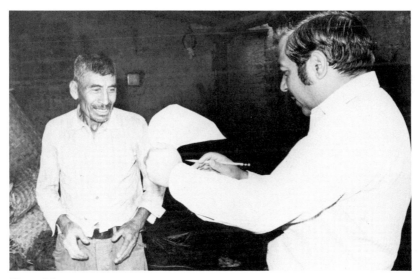

Figure 4.1
Census taker gathering information from the head of a family

cording to an established procedure that required from two to four weeks for the house to house visits, with an additional four weeks for verification of the data (figure 4.1). Data were obtained by an interview with the head of the family or other responsible adult and included information about names; sex; date of birth; family relationship; ethnicity; literacy; schooling; the wearing of shoes; quality of housing; environmental sanitation; ownership of animals, land, and home; and the uses to which cultivatable land was put.

Proper recording required a familiarity with local customs, some knowledge of the Cakchiquel dialect, and tact. This last was most important in view of the long-standing Indian fear about possible loss of land and property to ladinos, urban entrepreneurs, or the government.

The quality of the information from each census was verified by comparing actual enumerations with differences accounted for by births and deaths during intercensal periods, as recorded by the staff. Cross-checking was also done with the Official Register of the County Municipality in the neighboring village of Santiago Sacatepéquez.

The current census or intercensal extrapolations characterized the study subjects and their environment and provided the basis for determining rates of birth, death, and population growth and for creating the Socioeconomic Index.

Target Population
Although observations of one kind or another were made on practically all inhabitants of Santa María Cauqué, certain population groups were subject to

Table 4.2
Cohorts of Newborns Observed During the Study

	Number of live-borns in the cohort	Number of newborns by years of completed observation							
		1st	2nd	3rd	4th	5th	6th	7th	8th
1964	37	6, 31	2, 29	29	1,1 27	27	27	27	27
1965	54	3,1 50	1, 49	1, 48	2, 46	46	46	46	
1966	50	3, 47	6, 41	2, 39	0,1 38	0,1 37	37		
1967	60	14, 46	5,1 40	40	0,1 39	39			
1968	60	6, 54	1, 53	1, 52	1, 51				
1969	61	9, 52	1, 51	1, 50					
1970	67	5,1 61	61						
1971	63	3, 61							
1972	6								
Total	458	353	308	253	197	149	110	73	27

Note: Numbers to left of comma indicate newborns lost due to death; those to the right indicate newborns lost to migration. Lower numbers represent newborns completing year of study.

intensive study. They included all pregnant women and their newborn infants, the latter recruited into cohorts according to the time of birth. A requirement for enlistment in the study was the observation of the mother at an early stage of gestation and a promise of family collaboration in the investigation. This was difficult to obtain from the few ladino women of the village.

Pregnant Women   A total of 205 women experienced 469 pregnancies during the study. Two ladino women, married to ladino brothers living in the village, delivered three single live-born infants in urban clinics, and were excluded from the study and analysis because (a) cooperation during pregnancy was poor; (b) the infants were born outside the village; (c) information was incomplete; (d) the women were not native to the village; and (e) their socioeconomic and cultural status was significantly above that of the predominantly Indian population of the village; indeed, they were essentially of the Guatemalan urban middle class. A third ladino woman married the most progressive and educated Indian of the community; she gave birth to her first child in a city clinic, and likewise was excluded. Later, she entered the study and eventually contributed three pregnancies. Also excluded were two non-resident mothers who delivered single infants in the village and left with the children one to two weeks later.

After these exclusions the study population of pregnant women consisted of 203 women having 465 pregnancies. No losses to observation or withdrawals occurred in this group. Information was not always complete but basic items were obtained for each pregnancy.

Cohorts of Newborns Of the 465 pregnancies, 14 ended in fetal deaths (stillborn), 5 resulted in the birth of twins, and 446 were singleton infants. All liveborn infants were included in the annual cohorts, each identified by the year the babies were born (table 4.2). This population was the base from which survival and other analyses were computed. Not all liveborns, however, were available for the full complement of studies. In some few cases the family chose not to collaborate, with the result that birth weights were not collected nor the newborn examined. This was rare among Indians and more frequent among ladinos who, however, constituted only 4.4 percent of the population. Indians were highly cooperative. An occasional noncollaborating Indian family was encountered, mainly in the early days of the study, but it usually joined or reentered the study at a later date. Aside from an attrition of cohorts by mortality, seven children were lost by migration, all of whom were known to be living at the end of the study on 27 January 1972.

The 1964 cohort is small. The study did not begin until 11 February with the birth of the first cohort child; indeed, until then only one child had been born that year. The low number of births in 1964 relates to a smaller cohort of parents especially in the age group less than twenty years old. This in turn is traceable to epidemics that struck the village in the early 1940s. The first six children born in 1972 are also included in the newborn population to complete a full eight years of observation, from 11 February 1964 through 27 January 1972.

Data on physical growth were obtained for most children born during the eight-year period. The first 99, however, constitute a special group. They were consecutive births during the first two years, 11 February 1964 to 10 February 1966, and were studied more frequently in terms of physical growth and other variables. Of the 99, 45 were chosen for intensive study of diet, infection, illnesses, and growth, a group hereafter referred to as the "cohort children." The data derived from this group constitute the basis for most of the analyses presented on feeding, infection and colonization of the intestine, diseases, malnutrition, and physical growth. The selection was based mainly on a high degree of collaboration by the mothers. For about one-half of the selected cohort children, an occasional mother resisted some particular examination, but in almost all instances programmed items were completed. The remaining 54 of the special group are referred to as the "control

Table 4.3
Variables and Scores Employed in Computing a Socioeconomic Index

Land and Animal Resources		Housing Material		Sanitary Facilities		Education and Cultural Features[a]	
Land (cuerdas)		**Floor**		**Water supply**		**Literacy**	
10–98	3	Tile, cement	3	Home facility	3	Read, write	3
1–9	2	Earthen	1	Communal	1	Illiterate	1
None	1						
Livestock		**Walls**		**Feces disposal**		**School, primary**	
Cattle and hogs	3	Adobe, cement	3	Toilet, latrine	3	> 3 grades	3
Hogs only	2	Stalk, bajareque	1	None	1	1–3 grades	2
None	1					None	1
Poultry		**Roof**		**Garbage disposal**		**Shoes, sandals**	
10–98	3	Metal	3	Fertilizer	3	Shoes	3
1–9	2	Tile	2	Buried, burned	2	Sandals	2
None	1	Straw, palm	1	Discarded	1	None	1

[a]These refer to the head of the family, usually the husband.

children." They were born in the same period from similar parents, but lesser cooperation occurred. No differences were noted in physical anthropometry between the cohort children and the control children.

The separation of the cohort and control groups was effected after eighteen months of study. The cohort children were survivors by that age. Ten deaths occurred in the other group. The mean birth weight and the proportion of low birth weight infants, however, was very similar in both groups of children. Aside from the few withdrawals because of migration and a few additional deaths, no losses to observation occurred among the cohort and control children during the study period; nor were there withdrawals among the other yearly cohorts except through death or migration.

Through the fortuitous combination of a cooperative population and an efficient and highly qualified field staff, a unique situation occurred in which practically all members of a population at risk were studied prospectively.

Socioeconomic Index
The three censuses made during the study were examined to see if families contributing pregnant women and infants to the cohorts could be grouped into definable categories. The data closest to the birthday of a child were used to compute the Socioeconomic Index (SECI), as follows.

Of all variables investigated, 12 were selected to constitute the index, first, because the information was complete for most of the families and, second, because the item served for a reasonable gradation of socioeconomic characteristics (table 4.3). These variables were arranged in four classes—land and animal resources, housing material, sanitary facilities, and education and cultural features—with arbitrarily assigned scores of 1 to 3 for each category within which a variable occurred, using a procedure similar to that of Arroyave et al. (1970). A score of 1 indicated lowest value as in, for instance, a lack of land, which in this agricultural society almost invariably meant that the man worked as a hired laborer for other villagers. The score of 2 for land was allotted to families with one to nine cuerdas, an amount barely sufficient to support a family. Ten or more cuerdas characterized the small group of families with greatest production potential. Similar reasoning was applied in scoring other variables, except that scores of either 1 or 3 applied to floor and walls, water supply, feces disposal, and literacy, because intermediate categories did not exist.

The SECI of a family was the sum of all its scores, the minimum being 12 and the maximum 36. The observed values were 15 and 35. Their distribution was within a wide range of values, useful in appraisal of maternal and child characteristics.

Other special censuses were also made, three on feces disposal and one on availability of electricity. They were carried out by the same field worker responsible for the general population censuses. The censuses on feces disposal were for the same years as the general censuses; in addition to the interview, they included direct inspection of the facilities and adjoining premises. A similar survey made in 1960, before the Cauqué study began, provided a useful comparison. The electricity census was based on enumeration of light bulbs; the few electrical appliances all belonged to ladino families.

Enrollment and Observation of Cohort Populations
Pregnant Women   Earlier field work had indicated that enrollment of women as they became pregnant during the study (1963 to 1972) was the best means to recruit newborns. The enrollment of pregnant women was a continuing process dependent on repeated contacts with village women of reproductive age by midwives, nurses, field workers, and occasionally the physician himself. Over the years the attendance of pregnant women at the clinic progressively had improved so much that enrollment in the study was possible soon after conception. At least one visit subsequent to enrollment was intended each trimester. The findings at examination, recorded on precoded forms, covered identification of the mother, obstetrical history, physical anthropometry, and health status. Definitions of ensuing illness were in standard terms and could be obtained by request to INCAP.

After interview by the physician a physical examination included abdominal palpation and assessment of uterine height (figure 4.2). No gynecological examination was performed and observations took place with the woman fully clothed. To have done otherwise would have jeopardized study

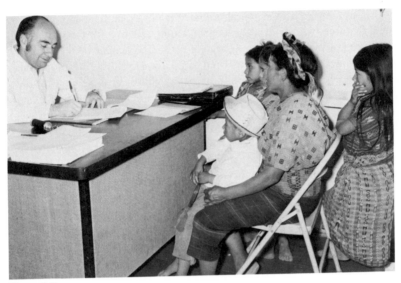

Figure 4.2
Mother and children visiting the prenatal clinic

participation. Anthropometric measurements were restricted to height, weight, arm and leg circumferences, and tricipital skinfold thickness. Physical examination included edema, measurement of pulse and blood pressure, and auscultation of the chest. Patients with active diseases had as much medical attention as the field station could provide.

No systematic laboratory tests were performed. Certain surveys of blood and feces were conducted for a general characterization of the population. Severe infections such as pyelonephritis, cellulitis, or dysentery often were studied bacteriologically. No general or specific programs of health education were instituted.

Through arrangement with the family or the attending midwife, field nurses were notified of an impending or expected delivery and promptly visited the home to record the circumstances on precoded forms. Ordinarily the nurse remained until delivery, making full notes and examining the newborn infant.

Newborns The excellent cooperation of the two village midwives made possible the attendance of a staff nurse at almost every delivery, thus ensuring the opportunity to acquire almost complete records. The nurse alone was responsible for a record of the birth, complications, type of delivery, and other related events. She weighed the baby within thirty minutes of delivery, made an examination for gross abnormalities, determined health status, and collected umbilical cord blood and sometimes meconium. This field

Table 4.4
Program of Study, Cohort Children, 1964–1972

	Times studied
Growth	
Weight	at birth
	daily, first week of life
Weight, height, circumferences	within 24 hours of birth
of head and thorax	weekly, neonatal period
	fortnightly, 1st to 12th month
	every 4 weeks, 2nd and 3 years
	every 3 months, 4th to 7th years
X-ray of hand	every 6 months, beginning at 6 months
Diet	
Feeding practices and nutrient intake	weekly, birth to 3 years; if weaned, up to 3 months after complete weaning (usually in 2nd or 3rd year)
Infection	
Fecal specimen	weekly, birth to 3 to 5 years
Feces or other specimen	when certain diseases were present, birth to 5 years
Health	
Physical examination	weekly, neonatal period
	fortnightly, 1st month to 5 years
Morbidity surveillance	weekly, birth until 3 to 5 years
Clinical examination	whenever symptoms were present, birth to 5 years
	at death

procedure was crucial for knowledge about the exact time of birth and the condition of the fetus (stillborn, live-born, or dead shortly after live birth). The procedure assured early and effective enrollment of newborn infants in the study.

The staff physician performed a complete anthropometric and pediatric examination, normally within twenty-four hours of birth. Anthropometric measurements included a second determination of weight, and measurements of length, and head and thorax circumferences. Pediatric examination included an appraisal of general appearance, skin, ears, eyes, heart, lungs, bones, and reflexes. Body temperature, diseases and disabilities, overt congenital malformations, convulsions, and other abnormalities were recorded. The apgar score was not determined. Observations were of a clinical nature, utilizing basic tools of tongue depressor, otoscope, stethoscope, percussion hammer, scale, and infantmeter.

Every child born in the village during the study was observed prospectively for physical growth, including weight and height, from birth to whatever age it had attained when the study ended. Many children also had measurements of head and thorax circumference.

The special group of cohort children was studied more intensively according to the program outlined in table 4.4. The control children were studied similarly, although not so completely as the cohort group; for instance, not all had complete morbidity, dietary, or microbiological observations.

The extensiveness of the data collected in the Cauqué study was possible because information on maternal characteristics and birth weight was available for practically all infants, on postnatal physical growth for almost all children born in the village, on prospective diet and morbidity for about 60 children, and on a comprehensive list of variables for all 45 cohort children. Furthermore, survival of every child born in the village during the study was determined for as long as the study continued. Special studies on intestinal infection during the neonatal period were made for about 100 newborns, and intestinal colonization and development of bacterial flora were recorded at short intervals for 12 children during infancy.

The techniques used in field epidemiology incident to measurement of growth, diet, morbidity, and infection are discussed below.

Physical Anthropometry

Anthropometric measurements were done according to standard norms. The physician and a nurse were directly responsible for all measurements. Before the study began they were tested in two standardization exercises, employing 20 children. Standard errors were calculated for each of the four variables investigated, namely, weight, length, head circumference, and thorax circumference. Measurements during the exercises and during the whole of the study were collected in duplicate. Standard errors were not permitted to exceed 15 grams for weight, and 0.5 centimeters for the other three variables. If the duplicate measurements differed by more than two standard errors, a second set of measurements was made.

All new field workers assigned to these examinations were subjected to the same tests, irrespective of previous training and experience. Even those of proved capacity in accurate measurements were required to requalify annually during the first three years of the study.

Pregnant Women   Barefoot but clothed, mothers at midpregnancy were weighed at the clinic on a Detecto scale. Observed weights were not corrected for clothes, which were estimated to weigh about one kilogram. All village women wear clothes of similar size, fabric and weight, and the number of garments worn does not change during the several stages of pregnancy. Height was obtained with a rigid scale (figure 4.3a), arm and leg circumferences with a nonelastic tape measure, and tricipital skinfold thickness with a Harpender caliper.

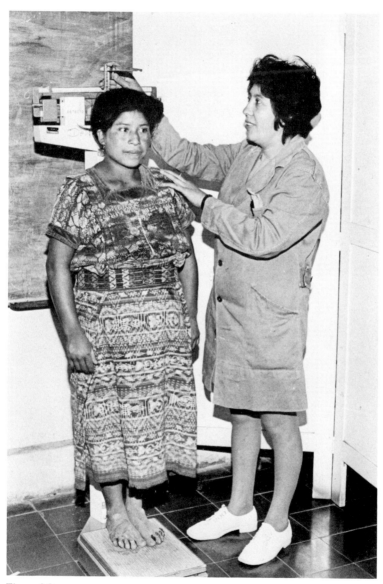

Figure 4.3a
Determination of weight of pregnant woman

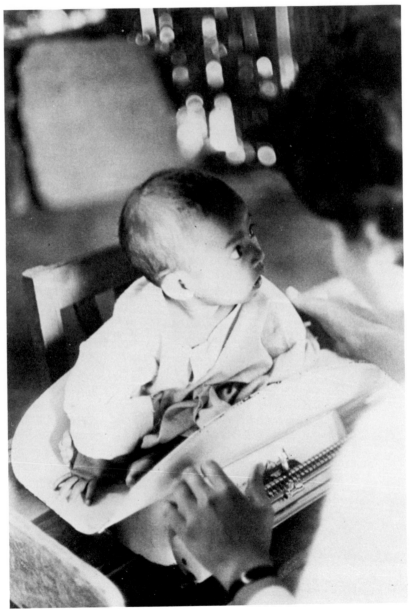

Figure 4.3b
Determination of weight of infant

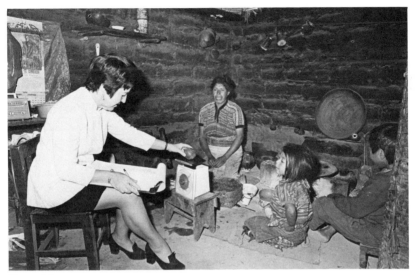

Figure 4.4
Dietician weighing a fruit as part of a routine visit to a typical home

Children   Children were measured either in the home or at the clinic. In homes both a Seca balance and an infantmeter were placed in a single area and position specifically chosen for the purpose, to avoid errors through placing the balance on unlevel areas (figure 4.4). In the first years mothers were provided with two infant gowns of known weight in which to hold the infant during measurements. Later, infants and children were weighed with clothes, and the weight of the apparel was subtracted. Mothers were notified one or two days in advance of a visit by the physician. Two balances and two infantmeters were available, one used at the clinic and another that could be transported to the home; both were periodically checked for accuracy.

Diet and Feeding Practices
Dietary considerations refer to food intake of women during pregnancy and to breast feeding and food supplements of infants and young children.

Pregnant Women   Dietary studies were conducted in 1967 and 1971, both using the method of a one-week daily record of food intake. The one-week recall method, so successfully used for children, proved unsatisfactory for women either because they were not sufficiently interested or because they were unable to recall what they had eaten during the previous week; reliable information was restricted to the most recent three days. The one-week daily record was therefore substituted.

     Observations required two visits per day to each woman from Monday to Friday and a further visit the morning of the subsequent Monday to record food consumption over the weekend. The dietician, who enjoyed an excellent rapport with the villagers, usually visited a home between ten and eleven in the morning and exchanged the requisite polite greetings and candid village gossip (figure 4.4). The survey then developed in an informal and relaxed manner that assured cooperation and reliable results. The professional purpose of the visit was to note remains of the breakfast meal, to ask about the food being prepared for midday, and to observe what was under way. During the afternoon visit, around 3 P.M., the dietician determined the food consumed at the preceding meal, recorded the weight of foods being prepared for supper, and noted the recipes employed. Hanson scales were used to weigh food in grams.

The main foods eaten daily were weighed during the visits. Maize is prepared by an elaborate process that eventually ends in tortillas remarkably uniform in size from home to home. Average weights of tortillas were determined for each home, however, because of occasional between-home variations in size. Recipes of every individual dish were investigated according to what items were involved and whether the food was a main dish, for example, rice with tomato, onion and green pepper, or a gravy or sauce. The average weight of common village units of bread, vegetables, fruits, tubers, or edible leaves also was determined.

Amounts of food eaten were recorded in household measuring units such as spoons, ladles, chunks, or units; these were then converted to grams of the various nutrients consumed daily during one week. The nutritive value of the diet was obtained by computer after making available the equivalences in terms of calories and individual nutrients per 100 grams of each food. Equivalences were those of the Central American Food Composition Table which lists about 560 food items (Flores et al., 1960).

Nutrient intake was expressed as mean daily consumption of calories and individual nutrients per woman per trimester of pregnancy. These intakes were compared with estimated daily recommendations of calories and nutrients for women 18 years old or more, of comparable weight, in the second or third trimester of pregnancy according to the National Research Council (NRC), Food and Nutrition Board (National Academy of Sciences, 1968). Also, comparisons were made with recommendations adapted by INCAP (Menchú et al., 1973) for Central American women 20 to 39 years old, of comparable weight, and also in the second and third trimester of pregnancy (table 4.5). INCAP recommendations are significantly larger for calories, iron, and total retinol than the values recommended for well-nourished industrial societies. This has to do with the greater caloric needs of Central American women due to physical activity and frequency of infections. The larger recommendation for iron is to compensate for its reduced availability in the common diet of poor rural women.

Table 4.5
Daily Nutrients Recommended for Women by Trimester of Pregnancy

	NRC	INCAP	
	2nd and 3rd	1st	2nd and 3rd
Total protein, g	65	45	60
Vitamin A (retinol), μg	750[a]	750	900
Thiamin, mg	1.2	0.9	1.0
Riboflavin, mg	1.8	1.2	1.3
Niacin, mg	15	14.5	15.8
Ascorbic acid, mg	60	30	50
Iron, mg	18	28	28
Calcium, mg	1,200	450	1,100
Calories	2,200	2,200[a]	2,400[a]

[a]FAO/WHO, 1967.

Infants and Young Children   Dietary observations began at birth and continued for the next three to four years, in general, until about three months after completed weaning. Weekly home visits took place according to a plan made with the mother for initial and subsequent contacts. By a single recall interview, the dietician and a field worker collected information on the child's diet for the preceding seven days. Observations included feeding practices, for example, how early in life was the breast offered, how frequently were herbs or foods given to the child during lactation, and so forth. The one-week recall dietary history recorded all fluids and solids; the amounts in units, spoons, tablespoons, ladles, or chunks; and the frequency of feeding per day and per week. The weekly observations provided the opportunity to identify introduction of new foods into the diet. The programmed weekly visits undoubtedly stimulated the interest of the mother and enlarged her experience about breast feeding. The field worker, on the other hand, acquired experience in recording the complex dietary habits of different families.

Food units were weighed using Hanson scales. The average weight of tortillas and the capacity of spoons, plates, and cups for the most common food items was investigated in individual homes, as was done for the mother's diet. Also, average weights were determined for bread, fruits, and vegetables as usually obtained in the village.

All foods recorded as units were converted into grams by computer, and eventually into calories and individual nutrients, to be expressed as mean daily intake per child per unit of time—week, month, or trimester.

The contribution of maternal milk to the total nutrient intake was not determined, primarily because of logistic and cultural difficulties. A field worker would have had to be posted at the mother's side around the clock

Table 4.6
Mean Daily Nutrient Intake of 12 Preschool Children, by Three-Day Daily Record (A)
and by One-Week Single Recall (B), 1967

Child Number	Age (Year, Month)	Feeding[a]	Calories		Total protein, g		Vitamin A, mg		Vitamin C, mg	
			A	B	A	B	A	B	A	B
3	3,1	W	1,044	926	27.3	27.1	0.258	0.986	29	65
12	2,10	Bf	1,061	852	27.3	17.7	0.130	0.036	14	4
15	2,9	W	902	1,090	24.2	34.1	0.180	0.512	17	56
16	2,8	W	576	573	15.7	18.5	0.143	0.118	6	· 8
17	2,8	Bf	1,276	726	33.7	24.7	0.379	0.388	24	22
20	2,8	W	772	886	19.2	22.8	0.490	0.592	47	67
35	2,5	W	742	933	26.9	31.2	0.444	0.292	16	6
42	2,3	Bf	827	907	21.7	23.0	0.145	0.470	14	25
49	2,0	Bf	523	571	18.5	19.0	0.094	0.066	2	16
50	2,1	Bf	953	1,100	28.8	30.6	0.571	0.750	56	72
67	1,8	Bf	572	592	14.1	13.1	0.094	0.186	2	7
75	1,8	Bf	637	749	17.3	18.0	0.392	0.255	18	11
		t	0.0274		0.2751		1.527		1.9964	
		r	0.5085		0.6336		0.4963		0.8127	

[a]W = weaned. Bf = still breast-fed.

to weigh the child before and after each feeding (Martínez and Chávez, 1971). The prevailing custom of offering the breast many times each day would thus require a substantial number of workers to obtain prospective data on a meaningful number of children. Evaluation of food supplements was important nevertheless, mainly because it extended throughout the whole weaning process and for several months thereafter.

The one-week dietary recall method used in the Cauqué study was compared with the more usual technique of the three-day daily record (Flores et al., 1964), to determine if the results were significantly different. Twelve children born to the study were selected for the comparison. Nutrient intake was determined by the two methods during alternate weeks. Data were processed blindly. The results in table 4.6 show a good correlation between the two methods, particularly with regard to estimates of protein and ascorbic acid. The paired t test reveals no differences in estimates of calories and total protein between the two methods, although variations were evident in regard to vitamin A and ascorbic acid. The findings indicate that both methods have an equal capacity to estimate the components of the diet. It is judged that prospective observations by the one-week recall method result in similar information to that obtained through the more time-consuming three-day direct record method. This data proved reliable for a variety of analyses.

Table 4.7
INCAP Recommended Daily Nutrient Intake for Infants and Young Children of Central America, 1973

	Amount of nutrients per age group			
	1 yr	2 yr	3 yr	4-6 yr
Total protein, g	24	28	30	33
Vitamin A (retinol), μg	250	250	250	300
Thiamin, mg	0.5	0.5	0.6	0.7
Riboflavin, mg	0.6	0.7	0.9	1.0
Niacin, mg	7.6	8.9	10.2	11.6
Ascorbic acid, mg	20	20	20	20
Iron, mg	10	10	10	10
Calcium, mg	450	450	450	450
Calories	1,150	1,350	1,550	1,750
Mean weight, kg	11.4	13.8	15.8	19.5

The observed mean nutrient and caloric intakes were compared with INCAP recommendations for infants and young children as recently revised (Menchú et al., 1973). The recommendations in table 4.7 are for children of the area and take into account increased nutrient demands because of known deficiencies in diet and in environment such as acute infections. Comparisons were made, taking into consideration either the age or actual weight of the child.

Disease and Injury

Surveillance of the illnesses and disabilities of pregnant women and of cohort children was facilitated by the excellent relations between field workers and villagers, which were strengthened through weekly home visits. Maternal morbidity was recorded in the course of regular visits to the clinic by pregnant women, or discovered and notified in connection with the home visits. The Cauqué study did not especially emphasize data on intercurrent illnesses during pregnancy. The figures obtained are believed to be underestimates. Nevertheless, all illnesses reported or discovered were recorded on precoded forms, and diagnosed according to a list of diseases, syndromes, signs, and symptoms established for the study (Morbidity Code, appendix C).

The main emphasis was on the illnesses and injuries of the cohort children. Observations extended from birth to age three or longer. The procedures now stated refer to that group.

Case Finding The main reliance was on the weekly home visits for routine collection of dietary data or obtaining fecal specimens. The latter frequently required repeated visits during the week until the material was procured.

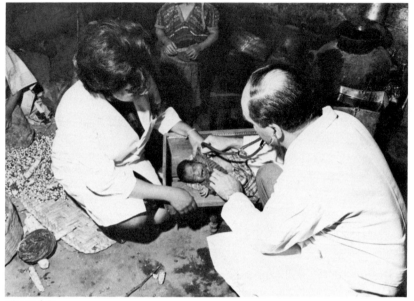

Figure 4.5a
Physician and nurse examining an ill infant

Word about disease and injury also came from visits of parents (mainly the mother) or other relatives to the Health Center. The result was that most cases were identified within three days of onset.

Diagnosis   The nature of a disease was established by a staff physician through clinical examination, preferably in the home, less frequently at the clinic (figures 4.5a, b). Once an indisposition was recognized, the child was examined every other day until the disability ended in recovery or death. If the disease was serious, daily visits were made. Such close supervision not only favored prompt identification of the illness and recognition of complications, but also established associated pathological conditions. Treatment and supervision were thereby much favored. Institution of the prescribed therapeutic measures and aid during evolution of the process were the responsibility of the nurses. At its end, each case was reviewed by the physician and the diagnosis assessed on clinical grounds.

Severity   Case severity was evaluated in terms of outstanding symptoms, fever, anorexia, vomiting, number of stools per day and their characteristics, and dehydration. Rectal temperatures were recorded twice daily through home visits by the nurses.

Illnesses and injuries defined on clinical grounds, as well as major symptoms, were classified according to the Morbidity Code (appendix C), which

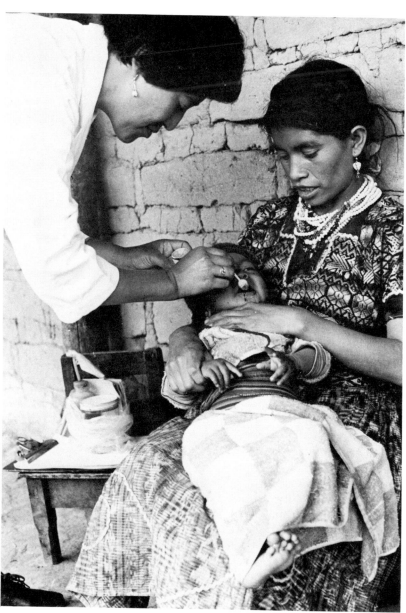

Figure 4.5b
The nurse administering a syrup

Table 4.8
Typical History of an Episode of Illness in a Cohort Child, 1965

| | | Date | | Duration, |
	Code	Onset	Last day	days
URI	0101	08-10-65	08-16-65	7
Diarrhea with mucus	0211	08-12-65	08-19-65	8
Vomiting	0203	08-12-65	08-13-65	2
Fever (rectal °C)				
38.5-39.4	1402	08-10-65	08-12-65	3
37.5-38.4	1401	08-13-65	08-13-65	1
Bowel movements				
7-9	1502	08-12-65	08-13-65	2
10-12	1503	08-14-65	08-16-65	3
4-6	1501	08-17-65	08-19-65	3
Anorexia	1601	08-10-65	08-16-65	7
Aspirin	1703	08-10-65	08-13-65	4
Kaolin-pectin	1702	08-12-65	08-19-65	8

Dates of episode: 08-10-65–08-19-65
Duration of episode: 10 days

summarizes all entities recognized during seven years among the cohort children.

Treatment   A stock of relatively few drugs, fluids, prescriptions, and placebos permitted treatment of most of the illnesses that came to the attention of the field staff (appendix C).* Treatments at the Health Center became accepted and mothers occasionally would aid in their administration.

Records   Two precoded forms served to record morbidity, a clinical form and a transfer form. On the clinical form symptoms were recorded daily according to systems and organs. When the patient could not be observed daily, information was obtained from the mother or other close relative.

The day symptoms appeared was considered the first day or onset of a disease. The last day was the final day that symptoms were present. Duration was the period inclusive between the first and last days. Diseases or symptoms often appeared in sequence when the last day of the first event coincided or succeeded the onset of the second event. Thus, two or more linked diseases or symptoms occurred frequently and constituted an episode. An episode was the continued period between onset of a first disease or symptom and the last

* The clinical guide to an established diagnosis, as well as the guide for treatment, can be obtained by writing to INCAP.

day of the last linked disease or symptom; the combined days corresponded to the duration of the episode. When clinical manifestations were interrupted by one or more days of apparent health, two episodes were assumed. To illustrate, table 4.8 presents an example from the study. Such happenings were not at all unusual, nor was the example the most complex episode. Diseases and symptoms within an episode were numbered sequentially as they appeared, and likewise, the episodes of a particular child as they occurred in his life experience. The morbidity file is among the most extensive records of the Cauqué study.

To characterize an episide realistically, the transfer form was used. Each part of the episode (i.e., diseases and symptoms) was recorded on a special form, and later card punched; thus, one episode could be represented by many cards, linked to each other by a code that permitted recognition of the episode as an independent entity. In the example of table 4.8, the episode involved eleven cards: two representing illnesses (URI and diarrhea); seven characterizing severity (vomiting, fever, number of bowel movements, and anorexia); and two the treatment used.

Infection

Studies of infection focused almost exclusively on the intestinal tract. More limited investigation was made of respiratory and skin diseases.

Feces   The study of intestinal infection and microbial colonization of the gut was a fundamental part of the Cauqué study. This comprised: (a) weekly examination of childhood feces from birth to three to five years of age for microbial and parasitic invaders; (b) weekly or bimonthly investigation of indigenous fecal bacteria during the first three years of life; and (c) the isolation of fecal pathogens from children with diarrheal disease and other morbid events.

Feces, and less frequently rectal swabs, were collected in the home or occasionally at the clinic by nurses or field workers. Feces were placed in half-pint cardboard boxes delivered in advance to the mothers by the nurses (figure 4.6a). Before the study began, collection of feces met with resistance from a number of villagers who were concerned with the ultimate fate of the specimens. They indicated their desire that stool samples remain in the village for incineration. Thus, a furnace was designed and constructed for the purpose and installed in front of the clinic. The furnace was later placed in the Municipal Building. Later in the afternoon specimens already processed were disposed of, often in the presence of officials of the village. After several months the practice became an established tradition and villagers were no longer suspicious.

Often the nurse waited while the mother transferred the material from the diaper to the container. For the transfer, mothers were instructed to use the

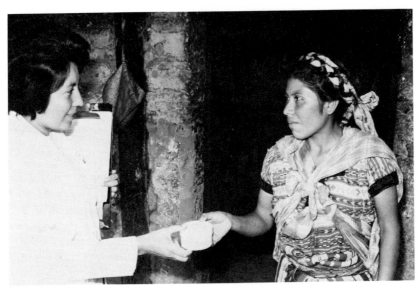

Figure 4.6a
Collection of sample of feces

sterile tongue depressors provided by the nurse. Frequently, specimens were not obtained on the prescribed day, a circumstance that required persistence on the part of the nurse or field worker as well as repeated visits. The close surveillance nevertheless was effective, and collection of specimens was highly satisfactory. The secured boxes were labeled and transported rapidly to the field laboratory for processing. The whole operation took no more than thirty minutes, a time short enough to guarantee recovery of such labile agents as anaerobes and shigellae.

Other Specimens   Biological materials such as urine, vaginal secretions, or pus intended for investigation of pathogens were generally collected in the clinic and processed immediately. Other specimens included umbilical cord blood and breast milk (figure 4.6b), collected in the home. Venous blood generally was collected at the clinic.

LABORATORY PROCEDURES

Our policy that all laboratory investigations be performed under the best possible conditions required that many procedures be carried out in the field with fresh specimens. Techniques and methods used in the field laboratory and at the base laboratory in Guatemala City are described in this section.

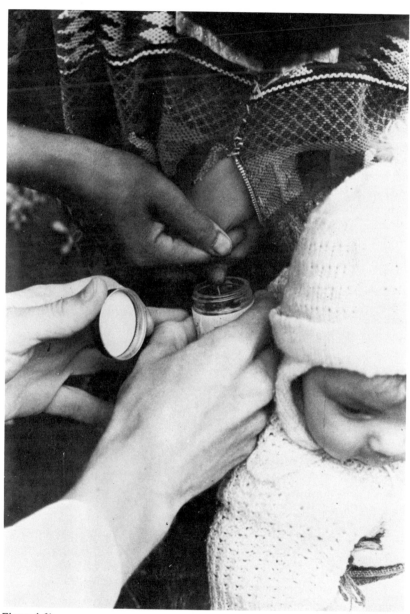

Figure 4.6b
Collection of sample of breast milk

Field Laboratory

Processing of Fecal Samples   Fecal samples from young children comprised most of the specimens collected in the field. A form was used for each sample to record the characteristics of the feces, physical appearance, color and consistency, and the presence of blood and mucus, along with the child's identification number, health status, specimen number, date of collection, and other relevant variables. The approximate hydrogen ion concentration was determined with litmus paper, and tests for occult blood were made with guaiac reagent. Initial processing was under a hood in the field laboratory as follows: (a) inoculation of *Salmonella-Shigella* (SS) and MacConkey agars and selenite and tetrathionate broths, the latter with brilliant green and iodine (Edwards and Ewing, 1962), by means of cotton swabs or bacteriologic loops; (b) inoculation of Levine-eosin methylene blue agar (L-EMB) containing 1 percent of commercial chlortetracycline (Weld, 1953), using cotton swabs; (c) by means of wooden applicators, preparation for virus examinations of a 20 percent fecal suspension in Hanks' balanced salt solution (Lennette and Schmidt, 1964) with 2 percent skimmed milk and a final concentration of 2,000 units of penicillin, 500 μg of streptomycin, and 20 μg amphotericin B per ml; and (d) preparation of a fecal suspension for investigation of parasites, a 25 percent suspension in polyvinyl alcohol-Schaudinn fixative (PVA) and a 50 percent suspension in 5 percent formalin (Mata, 1969).

Bacterial and Yeast Cultures   Agar and fluid media (except L-EMB) promptly were incubated at 37°C aerobically for 18 hours; the L-EMB medium at 37°C in a candle jar for five to seven days. After 24 and 48 hours incubation subcultures were made from selenite and tetrathionate broths on SS and brilliant green agar plates and then incubated at 37°C for 24 hours.

Techniques for isolation of enterobacteriaceae followed standard and accepted procedure (Edwards and Ewing, 1962). Inoculation of plates with swabs carrying as much as 0.3 gram of fresh feces, or of broths in amounts of 0.5 to 1 gram provides a reliable means to detect most *Shigella*, enteropathogenic *Escherichia coli* (EEC), and *Salmonella*. *Shigella* may be found in concentrations of 10^3 and 10^6 per gram of wet feces from carriers and cases respectively (Dale and Mata, 1968); *E. coli* reaches levels of 10^6 to 10^{10} bacilli per gram under both normal and pathologic circumstances (Mata et al., 1972a).

Six to ten nonlactose fermenting colonies suspected as *Shigella* or *Salmonella* were transferred from the primary and secondary agar plates to triple sugar iron agar (TSI) and incubated at 37°C for 18 hours. Also, ten lactose-fermenting colonies were transferred from MacConkey agar to nutrient agar.

Suspicious colonies from TSI agar were tested by slide agglutination with polyvalent and type-specific *Shigella* and *Salmonella* sera. *Shigella* cultures were tested for motility (semisolid agar), citrate utilization (Simmons),

Table 4.9
Quantitation of Gastrointestinal Bacteria

Agar medium		Bacterial group	Incubation	Range of bacterial count, log 10
BC-1 BC	Schaedler's base BC-1 + placenta + neomycin	Bacteroides, clostridia, bifidobacteria, lactobacilli, streptococci, veillonellae	48 hours Anaerobic	4–12
BC-1		Gram-negative bacilli Gram-positive cocci	48 hours Aerobic	4–11
MS	Manitol-salt	Micrococci, bacilli	24 hours Aerobic	4–9
H	Peptone-glucose + antibiotics	Yeasts	5 days Candle jar	3–9
T7T	Tergitol 7 + tetrazolium	Gram-negative bacilli	24 hours Aerobic	4–11
SS MC	Salmonella-Shigella MacConkey	Gram-negative bacilli	24 hours Aerobic	

Note: Adapted from Dale and Mata (1968), and Mata et al. (1971b).

splitting of urea (Christensen), and utilization of xylose, mannitol, and rhamnose (purple broth base with 0.5 g percent sugar). The *Salmonella* cultures also were tested for urease (Christensen) and cyanide tolerance (KCN broth) (Edwards and Ewing, 1962).

Lactose fermeters transferred to nutrient agar were tested by slide agglutination with EEC-OB sera after an 18-hour incubation. If agglutination occurred, cultures were retested with specific sera, and if still agglutinating, the O antigen was titrated after boiling the culture for one hour. Cultures with a titer of 1:320 or more were considered confirmed as EEC (Edwards and Ewing, 1962). All strains so characterized were tested for indol, methyl red, Voges-Proskauer, and citrate.

Serotyped strains were inoculated into stock agar in tubes stoppered with corks embedded in paraffin, and stored in the dark at room temperature (20-28°C).

The L-EMB plates were removed from candle jars five days after inoculation and transported to the base laboratories for examination.

All bacteriologic media were from Baltimore Biological Laboratory (BBL), except the stock agar and purified agar and sugars (Difco). All diagnostic sera were from BBL and Lederle.

Fecal specimens for isolation and characterization of indigenous intestinal bacteria had priority and were processed within thirty minutes of evacuation. The details of processing and culturing are given elsewhere (Mata and Urrutia, 1971). Briefly, no more than ten minutes elapsed between crumbling the sample and closing the anaerobic jar. The basic medium was Schaedler's agar (Schaedler et al., 1965) modified by inclusion of 1-percent-trypticase soy (Mata et al., 1969a). This medium and variations and media for facultative bacteria were streaked with log-10 dilutions of feces prepared in charcoal-adsorbed water (Schaedler et al., 1965). The media, dilutions, and incubation characteristics are summarized in table 4.9.

Cultures were examined in the field, the colony count estimated, and Gram stains of representative colonies prepared. Cultures were transported to the base laboratories for definitive counts and the characterization of bacterial groups.

Viral Suspensions   Fecal suspensions prepared in the field in modified Hanks' solution were frozen promptly at -15°C and so maintained for several hours until transported under refrigeration to headquarters for storage without delay at -60°C. Virus isolation was done at the base laboratories.

Suspensions for Parasites   Suspensions were transported to the base laboratories for identification of parasites. The preparations were kept at room temperature.

Processing of Other Specimens   Throat swabs, pus, blood, and other clinical specimens were collected and cultured on blood agar. Urine specimens were inoculated (dilutions 10^{-2} and 10^{-4}) on blood agar and MacConkey agar plates and cultures identified as described before. Isolation and identification of common pathogens (entrobacteriaceae, staphylococci, streptococci) was done in the field. Certain organisms (*Mycobacterium, Diplococcus*) were confirmed at the base laboratories.

Umbilical and venous bloods for serological or immunologic study were collected and stored in the refrigerator for no more than 24 hours; serums were obtained by centrifugation in the cold under aseptic conditions and stored at -20°C until tested.

Base Laboratories
Microbiology   *Enteric Viruses*   Fecal suspensions were thawed and centrifuged twice, first for 15 to 20 minutes at 1100 X G to eliminate gross matter, and then for 30 minutes at 3000 XG to produce final supernates; both centrifugations were at 4°C in a Servall centrifuge. The clear supernates were inoculated with two tubes each of (a) primary human amnion (Dunnebacke and Zitcer, 1957), (b) primary human kidney *post mortem* (Youngner, 1954), and (c) HEp-2 cells (Moore et al., 1955). Cell cultures were established and grown in Melnick's medium (Melnick, 1956) with 5 percent calf serum for kidney and HEp-2 cells and 20 percent calf serum for amnion cells (Weller and Neva, 1962).

Test tubes with screw caps were used. Cultures were inoculated as soon as confluent monolayers were observed. For maintenance, Melnick's medium in Earle's balanced solution (Lennette and Schmidt, 1964) with 3 percent calf serum was used. All cell culture fluids contained a final concentration of 100 units of penicillin, 100 μg streptomycin, and 2.5 μg amphotericin B per ml.

Volumes inoculated were 0.05 to 0.1 ml per tube. The total inoculum per specimen was 0.3 ml, thus providing an opportunity for isolation of viruses at a concentration of 10^3 $TCID_{50}$ or more per gram of wet feces. The inoculum was placed on the monolayer and left for adsorption for about one hour before medium was added. Cultures were incubated at 37°C in racks with 5° inclination and checked four hours later. If the monolayer showed evidence of cytotoxicity, a frequent occurrence with fecal extracts from young children, the culture fluid was replaced. Cultures still toxic the following day had another fluid replacement. If monolayers were degenerated, the inoculation was repeated, and the fluid replaced within one hour, and again four hours later.

Tubes were observed daily during the first week of incubation, and every two days thereafter (figure 4.7). The medium was replaced every three to four days. HEp-2 cells were held for two weeks, while amnion and kidney cultures were maintained for two to four weeks. Cultures with beginning cytopathic effect (CPE) were observed daily, and when the CPE was 3+ or 4+, the fluids were harvested and stored at −60°C in one dram vials.

Selected specimens were inoculated into litters of at least nine pooled infant mice (less than one day old Swiss, Webster strain). The volume injected was 0.075 ml per mouse (three 0.025 ml doses, intraperitoneal, subscapular, and intracerebral) (Lennette and Schmidt, 1964). The total inoculum (0.5 to 0.7 ml per litter) permitted isolation of paralytogenic agents excreted in concentrations of approximately 10^3 $TCID_{50}$ per gram of feces.

All viral isolates were passaged once undiluted, once in the cell system from which they were primarily isolated and also in the other cell systems. The CPE generally appeared more rapidly than upon primary isolation. These passages served to confirm the isolation, to raise the virus titer, and to allocate the isolate within a presumptive category, according to CPE and host susceptibility, as indicated in table 4.10.

Viral identification was limited to typing of enteroviruses isolated in the first week of life and to type characterization of polioviruses isolated from cohort children during the first six months of life. Adenoviruses were characterized as to group only.

Identification of enteroviruses was by neutralization test using 10 pools of serums (Lim and Benyesh-Melnick, 1960) in human kidney cells. Polio-like isolates were typed by neutralization tests using HEp-2 cells. Group characterization of adenoviruses was by complement fixation (Lennette and Schmidt, 1964).

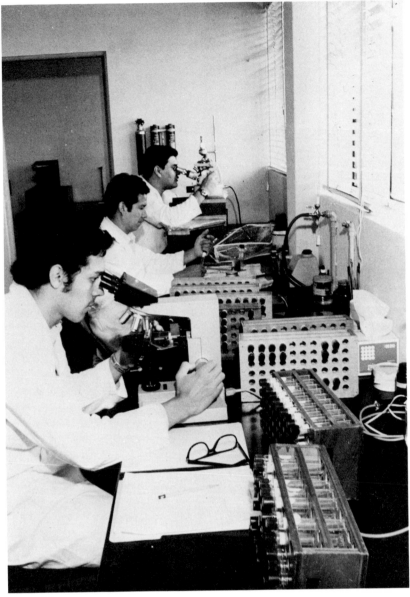

Figure 4.7
Virus and tissue culture unit at INCAP headquarters

Table 4.10
Presumptive Grouping of Virus Isolates, 1964–1972

Cytopathic effect	Replication in			Paralysis in mice	Presumptive identification[a]
	Amnion	Kidney	HEp-2		
Adeno-or					
Herpes-like	+	+	+		Adeno, Herpes
Entero-like	+	+	+		Polio
	+	+	+	spastic	Coxsackie B
	+ (-)	+ (-)	+ (-)	flaccid	Coxsackie A
	+ (-)	+	-		Echo

[a]Isolates of different behavior were found, but not included in the table.

All reagents were from the Reference Research Reagents Branch of the National Institutes of Health.

Enteric Bacteriology   Selected strains of *Shigella* and EEC were sent periodically to the Center for Disease Control (CDC) in Atlanta, Georgia, for verification. All *Salmonella* were typed there.

Bacteriology of the Indigenous Intestinal Microflora   All cultures made in the field were brought to the base laboratories for study after they had been incubated and examined in preliminary fashion shortly after removal from the incubator.

The definitive study was of colony and microscopic morphology, oxygen tolerance, and final estimation of the relative proportions and concentrations of bacteria. The procedures, diagnostic criteria, and other technical details have been described elsewhere (Dale and Mata, 1968; Mata et al., 1969a; Mata et al. 1971b; Nelson and Mata, 1970). Concentrations were expressed as log 10 per gram of wet feces.

Yeasts   The L-EMB agar plates were examined after five days incubation in candle jars. Colonies with star appearance were considered *Candida albicans* (Weld, 1953). Colonies on the plate representing the various morphological types were transferred to Sabouraud agar tubes and also tested in human serum for tube germination using microtiter disposable trays. Germinating yeasts were considered *C. albicans*.

Intestinal Parasites   Qualitative investigation was by trichrome-stained smears (Weatley, 1951) and in mounts obtained after ether-formalin concentration (Ritchie, 1948). Each trichrome slide was examined microscopically under oil for twenty to thirty minutes; the concentrated material was examined for five to fifteen minutes under high dry lens.

Serological Procedures   Serological analysis was restricted by an inability to collect blood systematically from all children. Investigations were made, however, on umbilical cord sera and on sera from children and women.

Antibodies to the following infectious agents were investigated: *Treponema pallidum*, *Salmonella* and *Shigella*, *Brucella*, herpesviruses, cytomegaloviruses, enteroviruses, rubella virus, reoviruses, and *Toxoplasma gondii*.

For syphilis the USR (Bossak et al., 1960), VDRL (Harris et al., 1946), and FTA-ABS (Deacon et al., 1966) techniques were used, employing BBL and CDC reagents. The tube agglutination test was used for *Salmonella D, d,* and *Vi* antibodies with Lederle reagents. *Shigella* passive hemagglutinating antibodies to the 0 polysaccharide were studied by microtechnique as modified at INCAP (Cáceres and Mata, 1970); antigens and reference sera were prepared at INCAP. The Huddleson slide agglutination test was used for *Brucella* antibodies, employing antigen provided by the US Department of Agriculture. Complement fixation for herpesviruses and cytomegaloviruses (Casey, 1965) was performed at the Department of Epidemiology and International Health, University of Washington, Seattle, Washington. For IgM antibody to cytomegaloviruses (CMV) in umbilical cord serum, the fluorescent antibody technique was used (Hanshaw et al., 1968) with antigen prepared at INCAP with the AD-169 CMV strain; anti-IgM fluorescent serum was from Hyland. Antibodies to polio and other enteroviruses were investigated by neutralization test (Wenner, 1964). Rubella antibodies were studied by the hemagglutination-inhibition test (Palmer et al., 1970), using microtiter equipment, chick cells, and antigen from CDC. Reovirus antibodies were tested by micro hemagglutination-inhibition test (Rosen, 1964) with antigen prepared at INCAP. Toxoplasma IgM antibodies in cord serum were investigated by the fluorescent antibody procedure (Remington, 1969) employing anti-IgM fluorescent globulin from Hyland and quenching with Evans blue. *Toxoplasma* antibodies in serum from adults were investigated by the dye-test at the Department of Pathology, the University of Kansas School of Medicine, Kansas City, Kansas.

Furthermore, umbilical cord serum and postnatal serums collected from individuals of all ages, were tested for three immunoglobulins (G, M, and A) by radial immunodiffusion (Mancini et al., 1965) employing Hyland reagents (Lechtig and Mata, 1971). Immunoglobulins in colostrum and milk were investigated by the same techniques, and for secretory IgA, an 11-S serum was used for standardization (Wyatt et al., 1972).

Hematology   For stated reasons relating to the difficulty and risks in collection of blood specimens, hematologic studies were restricted to hemoglobin, hematocrit, and differential white-cell counts.

PROCESSING AND ANALYSIS OF DATA

Collection of Data

When the Cauqué study first took form and during its early planning phases, there was little appreciation of the amount and complexity of the data such a study would generate, leading, as it did, to the accumulation of the one of the largest bodies of epidemiological data derived from single individuals or any population of its size.

The following factors were crucial in data collection: (a) registration of data in precoded forms; (b) systematic editing of forms; (c) transfer of data to cards and eventually to tapes; and (d) classification, verification, and interpretation of the information.

Obviously, before steps (a) through (d) could be undertaken, the pertinent procedures had to be established in the field and laboratory, tested for accuracy, and evaluated for efficiency. Protocols organized into a condensed standard operating procedure were made available to all staff members having a part in data collection. Group and individual staff meetings were held periodically to instruct in special features of data recording and to clarify problems arising during field and laboratory study.

The forms originally designed for the Cauqué study were based on those employed in the International Atherosclerosis Project (INCAP-LSU, 1962) but with subsequent desirable alterations during the course of observations. This was done to facilitate data handling for analysis by a Conversational Computer Statistical System (CCSS) (Kronmal et al., 1970), an assemblage of programs successfully used in exploration and interpretation of long-term biological studies such as the Virus Watch (Fox et al., 1972).

In order to minimize errors in transcription, data collection avoided the use of intermediary record sheets or forms. Field workers, technicians, nurses, the physician, and other staff members recorded data by pencil directly on the precoded forms. A professional staff worker or a data clerk edited the forms at daily or longer intervals according to the nature of the data. Contemporary editing throughout the Cauqué study provided a mechanism that maintained interest among staff members responsible for the original data; in a way, it substituted for the more laborious and often unjustifiable quality control.

The volume of edited forms to be transferred concurrently to IBM cards was so large during the final three years of the study that it required massive data handling.

The subsequent discussion was written jointly with R. A. Kronmal, Claire Joplin, and Juan J. Urrutia.

Preliminary Analyses

In the course of the study several findings became obvious from inspection of clinical growth charts and from their epidemiological interpretation through data tabulated by hand, by mechanical calculator, or by portable computer (Mata et al., 1967a). Thus, basic information was obtained on fetal and post-natal growth (Mata et al., 1972b), infant mortality (Mata et al., 1972c), microbial colonization of the intestine (Mata and Urrutia, 1971), intestinal infection (Mata et al., 1969b), and intereactions between malnutrition and infection (Mata et al., 1971c).

The effort was important to maintain the interest and the efficiency of field and laboratory staff, to release preliminary results, and to promote funding of the study; by necessity it was limited in scope and depth and was not conducive to correlations of the different kinds of data. The move to more comprehensive analyses was unavoidable.

Computer Analyses

Early in 1971 the services of Drs. John P. Fox and Richard A. Kronmal of the University of Washington were requested through the Pan American Health Organization for consultation on the status of the Cauqué study at all levels, and particularly regarding analysis. The conclusion was that the IBM 1620 facility at INCAP could not ensure efficient processing of the more than 5 million numbers on 300,000 cards. A decision was made to process the data on computers available at the University of Washington.

In order to accomplish processing at the University of Washington, the information on IBM cards was transferred to tapes by the IBM 360 at the Banco de Guatemala in Guatemala City. Five copies were made, of which two were hand carried to the University of Washington, and three were stored at INCAP.

A final edit of the data on the tapes was made by a listing prepared at the Boeing Computer Facility, Seattle. Some missing or repeated numbers and other mistakes were discovered at this level, but the set was judged of excellent quality for immediate use.

The processing and statistical analysis of these data required highly sophisticated computers and programming. A large part of the data related to the group of cohort children around whom the study centered. Each child averaged more than 2,000 cards including more than eight different basic records.

Data processing was accomplished on the General Automation SPC-16/50 computer using disk packs of 14 million words for storage and retrieval of data. The Conversational Computer Statistical System (CCSS) served for file handling, data screening, and the statistical computations.

The CCSS is a set of programs designed for processing data from large-scale prospective studies (Kronmal, 1974). It contains programs for checking, sorting, and maintaining complete data files generated from such research, as well as programs for display and analysis of complex data, examples of which illustrate the various chapters of this book. Among the programs are one for general purpose tabulation, one for statistical summary, one for retrieval and listing, one for estimation of probability density and cumulative distribution functions, and one for generation of scatter diagrams. In addition, the package permits summarization of data belonging to multiple records derived from individual persons, resulting in records of uniform size suitable for the more complex statistical analysis inherent in other systems of package programs. In the Cauqué study many such summary records were created and analyzed using the Biomedical Computer Programs (BMD) and the Statistical Package for the Social Sciences (SPSS). The latter were the product of a Control Data 6400 computer as described in the *CDC 6400 Users Guide* (University of Washington, 1973).

Data Files

The principal aims in analysis of these data were to provide the best possible description of the collected information and to explore interactions between two or more of the variables investigated, mainly those measuring growth, nutrition, and infection. As the work of final analysis got under way, it was immediately evident that the complex and impressive volume of information had to be reduced to numbers that were more readily manageable. The approach was to select and summarize into as few variables (or indices) as possible the time-dependent course of key variables that described the growth, diet, and health of children.

Permanent files immediately available to the processing programs were set up on computer disks. A standard routine was followed toward the goal of one large file containing all pertinent information on each person studied. A file was cleared and markers set in preparation for the sorting of data. A marker was set to designate the first card of each new identification code. A general program was written in accord with a three-digit code assigned to each child at birth.

All valid codes were specified for a discrete variable and a valid range was specified for each continuous variable. Missing value codes also were assigned before data were sorted into the file. As they were sorted in, each card received an initial screening and all card with nonvalid codes were rejected. A listing of cards with the rejected variable marked was made automatically, in order to account for all cards.

Entry of multiple records became possible through the inclusion of sort variables; the date often served for this purpose. Secondary screening was performed by descriptive statistics (mean, standard deviation, number of observations, number of missing values, minimum and maximum) and by numeric and alphabetic listing. In some instances strata (data subsets defined by the values of one or more variables, such as sex) were defined and examined separately. The technique of Boolean restrictions was used to define the strata. Once the file of a single record type had been checked and corrections made, it could be sorted and merged with other files for joint processing. The following files were set originally for data of this investigation.

Census File   For each of the four censuses taken in Santa María Cauqué in 1959, 1963, 1967, and 1971, a file was created, using the family number as the identification variable and the individual number as a sort variable. From these a second file was created with one record per family per year.   Tabulations included bar graphs and descriptive statistics on both family and individual variables.

Prenatal File   Each child born between 11 February 1964 and 27 January 1972 had a record. Descriptive statistics were calculated for all variables along with bar graphs for the discrete variables and either histograms or density plots for the continuous variables. Corrections were made for all nonvalid codes.

Newborn File   A newborn record existed for each child with a prenatal record. Descriptive statistics, bar graphs, histograms, and density plots were obtained. In this file, cards recording stillbirths were removed and twins included or excluded as desired, by use of a Boolean restriction.

Immunoglobulin File   This file contained values for umbilical cord IgM, IgA, and IgG for many newborns, along with date and cause of death in infancy or preschool age. Descriptive statistics also were calculated from this file, along with histograms on IgM, IgA, and IgG values. In addition, statistics were performed on these variables using various restrictions.

After screening, editing, and testing each file independently, the prenatal newborn and immunoglobulin files were combined into a single comprehensive file, and many cross-tabulations were performed. The merging of these files allowed descriptive statistics on immunoglobulins for strata defined by Boolean restriction on newborn and prenatal variables. Survival tables were derived for children with certain newborn and prenatal characteristics. The main variables for cross-tabulations were birth weight and gestational age.

Bacteriology File   This file held all records of samples examined primarily for enteric bacteria. Screening for bacteria codes was carried out and matched with names. Alphabetic lists were produced by chronological order and by child, arranged chronologically.

Parasitology File and Virology File These two files were prepared and handled in similar fashion to that just preceding.

Morbidity File Illness records of the Cauqué study pertain almost exclusively to the cohort children. After routine screening a file was created that matched illness cards with the prenatal, newborn and immunology records of each child. Variables were set up for loss of weight during illness, percent of weight loss, and a variable to measure nutritional status at the time of illness. Contingency tables were developed for weight loss in several diseases.

The morbidity, bacteriology, parasitology, and virology files were merged into a single comprehensive file arranged chronologically by child, indicating date of onset of each infection or disease episode, as well as duration and treatment of the event.

Anthropometric Files Two large files were established for anthropometric data. A preliminary file contained records of the cohort children only; they had been examined more frequently than the other 400 or more children. A second file was established for records of all pediatric examinations, including those of the cohort children and the twins. The latter file was designed to reject all cards where variables of weight, height, circumference of head, and circumference of thorax were not measured. This gave a smaller file for faster processing.

An additional file was set to cross-relate anthropometric variables with those of the prenatal, newborn and immunoglobulin files.

Diet File Dietary information was recorded weekly on cards for each of the cohort children. These records carry the amounts in units of food (spoonfuls, pieces, glasses, etc.), some of which vary from household to household. A program was written to change these units into calories and into grams of protein, fat, carbohydrate, vitamins, and minerals, 14 nutrients in all. Another program sums the data on foods consumed in one week and expresses the average daily intake for each child and each week. A new file was established to merge the dietary data with those of newborn and anthropometry.

Statistical Analysis and Biological Interpretation
Once the data were summarized and the statistics computed, the results were subjected to scrutiny, description, and interpretation. The next step was to correlate data on different variables. For instance, growth of individual children was characterized by fitting that data by the equation $y = a + bx + c \log(x)$; the parameters were estimated by the method of least squares. The fit of this mathematical model to the observed data was exceptionally close and a large volume of data on growth was thus reduced to three parameters,

namely a, b, and c. Each was later related in turn to other variables describing diet, infection, morbidity, and socioeconomic level.

Although the variability with dietary data was greater than with growth, the general pattern of nutrient intake over time could be described adequately by a linear function of the form $y = a + bx$. Parameters a and b of this function were used to relate diet and growth. Since calories, total protein, and other nutrients correlated highly with each other, probably as a consequence of the relatively few sources of food available to these children, calorie intake was used to represent the overall intake of other nutrients, although each nutrient was examined relative to the child's growth pattern.

The greatest difficulty was in the description of infection and morbidity. In order to summarize this information, the number of days or weeks a child was ill or disabled or infected with various microorganisms was used as an indicator of the degree of infection or morbidity, expressed as rates of illness or infection in specified periods of the child's life, for instance, the first year.

Still other variables were considered in the analysis of growth, such as height and weight of the mother, her socioeconomic status, and the particular process by which the child was weaned. These variables were analyzed both independently and in combination in an attempt to measure their relationship to growth.

In judging the results of the analysis it is necessary to appreciate that statistical tests were used for descriptive purposes only. "P values" therefore indicate the relative magnitude of observed differences or relationships and are not to be interpreted in the strict sense of statistical significance. Biological interpretation has dominated decision throughout this book. Statistical reasoning has entered into consideration, but always with a leaning toward common sense and logic, yet recognizing their potential drawbacks (Beveridge, 1950).

Investigations such as the Cauqué study are valuable in that they provide hypotheses and potential explanations for complex biological phenomena. Statistical analysis is the tool by which the investigator in such studies sees more clearly and in greater detail the complex interrelationships of the facts observed. As is true in all long-term observational studies, validation of the present findings must await verification through other observational studies in the same or similar settings or through interventions based on specific hypotheses generated by the study.

It is worth recalling that similar prospective studies continue in Santa María Cauqué, employing much the same techniques and essentially the same staff. Six months after the Cauqué study ended a nutrition intervention was implemented (Mata et al., 1972e) seeking evidence of experimentally induced changes through assessment of parameters that had been systematically established during the Cauqué study itself.

The data archive at the University of Washington contains the files of the original Cauqué study along with data pertaining to the new nutrition intervention. These materials are available for independent examination. The possibilities of further analyses are almost endless; the group responsible for collection and analysis of these data invites other investigators to undertake further work, as, indeed, has already occurred (Cherkin, 1974). Specific analyses by the field staff are presently under way to answer or explore questions raised by the nutrition intervention.

PART III
RESULTS

Chapter 5
Maternal Environment

The Santa María Cauqué mother is a product of the stoicism, endurance, and dedication of the Mayan Indian. Preparation for motherhood begins so early in childhood that by age seven girls have learned the intricate art of making tortillas, the single most important food of the Indian, and have begun to help in child rearing. The Indian girl's education in daily domestic chores continues so that by 14, when she may be married, she is able to assume the duties of a housewife (figure 5.1). Marriage, however, generally does not take place until one to three years later. The important aspects of sexual education, pregnancy, and childbirth are absent in the formal preparation of the prospective bride. These matters are learned about through experience, generally after marriage. In practice, the girl becomes pregnant within the first two years of marriage, enters motherhood at an early age, and gains experience in child care initially through exposure to her mother-in-law and subsequently through her own succession of pregnancies which span 20 years or more of childbearing.

Originally the Cauqué study made no provision for specific tests of hypotheses regarding the maternal environment, yet the information obtained about the mother and her immediate surroundings has proved fundamental to a satisfactory understanding of many characteristics of growth and survival of the newborn.

While the term maternal environment (matroenvironment) has long been used to describe physical, physiological, pathological, and obstetrical characteristics of the mother (Jurado-García et al., 1970), the concept is expanded here to include environmental influences affecting the mother, and

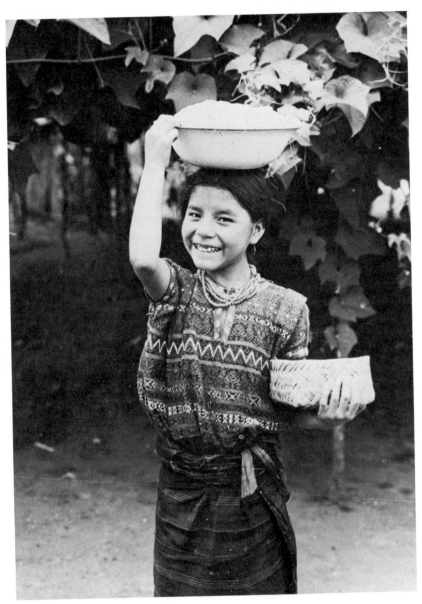

Figure 5.1
From childhood, the future mother helps with daily household chores

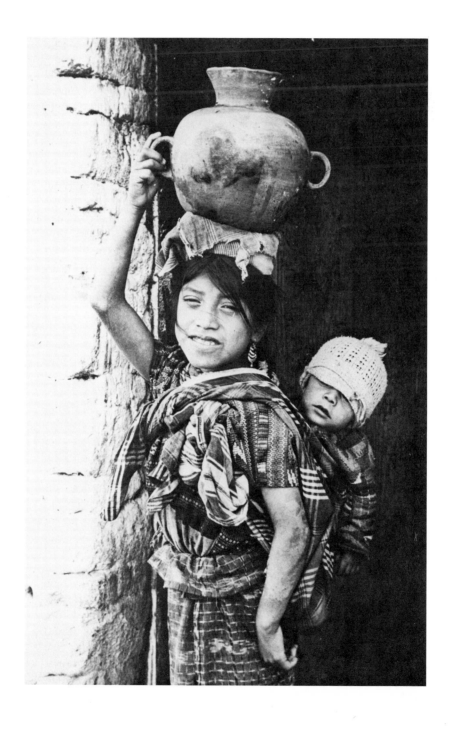

thereby the fetus, whether they originate in the home or from external sources. This is in accord with the concept that fetal growth and development are determined by interactions of genetic endowment and environmental stimuli—physical, biological, and sociocultural. The external environmental influences are those of the mother, and their effect on the prospective infant extends throughout infancy and childhood.

The biological emphasis of the Cauqué study is the principal reason for presentation of the following data. They relate to the 203 village women who contributed 465 pregnancies terminating in a live or a dead infant in Santa María Cauqué. Reference will be made to this population in total or as sub-samples of observed deliveries. The terminology is that ordinarily employed in modern usage (Niswander and Gordon, 1972). Pregnancy is marked by the presence of a developing embryo, evident by cessation of the menses. Duration of pregnancy (gestational age) is the elapsed time between the last menstrual period and termination of pregnancy, measured in weeks. An abortion is a pregnancy terminating at less than 20 weeks of gestation. If longer, it becomes a delivery either of a live (liveborn) or dead (stillborn) infant.

Age of the subject is the number of years of life at initial visit to the clinic because of a current pregnancy. Parity is the number of previous pregnancies terminating in delivery. A primipara (parity zero) is a woman with no prior pregnancy ending in delivery.

The objective of this chapter is to describe the mother in terms of her obstetrical experience, socioeconomic status, and anthropometric characteristics. The chapter also includes a description of diet and morbidity during pregnancy and an account of childbirth and maternal-infant interactions. All relate closely to the social and cultural environment of the community and are highly relevant to the health of fetus and infant. In the Santa María Cauqué study a description of the maternal environment in the village is the basis for understanding the welfare of the newborn; for discussion of maternal-fetal interactions; and for comprehension of child-feeding practices, infection, disease, nutrition, and growth.

Socioeconomic Level

Measurements of selected host and environmental variables permitted computation of an index useful in separating families into categories of differing socioeconomic status (table 4.3). This arbitrary index was calculated for each family at the approximate date of pregnancy, using the data of the nearest census. Information was available for 401 of the 465 pregnancies. Possible scores on the index were 12 through 36, but the observed limits of dispersion were between 15 and 35, indicating that even within a village structure of prevailing poverty women living under better conditions could be distinguished from those in worse conditions. Despite differences in capital, housing, education, and hygiene among pregnant women, almost all would be classed as poor by any usual standards of industrial societies. Useful comparisons were of families with regard to the number of domestic animals, the amount of land, sanitation practices, and educational level. As discussed below, the SEC Indexes were used in correlation analyses and in effecting arbitrarily grouped categories for comparison with a variety of maternal and infant variables.

Obstetric History

Among the 465 pregnancies information on motivation for visiting the clinic was available for 378; reasons given were: illness of mother (16, 4.2 percent), advice of midwife (31, 8.2 percent), promotion by clinic personnel (80, 21.2 percent), and the mother's own initiative (251, 66.4 percent). The civil status of the mother at the time of pregnancy for 465 pregnancy histories was: married (97.2 percent), common-law union (1.7 percent), and single (1.1 percent). For 181 women whose marital status was known at the time of the first visit to the clinic, figures were: married (97.2 percent), common-law union (2.2 percent), and single (0.6 percent). This, as well as other analyses, reveals that results were similar whether derived from tabulation of individual women or of pregnancies, an important consideration when dealing with prospective observations.

Information on abortion, stillbirths, and some other specific items was, however, less than for the series as a whole, in some instances by as much as one hundred cases.

A reliable duration of pregnancy was established for 416 (93 percent) of 446 pregnancies that terminated in delivery of a live singleton. Diagnosis was by date of last menstruation (28.5 percent), by measurement of uterine height (15.7 percent), or by a combination of the two (55.7 percent).

Fertility of village women is high. This would appear paradoxical in the context of the prevailing malnutrition but is accounted for by the long period of childbearing, each woman contributing approximately ten pregnancies to a society that, as yet, does not have the socioeconomic characteristics necessary for preventive medicine and disease control. Women enter motherhood at an early age and give birth to several children through a span of 20 to 25 years. In most instances spacing of pregnancies exceeds two years which undoubtedly is influenced by prolonged breast-feeding, and perhaps augmented by chronic malnutrition. Fertility, in fact, would be higher if breast-feeding did not provide a natural means for child spacing.*

---

* Village women who have successfully reared four consecutive born children through the critical first three years of life become interested in contraceptive measures. A family planning program of the Government of Guatemala has been in operation for the past three years in the Health Center of the neighboring village of Santiago Sacatepéquez. The program has not been evaluated; however, it has strengthened the concept that the

Table 5.1
Selected Obstetrical Characteristics, 458 Pregnancies, 1964–1972

Mother's age, years	Number of cases	Number of previous pregnancies	Outcome of preceding pregnancies:			Children at time of current pregnancy:	
			Deliveries	Abortions	Stillbirths[a]	Living	Dead
14	2	0	0	0	0	0	0
15–19	107	1.66 (0.79)[b]	0.57 (0.73)	0.10 (0.39)	0.19 (0.14)	0.35 (0.60)	0.22 (0.54)
20–24	124	3.31 (1.31)	2.10 (1.21)	0.20 (0.46)	0.10 (0.33)	1.55 (1.03)	0.57 (0.85)
25–29	70	5.77 (1.74)	4.21 (1.44)	0.54 (1.13)	0.23 (0.71)	3.06 (1.15)	1.17 (0.71)
30–34	86	7.81 (1.99)	6.18 (1.58)	0.64 (0.77)	0.33 (0.74)	4.53 (1.55)	1.67 (1.36)
35–39	52	9.35 (2.05)	7.63 (1.72)	0.73 (1.05)	0.25 (0.48)	5.35 (1.94)	2.31 (1.46)
40–43	17	12.24 (2.17)	9.12 (1.76)	2.12 (2.26)	0.24 (0.56)	6.17 (1.29)	2.94 (1.71)

[a]Included in deliveries.
[b]Mean (S.D.).

Table 5.2
Anthropometric Values, 171 Women, 410 Pregnancies, 1964–1971

Mother's age, years	Number of cases	Weight, kg	Height, cm	Arm circumference, cm	Leg circumference, cm	Tricipital skinfold, mm
14	1	58.4	142.2	26.5	31.5	14.0
15–19	80	52.2±0.7[a]	142.5±0.5	23.3±0.2	29.9±0.2	10.7±0.4
20–24	117	52.7±0.6	143.5±0.4	23.1±0.2	30.2±0.2	9.5±0.3
25–29	66	52.8±0.7	144.3±0.6	22.8±0.2	30.0±0.3	8.5±0.4
30–34	75	52.8±0.8	142.8±0.5	23.4±0.2	30.3±0.3	9.4±0.4
35–39	50	53.1±0.9	141.9±0.6	23.4±0.4	30.0±0.3	10.0±0.5
40–44	21	56.8±1.6	143.5±0.9	24.4±0.5	31.0±0.6	9.6±0.8
Mean		52.9	143.1	23.3	30.2	9.6

[a]Mean ± S.E.

Table 5.1 gives obstetric information for 458 (98 percent) of the 465 pregnancies, all having full information on the variables concerned; tabulation is by age of the mother. The data give evidence of the high fertility of the village population. For instance, 124 women from age 20 to 24 reported on the average a third pregnancy, an average of two deliveries, and 1.6 surviving children. Women 35 to 39 years old reported 9.4 pregnancies; 44 to 45 year old women still were delivering livebirths. Most village women lost one or more children by death.

The frequency of pregnancy and of delivery is reflected in birth intervals. The data for 361 cases (the remaining 104 were primiparae or had delivered stillborn infants) reveal that 79 percent of all births to multiparas were separated by intervals of 18 months to 3.5 years; for 49 percent the spacing of pregnancies was two to three years. Despite breast-feeding by all mothers for long periods 4 percent of subsequent births were within 9 to 12 months; for an additional 6 percent the interval was 13 to 18 months.

Physical Anthropometry
Outstanding features of village mothers are their relatively short stature and diminished subcutaneous fat, as evidenced by low body weight, observed small arm and leg circumference, and diminished skinfold thickness compared to well-nourished women. Since the stature of women is influenced strongly by malnutrition, infection, and other types of stress centered in infancy and childhood and extending into adulthood, the low values for height, skinfold thickness, and arm and leg circumferences are indicative of suboptimal

operation of family planning units may be feasible, after all, under poor environmental conditions, provided the population is sufficiently motivated and survival of children is ensured.

Table 5.3
Weight Increment of Women During Pregnancy, 1964-1971

Trimester	Number of measurements	Weight, kg	Mean weight increment, kg	
First				
6-8 wk	13	46.92 ± 1.76[a]		
12-14 wk	16	47.01 ± 1.46		
Second			4.77	
26-28 wk	90	51.73 ± 0.59		
Third				2.03
36-37 wk	91	53.64 ± 0.59		
38-39 wk	72	53.88 ± 0.78		

[a]Mean ± S.E.

maternal health and nutrition, and in turn contribute to low weight gain during pregnancy (Mata et al., 1971c). Table 5.2 distinguishes 171 pregnant women of Santa María Cauqué by size (height and weight), based on 410 (88 percent) of the 465 pregnancies. Pregnant women averaged 53 kilograms (116 pounds) in weight and 143 centimeters (4 feet 8 inches) in height. Weights are those determined to midpregnancy or towards its end, and mainly representative of the second and third trimesters of pregnancy. While weight, arm and leg circumference, and skinfold thickness are not necessarily indicative of an average prepregnancy state, the cited values, nevertheless, suffice in general description, first because nutrient intake is not significantly increased during pregnancy, and second, because changes in other anthropometric variables are not great during pregnancy.

Data obtained from 171 women provide ground for estimating the amount of weight increment during pregnancy (table 5.3), another indication of maternal health. The data represent measurements in 282 examinations, at different pregnancy stages. Several women evidently had more than one examination. An average gain of 4.8 kilograms was recorded by the beginning of the third trimester of pregnancy and an additional two kilograms by the end of the third. Total increments averaged 6.8 kilograms.

No significant differences by age were evident in the five assessed variables of table 5.2, except among women 40 to 44 years old, who appeared heavier. This question was explored further by examining the records of 110 women who had contributed at least two liveborn infants to the study. For analysis the sample was divided into three age groups (less than 19, 20 to 29, and over 30 years old each) containing, respectively, 33, 42, and 35 women. Weight loss or gain between two pregnancies was evaluated by the sign test. No differences were noted, indicating that the weight of village women, on the average, is rather stable throughout reproductive ages.

Table 5.4
Maternal Variables by Socioeconomic Index, 1964-1971

SEC Index	Age, years	Weight, kg	Height, cm	Arm, cm	Leg, cm	Tricipital skinfold, mm
15-20	26.3±1.1[a] (37)	50.7±0.8 (31)	141.6±0.9 (36)	22.7±0.3 (36)	29.9±0.3 (36)	8.6±0.5 (35)
21-25	25.1±0.6 (131)	52.6±0.6 (108)	143.2±0.3 (123)	23.4±0.2 (119)	30.3±0.2 (119)	9.7±0.3 (119)
26-30	27.9±0.6 (204)	53.5±0.5 (158)	143.3±0.3 (189)	23.4±0.1 (182)	30.2±0.2 (183)	10.0±0.2 (183)
31-35	28.4±1.4 (29)	53.8±1.3 (21)	143.9±0.8 (26)	23.2±0.8 (25)	29.5±0.4 (25)	9.0±0.7 (25)
F	4.389	2.409	1.980	1.826	1.284	2.391
d.f. (1,2)	3,397	3,314	3,370	3,358	3,359	3,358
P	< 0.01	> 0.05	> 0.05	> 0.05	> 0.05	> 0.05

[a]Mean ± S.E., below (number of observations).

Table 5.5
Relative Frequency of Foods in the Diet of Pregnant Women, by Trimester, 1971

Food	Trimester			
	First	Second	Third	Total
Tortilla	9.58	10.10	10.28	10.06
Bread	10.18	9.64	9.61	9.75
Beans	7.53	7.07	7.60	7.41
Coffee	5.70	5.27	5.59	5.51
Beef	5.70	5.12	5.36	5.37
Tomato	5.30	4.97	5.36	5.22
Beef broth	5.30	4.82	5.25	5.12
White sugar	4.68	4.37	4.13	4.29
Rice	4.07	3.92	4.02	4.00
Eggs	2.85	3.31	3.02	3.07
Noodles	2.44	3.16	3.24	3.02
Black nightshade, leaves	3.26	3.01	2.79	2.98
Onion, head	2.24	1.96	2.57	2.29
Other foods	31.17	36.28	31.18	31.91

Note: Figures show percentage of instances in which particular food was recorded among 113 dietary histories of seven days each. Percentages bear no relation to the actual amounts ingested.

Table 5.6
Consumption by Pregnant Women of Coffee, Black Beans, and Macuy, by Trimester, 1971

Food	Tri-mester	Number of women	Frequency (days per week)							Women eating food any time during survey
			1	2	3	4	5	6	7	
Coffee	First	28	0	0	0	0	0	0	26	28
	Second	35	0	0	0	0	0	1	34	35
	Third	50	0	0	2	0	0	1	47	50
Beans	First	28	2	3	1	6	12	2	2	28
	Second	35	3	1	4	4	9	8	3	32
	Third	50	0	4	13	7	11	11	4	50
Macuy	First	28	10	3	3	0	0	0	0	16
	Second	35	13	4	3	0	0	0	0	20
	Third	50	16	5	4	0	0	0	0	25

Maternal variables were also examined with respect to the socioeconomic index (table 5.4). No parameter examined, except that of maternal age, showed a relation to SECI by analysis of variance. It would appear, however, that women with the lowest SEC indices were smaller. Age of the mother evidenced a positive trend as a linear function of an increasing SECI ($P < 0.01$). Suggestive correlations between fetal or infant characteristics and maternal variables such as age, socioeconomic status, and parity always must be interpreted with caution, however, because these are often confounding variables.

Diet
Two dietary surveys of pregnant women were conducted, one at the middle of the study period (February to September 1967) and the other at its end (March to November 1971). In the first survey 33 women at various stages of pregnancy were interviewed once. The second survey was of 65 women, 13 studied only in the first trimester of pregnancy; 2 in the second; 17 in the third; 18 in both second and third; and 15 in all three timesters. Together, the surveys included 98 women and 146 one-week dietary histories, 33 in 1967 and 113 in 1971.

Of the several hundred different foods listed in the Central American Food Composition Table (Flores et al., 1960), approximately 100 were observed in one or another of the two surveys. Table 5.5 gives the relative frequencies of the foods most often consumed. The stated frequencies, however, do not necessarily bear a relation to amounts ingested or to nutritive value. Thirteen foods accounted for about two thirds of the total, and frequencies in their use were consistent throughout pregnancy. The pattern and frequency of consumption of these foods were examined by trimester of pregnancy. Tables

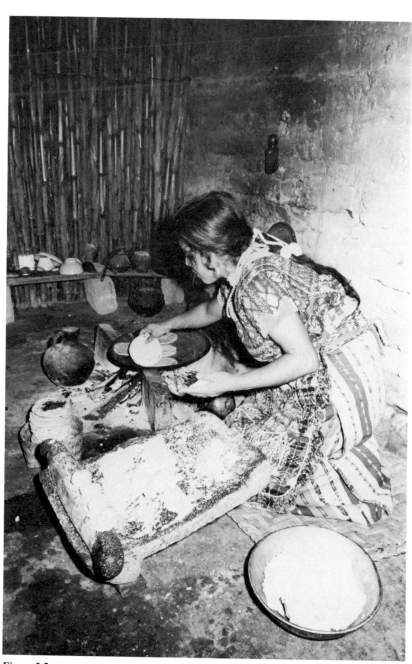

Figure 5.2
Young mother preparing tortillas

Table 5.7
Mean Daily Food Consumption by Pregnant Women, by Trimester, 1971

	Trimester		
Food	First (N = 28)	Second (N = 35)	Third (N = 50)
Tortillas	621[a]	624	595
Sugar, raw sugar	61	62	83
Beans	53	56	56
Vegetables	46	51	53
Bread	26	36	30
Meats	19	23	21
Fruits	22	24	15
Rice	8	9	9
Bananas, plantains	2	10	7
Eggs	6	6	7

[a]Grams per day per woman.

were set up for each food, (table 5.6) for coffee, black beans, and leaves of *macuy* (black nightshade). Foods such as coffee and tortillas almost invariably were consumed daily, others like beans and noodles were served irregularly during the week; and still others, for instance macuy, were served no more than three days a week, and usually only once. Most women partook of foods such as tortilla and sugar; other foods were consumed by a limited few. The diet of pregnant village women fundamentally consists of maize prepared as tortillas (figure 5.2). It should be noted, however, that maize in its preparation for tortillas undergoes important nutritional changes such as enrichment with calcium and loss in certain nutrients (Bressani et al., 1958a). Beans are the principal complement to maize, but are not consumed to the desired level. For economic more than cultural or behavioral reasons, animal protein is not an important component of the diet in pregnancy, although field experience indicates that women like and accept a variety of foods such as meats, cheese, and eggs.

Average food composition of the daily diet was remarkably similar in the two surveys in terms of grams of each important food. The findings of the 1971 study are shown in table 5.7. Five or six foods consistently contributed the bulk of the diet, of which tortillas, beans, and sugar were most prominent. In summary, the outstanding features of the diet are the relatively few foods consumed, the contribution by a few to most of the bulk, the predominance of foods of vegetable origin, and the virtual absence of animal protein.

Nutritive values from the 1967 and 1971 surveys are summarized in tables 5.8 and 5.9. Table 5.8 shows nutritive values of the mean daily food intake in

Table 5.8
Mean Daily Nutrient Intake by Pregnant Women, 1967 and 1971

	1967, third trimester (N = 18)	1971, by trimester First (N = 28)	Second (N = 35)	Third (N = 50)	Daily recommendation[a] NAS-NRC	INCAP
Calories	2,083 (503)[b]	2,047 (483)[b]	2,105 (480)	1,942 (524)	2,200	2,400
Total protein, g[c]	64 (18)	57.9 (13.6)	60.5 (14.4)	56.6 (15.6)	65	60
Animal protein, g	6 (6)	5.4 (2.5)	6.5 (4.2)	5.8 (2.8)		
Fat, g	19 (11)	18.6 (6.7)	21.6 (8.2)	19.5 (8.4)		
Calcium, mg	1,135 (341)	1,080 (291)	1,115 (306)	1,011 (359)	1,200	1,100
Iron, mg[d]	21 (8)	19.4 (7.2)	20.9 (8.0)	19.1 (7.4)	18	28
Retinol equiv., μg	253 (212)	165.7 (112.9)	160.4 (103)	154.7 (94.4)	750[e]	900
Thiamin, mg	1.3 (0.4)	1.1 (0.3)	1.2 (0.3)	1.1 (0.3)	1.2	1.0
Riboflavin, mg	0.7 (0.2)	0.6 (0.1)	0.7 (0.2)	0.6 (0.2)	1.8	1.3
Niacin, mg	13 (3)	11.3 (2.5)	12.0 (2.8)	11.4 (2.9)	15	15.8
Ascorbic acid, mg	51 (33)	34.4 (24.2)	36.8 (20.0)	36.3 (25.5)	60	50

[a] For pregnant women, more than 18 years old, second and third trimesters.
[b] Mean (S.D.).
[c] Mainly maize.
[d] Mainly from vegetable origin (beans and other pulses).
[e] FAO/WHO (1967).

Table 5.9
Adequacy of Diets of Pregnant Women in the Second and Third Trimesters, by Percentage of INCAP Recommendation, 1971

	Percentage of nutrition adequacy[a]									
	35 pregnant women, second trimester					50 pregnant women, third trimester				
	≤25	26-50	51-75	76-100	>100	≤25	26-50	51-75	76-100	>100
Calories	0	0	26[b]	49	26	0	6[b]	39	35	20
Total protein	0	0	14	34	51	0	4	25	22	49
Calcium	0	0	11	43	46	0	10	18	35	37
Iron	0	20	34	23	23	4	22	31	29	14
Retinol equiv.	71	29	0	0	0	86	14	0	0	0
Thiamin	0	0	3	23	74	0	2	6	27	65
Riboflavin	3	46	46	6	0	2	59	39	0	0
Niacin	0	6	43	37	14	0	10	45	41	4
Ascorbic acid	6	23	31	14	26	6	31	31	16	16

[a] Adequacy as percentage of requirement for pregnant women, second and third trimester, 53 kg, 20+ years old.
[b] Percentage of women falling in this category of nutrient adequacy.

Table 5.10
Mean Daily Nutrient Intake by Prepregnant and Lactating Women, 1972

	Prepregnant (N = 10)		Lactating (N = 10)		INCAP daily recommendation	
					Prepregnant	Lactating
Calories	1,881	(325)[a]	2,078	(627)	2,050	2,600
Total protein, g	54	(10)	59	(17)	45	68
Animal protein, g	7	(3)	5	(3)		
Calcium, mg	1,005	(240)	1,075	(292)	450	1,100
Iron, mg	21	(5)	18	(6)	28	28
Retinol equiv., μg	244	(108)	287	(192)	750	1,100
Riboflavin, mg	0.5	(0.1)	0.6	(0.1)	1.1	1.4
Ascorbic acid, mg	28	(19)	29	(18)	30	50
nDpCal %	6.9	(0.5)	6.8	(0.6)	4.5[b]	5.0[b]

[a]Mean (S.D.).
[b]Swaminathan (1970).

various trimesters of pregnancy. In the 1971 survey there was some indication of an overall decrease in intake of calories, protein, vitamin A (retinol), and ascorbic acid. Estimated optimal requirements for women of the area (18 years old and over, healthy, 53 kilograms, third trimester of pregnancy) are included in the tables for reference. A deficiency in calories and animal protein and a marked deficiency in vitamin A and riboflavin are evident when observed means are compared with the recommendations. Standard deviations are large, however, and imply that some women consumed as much or more of the recommended amounts while others fared worse than indicated.

To overcome the recognized limitation of presenting average values, a more precise description of the diet of women was set, according to levels of adequacy of nutrient intake, at arbitrarily determined intervals of 25 percent of INCAP recommended levels (table 5.9). This revealed more explicit differences in the degree of deficit of the various nutrients. Deficiency in total retinol and riboflavin was greater than for any other single nutrient since a greater proportion of women failed to meet even moderate levels of the requirement. Intake of calories, total protein, calcium, and niacin appeared inadequate, although deficits were not as marked as for vitamin A and riboflavin. The deficit in iron is serious; its source is mainly beans and other pulses and therefore is not readily absorbed. The nutritional deficiencies noted appear accentuated in the third trimester of pregnancy. The diet of prepregnant and lactating women of Santa María Cauqué has a similar composition to that of pregnant women. Lactating women did not increase their intake in a significant manner (table 5.10) and their daily diet shows marked deficits in calories, vitamin A, and riboflavin as well as deficits in iron and ascorbic acid. Protein did not appear deficient; the nDpCal percent values

Table 5.11
Correlation of Nutrient Intake Between Second and Third Trimesters of Pregnancy,
33 Women, 1971

	Slope (b)	Correlation coefficient (r)	P
Calories	0.7203	0.7828	< 0.001
Total protein	0.6237	0.6337	< 0.001
Carbohydrate	0.6920	0.7718	< 0.001
Fat	0.4178	0.4035	< 0.05
Calcium	0.7210	0.6962	< 0.001
Phosphorus	0.6678	0.7105	< 0.001
Iron	0.2791	0.2870	< 0.1
Retinol equiv.	0.2662	0.3753	< 0.05
Thiamin	0.5393	0.5950	< 0.001
Riboflavin	0.3281	0.4817	< 0.01
Niacin	0.5487	0.6459	< 0.001

were adequate. This observation is important in view of the fact that breast milk represented the only source of food for infants in the first few months of life.

Other negative factors in the diet are due to irregularities of food availability throughout the year because of droughts, food price fluctuations, and changes in yield of the land.

Finally, although not quantified, poor food hygiene requires mention because of its relation to diarrheal disease. The inadequate environmental sanitation and the ways in which foods are stored, prepared, and eaten favors spoilage and contributes heavily to the transmission of intestinal pathogens.

Nutrient intake varied little during pregnancy. This is important because of the relatively limited weight gain during gestation and the high incidence of infants with low birth weight. The observed stability could be due, however, to individual variations within the sample of mothers, in either direction, in a random fashion, or to inherent variations in methods of collecting the information. To answer this question the diet was examined prospectively. A significant correlation was noted for calories and most nutrients (table 5.11). This additional evidence supports the view that women with the worst intakes in the second trimester tended to continue this way in the third, and that those who were eating better in the second trimester did so in the third as well.

Overall, dietary intake was rather constant throughout pregnancy with no evidence of significant changes in quality, quantity, or pattern of intake. The diet of the mother, however, is biologically inadequate because it is limited to a few food items, with maize contributing about 60 percent of the total; it is also bulky, has low digestibility, and shows an overall deficit in calories,

Table 5.12
Prevalence Rates for Enteric Infectious Agents among Mothers of Cohort Children,
1964-1965

Number of women examined	Agent identified	Percentage of women infected
24	*Entamoeba histolytica*	54
	Entamoeba coli	92
	Dientamoeba fragilis	8
	Giardia lamblia	8
	Ascaris lumbricoides	83
	Trichuris trichiura	58
	One or more parasites	100
116	*Shigellae*	9
	Salmonellae	5
	One or more enteropathogenic bacteria	14
32	Enteroviruses (polio, coxsackie, echo)	25
	Adenoviruses	3

Note: Determined by single fecal specimen during asymptomatic periods.

animal protein, vitamin A, riboflavin, and iron, deficiencies similar to those originally described for this village in 1950 (Flores and Reh, 1955).*

This observation must be taken into consideration when correlations with fetal growth are made in later chapters. The background health of the woman before she becomes pregnant could well be more important for fetal development than the actual diet during gestation.

Infection

Exceedingly high rates of infection and infectious diseases were observed among village women, greater than those revealed by studies in industrial countries (Sever, 1966; Niswander and Gordon, 1972). Ongoing microbiologic and serologic prevalence studies in Santa María Cauqué showed a similarly high incidence of enteric infectious agents, in large part unassociated with clinical signs or symptoms (Mata et al., 1972b) (table 5.12). These results, based on examination of feces, suggest that investigation of other materials also would unveil an equally high prevalence of infectious agents, for instance in upper respiratory and genital tracts and the skin.

The extreme burden of infection experienced in this rural setting throughout life is also reflected in highly elevated levels of serum immunoglobulins. For instance, village adults have mean concentrations (mg/ml) of 1.9 IgM,

* The findings apply to Guatemalan rural populations in general, as well as to rural areas of other Central American nations (Flores et al., 1973; INCAP-CDC, 1972).

Table 5.13
Prevalence of Antibodies to Selected Infectious Agents in Women of Childbearing Age,
1964-1971

Agent, dilution, technique[a]	Number of women tested	Number and percentage with antibodies
Poliovirus 1, N, 1:8	50	50 (100)
Coxsackievirus Bl, HI, 1:10	93	59 (55)
Echovirus 3, HI, 1:10	93	29 (27)
Reovirus 1, HI, 1:10	93	15 (14)
Rubella virus, HI, 1:8	48	24 (50)
Toxoplasma, D-T, 1:16	22	11 (50)
Brucella, A	200	1 (0.5)
Treponema pallidum, FTA-ABS	200	0

Note: N = neutralization; HI = hemagglutination-inhibition; D-T = dye test; A = slide
agglutination; FTA-ABS = fluorescent antibody-absorbed.
[a]Test and dilution at which a case was considered positive.

2.42 IgA and 15.3 IgG (Cáceres and Mata, 1974). These values are considerably greater than for populations living in better sanitary conditions (Cáceres
and Mata, 1974) and are comparable to levels reported for other preindustrial
nations (Rowe et al., 1968).

The presence of antibodies also demonstrates that a large proportion of
village women are exposed to many infectious agents. Table 5.13 illustrates
the serological status of village women to selected antigens. Despite the fact
that polio vaccine had not been introduced, all the women examined
possessed antibodies to Type 1 poliovirus and most to Types 2 and 3. Antibodies to other infectious agents were less prevalent, e.g., to the virus of
rubella and to *Toxoplasma*. The presence of susceptibles to rubella could
relate to a relative isolation of the villages (Mata et al., 1974a). In the case of
Toxoplasma, transmission rather surely is by cat feces, since meat consumption is low.

Although a variety of antibodies is highly prevalent, indicating active transmission of the corresponding infectious agents, many women reach reproductive ages without immunity to some of the common infections of the region,
either because the protection after an attack is short-lived or because of
existing antigenic differences. They are susceptible to infection if exposed, a
matter of rather certain probability, because of their close association with
small children and their housekeeping responsibilities and because of environmental conditions that favor dissemination of agents introduced from the
outside or those already present in the village. The susceptibility and greater
exposure of women to infection has indirect and direct effects on maternal
welfare and fetal growth and development (Mata et al., 1974a), effects not
yet fully appreciated by health workers, particularly in developing nations.

Table 5.14
Frequency of Infectious Diseases During Pregnancy, 365 Women, 1964-1971

Number of episodes	Frequency		
	Number of pregnant women	Percentage ill	Accumulated percentage
0	106	29.0	
1	114	31.2	71.0
2	80	21.9	39.7
3	58	15.9	17.8
4	6	1.6	1.9
5	1	0.3	0.3
Total	365	99.9	

Frequent infection and inadequate diet are major factors that lead to the deterioration of nutritional status and undoubtedly affect the mother and fetus (Lechtig et al., 1972b; Charles and Finland, 1973; Mata 1974) through reduced intake, increased nutrient losses and demands, nutritional wastage, and metabolic alterations (Beisel, 1972). Furthermore, the prevailing malnutrition of the mother is reflected in a diminished immune response, particularly of the T-cell (Awdeh et al., 1972; Mata and Faulk, 1973). The probability of direct injury to fetal growth and development increases with augmented maternal infection and raises the incidence of abortion, fetal growth retardation, premature delivery, and other abnormalities, an observation that deserves serious consideration (Mata, 1974).

Morbidity
Although village childbirth and obstetrical practice appear primitive, inadequate, and dangerous to the westerner, complications of pregnancy common in industrial societies, namely pre-eclampsia and eclampsia, were not observed in any patient in Santa María; one had a mild edema of the legs. The frequency of abortion in Santa María Cauqué has been estimated at around 20 per 100 pregnancies (preliminary results of an ongoing study), and stillbirths averaged three per 100 pregnancies during the eight-year period. These figures are not strikingly greater than those reported in industrial societies (Greenhill and Friedman, 1974). No case of puerperal fever was recorded in the series, however, and no deaths of the mother during childbirth or puerperium occurred during the study; delivery in general was uneventful.*

* The absence of puerperal fever must be due to fewer nosocomial pathogens in the home environment; puerperal fever is related to hospitals and attendants who harbor the infectious agents. Why puerperal fever of endogenous origin does not occur is unknown.

Table 5.15
Infectious Disease Syndromes Recorded in 365 Pregnancies, by Trimester and Number
and Percentage of Pregnancies, 1964–1971

	Trimester		
	First	Second	Third
Upper respiratory disease	69 (18.9)[a]	96 (26.3)	113 (30.9)
Bronchitis	7 (1.9)	9 (2.5)	11 (3.0)
Laryngotracheobronchitis	1 (0.3)	6 (1.6)	6 (1.6)
Otitis media	0	3 (0.8)	3 (0.8)
Pneumonia	0	2 (0.6)	1 (0.3)
Conjunctivitis	1 (0.3)	0	1 (0.3)
Fever of unknown origin	1 (0.3)	0	0
Diarrhea	18 (4.9)	18 (4.9)	30 (8.2)
Dystentery	5 (1.4)	4 (1.1)	4 (1.1)
Cystitis and pyelonephritis	7 (1.9)	7 (1.9)	5 (1.4)
Hepatitis	0	2 (0.5)	4 (1.1)
Skin infection[b]	11 (3.0)	3 (0.8)	11 (3.0)
Tenosynovitis	0	1 (0.3)	0

[a]Number (percentage of pregnancies).
[b]Includes impetigo, cellulitis, and abscess.

Most intercurrent illnesses during pregnancy were of infectious origin.
Complete records were available for 365 (78.5 percent) pregnancies during
the study. The remaining 100 records were incomplete and excluded. The
main body of information was collected by a physician through interviews
during scheduled prenatal clinic visits but also during home visits of illnesses.
Some episodes were identified retrospectively since visits to the clinic usually
were one or two per trimester. Some information, of a magnitude that cannot
be assessed, likely was lost through failure of recall.

The frequency of illnesses, particularly infectious diseases, was decidedly
high. Table 5.14 shows only 29 percent of all pregnancies as free of reported
illnesses; the remainder had from one to as many as five different attacks. The
frequency was rather similar by trimester, but with a trend toward more illnesses as the gestational period advanced. At least one illness occurred in 31
percent of first trimesters and the frequency reached 44 percent in the third.
Two independent episodes were recorded in 2.5 percent of first trimesters
and in 4 percent of thirds. The report of the Collaborative Perinatal Study in
the United States showed a frequency of infection and infectious disease
during pregnancy that was materially lower than in the village women of
Santa María Cauqué (Sever, 1966; Niswander and Gordon, 1972).

The most important infectious disease syndromes are listed in Table 5.15
by trimester of pregnancy. A high frequency of infectious diseases, some of

considerable severity such as dysentery, pneumonia, and pyelonephritis, was a consistent observation throughout gestation. A large proportion of pregnant women had at least one attack of diarrhea or dysentery or of an acute respiratory disease (pneumonia, bronchitis, laryngitis). The gross frequency of symptomatic urinary tract infection was 5 per 100 pregnancies.

The observed rates for infectious disease probably underestimate the true situation because complete identification of mild bacteruria and minor infections of skin, throat, eye, and gastrointerestinal and respiratory tracts during widely spaced clinic visits was impossible, especially since women of developing rural areas, accustomed to disease throughout their lives, do not often complain and do not report signs or symptoms unless they are relatively severe.

The Birth Process
The village community considers childbirth a natural event with no particular hazard. Tradition permeates the process, likely accomplished in much the same fashion as it was in ancient Mayan days, with knowledge passed from one generation of women and midwives to the next. Full information was obtained about all births in the village because through the entire Cauqué study a nurse was posted at the clinic around the clock, including weekends. Excellent relations with the midwives of the village enabled nurses to visit homes in more than 95 percent of births, during or shortly after delivery. Ordinarily the nurse did not attend or take part in the delivery; her instructions were not to interfere but to collect information and to enter it on a form designed for the purpose. Data from 297 deliveries directly observed by nurses are the basis of the following analyses.

Women perceived that delivery was imminent through onset of pains (95 percent) or by the appearance of bloody vaginal mucus (3 percent) or of vaginal fluid (2 percent). Localization of pains was reported as at the waist (59 percent) or abdomen (41 percent). Women notified the husband whenever he could be reached; if he was far away in the fields or in another village the midwife was the first to be informed. In 5 percent of instances neither husband nor midwife could be located promptly and notification was to the clinic nurse (4 percent) or to a relative (1 percent). Births occurred most often in early morning hours. Delivery was in the usual one-room home, next to the fire; in only 31 percent of deliveries were the quarters destined for delivery especially cleaned; ordinarily no special preparations were made. Delivery of the baby was either on a palm mat spread on the floor (95 percent) or on the bare dirt floor (4 percent); only four were in a bed (1 percent). In addition the midwife and husband and other relatives and neighbors often were present during delivery. Precise details of the birth process often were obscure because the woman remained clothed during delivery.

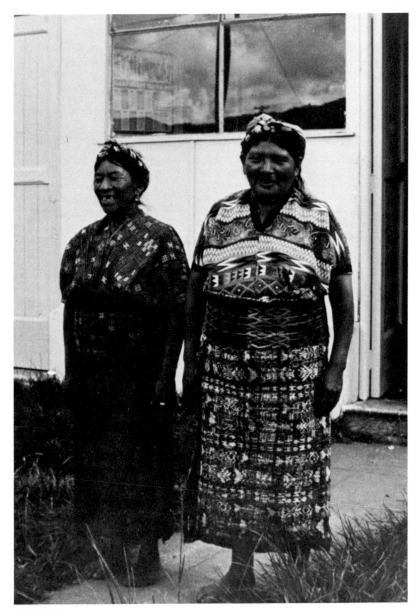

Figure 5.3
The midwives of Santa María Cauqué, to whom the study is greatly indebted. One wears
the typical red native *qüipil* (blouse) of Santa María Cauqué; the other that of the twin
villages of Santa Catarina Barahona and San Antonio Aguas Calientes.

Midwives usually were the sole source of antepartum advice about obstetrical procedure, and they provided all of the assistance received in labor (figure 5.3). No drugs were employed to precipitate or accelerate delivery. Verbal instructions and consolation, physical pressure to the abdomen, and superficial abdominal exploration were the main contribution of midwives. Verbal advice was given in 78 percent of deliveries, abdominal palpation in 6 percent, rectal examination in 5 percent, and abdominal and genital examination in 10 percent. There was no preparation for delivery by shaving, disinfection, enema, or otherwise; an accompanying passage of feces by the mother occurred in 295 of the 297 deliveries.

The position of the woman during childbirth as recorded in these deliveries was on the knees (90 percent), squatting (8 percent), and supine (2 percent). The preferred position on the knees seems to be a more favorable position than the orthodox recumbent position common to western medicine, especially for older women who may have diminished capacity in labor. The mother remained in the same position during birth of the placenta and thereafter rested on the bare floor, either on her side (95 percent) or on her back (5 percent).

Rupture of the membrane was spontaneous in the 408 deliveries for which this information was obtained. It occurred within 10 to 20 minutes preceding birth in 349 instances (85.5 percent), 20 to 60 minutes in 18 (4.4 percent), 61 to 120 minutes in 14 (3.4 percent), and 3 to 98 hours in the remainder (6.6 percent). The frequency distribution of time of rupture of membranes showed little or no relation to parity. The spontaneous rupture of the membrane shortly before delivery is protective to the child since premature iatrogenic rupture, in practice in hospitals for many years, has been found to increase compression and deformation of the fetal head (Althabe et al., 1969).

Duration of labor, estimated from the beginning of moderate pains, ranged from a few minutes to 19 hours, with a mode of 4 hours as established by 429 deliveries, a shorter time than stated in most textbooks. Few women had a labor of more than 8 hours.

Presentation and type of delivery was determined in 435 and 432 cases, respectively, of the 465 recorded deliveries. The predominating normality was cephalic presentation (99.3 percent of deliveries) and only 0.7 percent of deliveries were by breech presentation. Twins were born in three instances, and 429 were single births. Delivery in the home favors infant colonization with maternal indigenous bacteria. Since the *vernix caseosa* is not removed, colonization with such bacteria is facilitated (Rosebury, 1962). Other aspects of childbirth, however, could benefit from improved midwivery practices to the advantage of the newborn. For instance, regular exposure to heavy doses of maternal feces provides a source of infection with pathogenic agents; in fact, neonates have been found shedding enteroviruses (Mata et al., 1972b) and *shigellae* (Mata et al., 1969c) so early in life as to suspect fecal contamination at birth.

The midwife was the chief source of postpartum assistance to women. She cut and tied the umbilical cord in 98 percent of cases; the remaining few were cauterized with a hot metal instrument (a sickle or machete), a custom that has ancient roots. Dressings of gauze and alcohol were applied to 72 percent of cord stumps, 7 percent were not treated, and the remainder were covered with a dry cloth. No cases of tetanus neonatorum were recorded during the study period. Without exception, the placenta was burned in the home hearth, the ashes collected in an earthenware bowl, stored for several days, and then buried or scattered in the fields, purportedly to prevent misfortunes to mother or infant.

Maternal-Infant Interaction

Support to the mother is provided during and after childbirth by relatives and friends who take responsibility for the usual household chores and preparation of the temascal for the traditional postpartum steam bath.

The mother resumes her household duties one to three days after the birth but ordinarily remains within the house for the next two weeks. On the first two days after delivery, mother, infant, midwife, and occasionally a female relative, take a steam bath in the temascal lasting for 30 to 45 minutes. The bath has a variety of purposes: to clean the body, to stimulate lactation, to prevent colic in the child, and to promote the original size and position of the womb. The temascal is continued by mother and infant daily during the two-week period of confinement. The infant meanwhile is dressed with a diaper, shirt, coat and cap and wrapped in blankets that permit little movement of the arms and more of the legs (figure 5.4). Habitually, the child is carried on the mother's back or on her hip throughout infancy and a goodly part of early childhood and is rarely left alone.

While no systematic study of maternal-infant behavioral interaction was made, the relations of mother and infant are most intimate, involving physical contact from the moment of birth. If the mother had been nursing an older child throughout the present pregnancy, she offered the breast to the newborn without delay. In many instances the mother gives colostrum to her baby. Under other circumstances a foster mother, generally a friend or relative, or the grandmother of the infant as recorded in a few instances, serves in this capacity. As soon as her own milk thickens, the mother assumes full responsibility for nursing, which she accomplishes with much success. Mother and infant sleep together in a position favoring breast-feeding on demand during the night.

This natural mother-child relationship undoubtedly contributes to biological colonization of the newborn's skin and gut by indigenous bacteria;

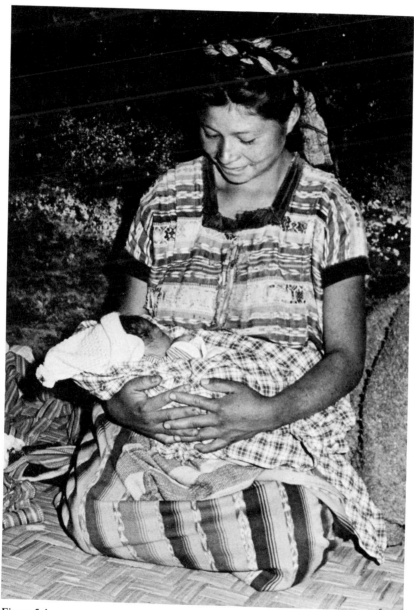

Figure 5.4
Mother and firstborn in the favored position for nursing and attending the baby

it clearly favors breast-feeding and contributes to childhood physical growth and behavioral development (Kennell and Klaus, 1971; Klaus et al., 1972; Kennell et al., 1974).

Chapter 6
The Newborn Infant

Characterization of the newborn infant is a fundamental part of a long-term prospective analysis of growth and health of children. This is particularly true in developing regions where fetal growth retardation (FGR) expectedly is greater in degree and more frequent than in industrial areas. Unfortunately, it is precisely in developing countries and mainly in their rural areas that information on fetal life and the newborn infant is at its lowest level. Even for the urban populations of the larger preindustrial cities, information is scarce and often inaccurate because existing statistics are so often rudimentary, routine, or handicapped by inexact methodology. This need not be the case, however.

The Cauqué study collected considerable information on the health status and care of the newborn infant by controlled techniques that permitted assessment of fetal growth and development and other infant characteristics over a span of eight years. Birth weight and gestational age were obtained for more than 90 percent of consecutive newborns. Subsequent pediatric evaluation satisfactorily agreed with observations on physical appearance and vitality obtained through interviews with the mother, midwife, and other attendants, a finding that should stimulate collection of similar information from other rural areas of Central America, with the aim of characterizing the frequency of high-risk neonates and the nature and magnitude of perinatal mortality and postneonatal growth and survival.

The chapter is organized into three sections: the first describes the newborn population and its characteristics at birth and physical anthropometry; the second section discusses the levels and significance of immunoglobulins in umbilical cord serum and the frequency of fetal antigenic stimulation and antenatal infection; and the third part is concerned with the incidence and implications of preterm and low-birth-weight infants.

The newborn population considered here was the result of 465 pregnancies that terminated in delivery of an infant either alive or dead. A live birth is the expulsion or complete extraction from the mother (delivery) of an infant of more than 20 weeks gestation who breathes or gives other signs of life, such as pulsations of the umbilical cord. Stillbirth is the delivery of a dead infant of more than 20 weeks gestation. Gestational age is the time in weeks between the date of last menstruation and the date of birth. Low birth weight (LBW) is any amount less than 2,501 grams; a preterm infant is one born at less than 37 weeks of gestation; a term-small-for-gestational age infant (TSGA) is of less than 2,501 grams birth weight, but of 37 weeks or more gestation; a term (full term) infant (T) is one whose birth weight is 2,501 or more and whose gestational age is 37 weeks or more.

Newborns: Characteristics and Anthropometry

The 465 deliveries resulted in 470 newborns in the course of the study, 11 February 1964 to 27 January 1972. Of these, 460 (97.9 percent) were singletons and 10 (2.1 percent) were twins; the twin rate was one per 100 deliveries or two per 100 newborns. Among the 460 singletons 446 (97 percent) were liveborn and 14 (3 percent) stillborn; all twins were liveborn. Among the 470 newborns 228 (49 percent) were male and 242 (51 percent) were female, a sex ratio of 0.94. Of live singletons, 204 (47 percent) were male and 227 (53 percent) were female.

The data on abortions were far from adequate; cultural beliefs and associated taboos interfere with an adequate recognition of these events even under optimal field conditions. An early recruitment of pregnant women for prospective surveillance permitted, however, an accounting of most stillbirths. Limited physical inspection of stillbirths with a determination of birth weight was possible for 6 of the 14 cases identified. Birth weights ranged from 1,192 to 2,946 grams. All observed instances of stillbirth suggested a pathologic condition. One had an elevated cord serum IgM (more than 0.19 mg/ml), and at least two exhibited overt anatomic malformations. As already noted, the birth of the child itself brings virtually no intervention by the midwife. The baby falls on the mat or floor or is received by the midwife, and if breathing appears normal, the cord is severed, and the child is placed next to the mother on some clothes or on a mat. For the next few minutes care is centered on the mother with advice, comfort, and reassurance. After birth of the placenta, the mother rests and the midwife turns to the child. Midwives and attendants showed interest in the cry, respiration, and physical appearance of the baby. The midwife was responsible for the initial care which, in 297 cases observed and recorded by the nurses, was as follows: 33 percent of the babies were cleaned while the remaining were left untouched; the child was wrapped in adult clothes or a poncho in 82 percent of the cases, and in 18 percent the child was left naked sometimes for as long as an hour until the mother had been cared for. The eyes were cleaned with a cloth (10.9 percent) or with the bare hand (1.7 percent) or were given eye drops (10.9 percent); in most cases the eyes were not touched. The mouth and nose of 11 percent and the genitals of 9 percent of the infants were wiped. If the infant appeared in poor condition or was breathing abnormally, the midwife might massage the body or open the infant's mouth with a finger and blow a spray of the local alcoholic spirits onto the baby's face.

There is virtually no emphasis on asepsis. From birth onward the newborn has ample opportunity for exposure to a variety of infectious agents of fecal origin. Despite the rigors of delivery, the risks of trauma for the newborn apparently were not greater than those in more advanced societies, as judged by neonatal mortality by birth weight. All liveborn infants of at least 2,750 grams birth weight and all mothers survived. Better-defined studies with emphasis on obstetrical, gynecologic, and physiological aspects of childbirth are essential, however, to determine improved practice.

The observer nurse made the first appraisal of the newborn and recorded outstanding features, some subject to personal judgment such as general appearance and vitality, and others better characterized as overt congenital defects. When the nurse was not permitted to examine the infant, information was from the mother (51.3 percent of cases), midwives (12.1 percent), relatives (2.3 percent), physician (1.4 percent), or other source (0.5 percent). The physical *appearance* of infants was normal for 395 (91.8 percent), fair for 27 (6.3 percent), while the remaining 8 (1.9 percent) were judged in poor condition and weak; 3 died shortly after birth. Crying was reported as immediate in 93 percent and delayed in 5 percent, while 8 babies (1.9 percent) exhibited only a moan and did not cry. Four died within 48 hours of birth. Respiration was normal in 92 percent of the infants, had to be stimulated in 12 cases (2.8 percent), appeared slowly in 21 (4.9 percent), and was undetected in 2 (0.5 percent). These latter two and one in whom stimulation failed died shortly after birth.

During his daily visit a physician subsequently evaluated each newborn; most medical examinations took place within 18 hours of birth. This physical examination was accomplished successfully in all but 5 of the 430 cases. Results of the evaluation were as follows:

Appearance: The pediatric examination showed that 93.7 percent had good physical appearance, 5.2 percent were fair, and 1.2 percent were rated poor. The last two categories combined give a number close to the 8.1 percent related above from the observations of relatives and midwives.

Skin appearance: Three infants (0.7 percent) were blanched, 12 (2.8 percent) were cyanotic, 23 (5.7 percent) showed varying degrees of jaundice, and 3

(0.7 percent) showed noninfectious desquamation. Infants with poor appearance or those cyanotic had a low survival rate. Neonatal jaundice faded within a matter of days.

Respiration: Two babies only groaned or moaned; 1 exhibited signs of asphyxia, and another was hypoventilated; 2 died within 12 hours.

Lungs: Two infants had an abnormal amount of mucus in the respiratory tract.

Heart: Two infants had bradycardia (less than 100 beats per minute).

Moro's reflex: This was unilateral superior in 95.5 percent of cases, bilateral superior in 0.5 percent, and absent in 3.9 percent.

Muscle tone: Twenty-two infants (5.4 percent) were hypotonic, and 1 atonic.

Birth injury: One child with a fractured hip died within 48 hours.

Congenital malformations: Nine infants had overt malformations such as polydactylia, clubfoot, hare lip, and preauricular papillomas, an incidence of 2.3 per 100 births, including both living and dead. The rate was probably greater because 8 stillbirths could not be examined.

The frequency of overt congenital malformations is still likely to be underestimated because diagnosis by necessity was limited to clinical methods, without benefit of techniques and procedures required to discover malformations of the circulatory, renal, nervous, and other systems. Nevertheless the figure falls within the range of globally reported rates for observations of newborns (Kennedy, 1967; Howie, 1970) and thus casts doubts on the suggested role of maternal and fetal malnutrition in the etiology of birth defects. The identification of only 3 congenitally malformed infants during the first four years of the study, in contrast to 8 during the second four years suggests that either methods of surveillance had improved over the years or the community had become more cooperative in activities of the field staff.

Data were obtained for all newborn twins except two. One pair could not be examined as newborns but were in good condition when first seen at age three weeks. They survived infancy and early childhood. A second pair, the smallest recorded babies born during the study (783 grams and 1,054 grams), were in poor condition at birth and died within four hours. No congenital malformations were found at birth among the five sets of twins.

Mean values and standard deviations for all liveborns (single births and twins) were: birth weight 2,533 ± 398 grams; birth length 45.6 ± 1.8 centimeters; head circumference 32.0 ± 1.5 centimeters; thorax circumference 29.9 ± 1.8 centimeters. Measurements of the four variables for single live births by sex are summarized in table 6.1. Differences by sex were significant in all four instances; males averaged about 100 grams heavier than females and had lengths and circumferences of head and thorax about 1 centimeter

Table 6.1
Anthropometry of the 430 Newborn, Single Live Infants, by Sex, 1964–1972

	204 males	226 females	F	P
Weight, g	2,598 ± 366 (1,225–3,562)[a]	2,501 ± 383 (1,194–3,374)	7.044	< 0.01
Length, cm[b]	46.2 ± 2.0 (39.5–51.0)	45.2 ± 2.2 (37.4–50.2)	23.844	< 0.0005
Head circumference, cm[b]	32.5 ± 1.3 (28.0–36.4)	31.7 ± 1.4 (24.8–35.1)	29.277	< 0.0005
Thorax circumference, cm[b]	30.0 ± 1.7 (24.2–36.0)	29.7 ± 1.7 (24.2–35.8)	4.249	< 0.05
Fetal age, weeks[c]	39.4	39.4	0	N.S.

[a]Mean ± S.D. (minimum–maximum values).
[b]Data for 202 males and 223 females only.
[c]Data for 416 infants only.

Table 6.2
Anthropometric Measurements of Eight Liveborn Twins, 1964–1972

Pair	Case numbers	Sex	Weight, g	Pair weight, g	Length, cm	Head circum- ference, cm	Thorax circum- ference, cm
1	124	M	2,657		47.4	33.0	30.4
	125	M	2,711	5,368	47.3	32.8	30.7
2	285	M	1,054		*	*	*
	286	M	783	1,837	*	*	*
3	302	F	1,749		40.1	29.0	26.3
	303	F	1,942	3,691	41.3	30.5	27.8
5	327	F	1,749		40.3	28.9	25.8
	328	M	1,600	3,349	41.0	29.4	24.3
4[a]	498	F	3,459		49.0	35.7	*
	499	F	3,106	6,565	48.5	34.9	*
Mean[b]			1,780		42.9	30.6	27.5
(S.D.)			(677)		(3.5)	(1.9)	(2.6)

[a]Measurements correspond to third week of life.
[b]Excluding pair 4.
*No measurements made.

greater than for females. Measurements of four sets of liveborn twins are given in table 6.2.

In general, infants were small compared with Guatemalan newborns from urban upper and from middle classes (Hurtado, 1962) and rural lowland ladino areas (Lechtig et al., 1972a; 1972c) although the latter differences were smaller. Similarly, the distribution of newborns by weight at intervals of 500 grams (WHO, 1961) shows a pattern distinct from that of industrial nations. The average birth weight for males and females was just above the 2,501 grams established arbitrarily to distinguish premature or low birth weight babies from normal newborns in technically advanced societies (WHO, 1950). While many village infants had weights below 2000 grams (7.6 percent) and practically none were of more than 3,500 grams (0.49 percent), in the United States the corresponding figures are 2.8 percent and 35.7 percent, respectively (US DHEW, 1972c).

The fixed biological behavior of the host population in Santa María Cauqué and the continued status quo of factors determining or influencing fetal growth are further evidenced by the remarkable uniformity in newborn size throughout the span of eight years, graphically illustrated in table 6.3. The important point here, once again, is that through effective field work a sizable portion of the newborn population can be measured adequately at birth, a consideration of importance in assessing the general health of a population even in rural and underprivileged areas of developing nations.

Table 6.3
Anthropometry of Single Birth Newborns by Study Year, 1964-1972

	Live born infants	Weight, g	Length, cm	Head circumference, cm	Thorax circumference, cm
1964	37	2,595 (360)[a] (1,510-3,313)	46.5 (2.2) (39.5-50.0)	32.4 (1.5) (28.4-34.9)	30.8 (1.8) (25.5-36.0)
1965	45	2,573 (376) (1,635-3,267)	46.4 (2.2) (39.0-51.0)	32.3 (1.4) (29.0-36.4)	29.8 (1.4) (29.0-36.4)
1966	46	2,506 (321) (1,344-3,135)	45.4 (1.9) (38.8-48.6)	31.9 (1.3) (27.9-34.9)	30.0 (1.7) (25.0-35.8)
1967	59	2,580 (389) (1,710-3,374)	45.7 (2.1) (39.8-50.2)	32.0 (1.3) (28.0-34.8)	29.9 (1.7) (25.7-33.6)
1968	57	2,510 (422) (1,357-3,903)	45.2 (2.2) (37.4-49.3)	31.8 (1.5) (25.5-34.2)	29.9 (2.2) (24.2-37.7)
1969	53	2,526 (448) (1,194-3,387)	45.1 (2.5) (37.8-49.6)	32.0 (1.9) (24.8-34.6)	29.8 (2.1) (24.3-34.2)
1970	67	2,558 (412) (1,225-3,562)	45.7 (2.1) (40.0-49.3)	32.2 (1.6) (26.4-35.6)	29.7 (1.8) (24.3-34.7)
1971	60	2,564 (328) (1,745-3,310)	45.8 (1.7) (40.2-49.8)	32.1 (1.2) (28.6-35.1)	29.7 (1.5) (26.1-32.8)
1972	6[b]	2,434 (163)	44.9 (0.6)	31.9 (1.1)	28.8 (1.2)
Total	430	2,549 (383) (1,194-3,903)	45.7 (2.2) (37.4-51.0)	32.1 (1.5) (24.8-36.4)	29.9 (1.8) (24.2-37.7)

[a]Mean (S.D.); below, (minimum-maximum values).
[b]The Cauqué study ended January 1972.

Levels and Significance of Umbilical Cord Serum Immunoglobulins

Unless the fetus is exposed to antigenic stimulation, significant synthesis of IgM and IgA does not occur, with the result that these immunoglobulins normally are not detectable at birth in significant amounts. Cases with umbilical and serum immunoglobulin levels above those in which fetal antigenic stimulation is suggested (Alford et al., 1969) were regularly observed among village newborns (Mata et al., 1972b; Lechtig and Mata, 1971) and deviated materially from the values characteristic of newborns in industrialized nations (Lechtig and Mata, 1971; Alford et al., 1969; Stiehm and Fudenberg, 1966; Stiehm, 1975). After the immunoglobulin levels of infants in the study are detailed, their relation to birth weight, gestational age, and congenital infection will be analyzed.

Of cord blood specimens from 401 deliveries collected during the study, 336 proved satisfactory for investigation after discarding specimens where calculation of IgM/IgA ratios indicated possible admixture with maternal blood (Lechtig and Mata, 1971) due to the inherent difficulty in collecting cord blood, particularly by untrained midwives. When the more stringent criterion was observed of eliminating specimens with an IgA concentration

Table 6.4
Immunoglobulin Concentrations in Umbilical Cord Serum (mg/ml), 250 Cases, 1964-1972

	Minimum	Maximum	Mean (S.D.)	Elevated levels (mg/ml)[a]
IgM	0.025	0.850	0.217 (0.147)	101 (40.4)
IgA[b]	0.035	0.090	0.036 (0.008)	
IgG	6.30	28.80	13.72 (4.07)	66 (26.4)

[a] IgM $\geqslant$ 0.20; IgG $\geqslant$ 15.00.
[b] By definition, all cases with IgA $\geqslant$ 0.10 mg/ml were not tabulated.

greater than or equal to 0.10 mg/ml, only 250 serums remained, and the description that follows is based on these 250 samples. By excluding cases with IgA greater than or equal to 0.10 mg/ml, some nonmixed specimens with truly elevated IgA may have been missed. On the other hand, probably none of the 250 cord serums had an admixture of more than 4 percent of maternal blood. Even in that event, the contribution of maternal IgM to the cord serum specimen would not have been greater than 0.20 mg/ml, the value arbitrarily accepted in discrimination of infants with fetal antigenic stimulation. The practice followed here is based on the known values of maternal serum immunoglobulins in village women.

The mean concentration of the three immunoglobulin classes IgM, IgA, and IgG in cord serum is shown in table 6.4; the distributions of IgG and IgM are indicated in table 6.5. A high proportion of infants (26 percent) had concentrations of IgG greater than 15 mg/ml. Eight percent of infants exhibited exceptionally high levels of 20 mg/ml or greater. This is the result of the considerably higher IgG values observed in adult women of the village (Cáceres and Mata, 1974) which in turn is related to intense antigenic stimulation to which the host is subjected in that environment.

The distribution of IgM seems to indicate that two populations of infants can be distinguished by this variable: one a large number of cases with low IgM values and another having a wide range of IgM values, many of them considerably elevated. Although 60 percent of infants had IgM levels below 0.20 mg/ml, the remainder had IgM concentrations indicative of fetal antigenic stimulation (Alford et al., 1969) and suggestive of prenatal experience with infectious agents. Possible explanations are that IgM was synthesized as a result of stimulation with allotypic antigens; this is unlikely, however, in view of the homogeneity of the population and the high rate of endogamy. It could also result from placental leaks, a possibility presumably excluded by the high incidence of elevated IgM demonstrated in another ongoing prospective study in four lowland Guatemalan villages that employed venous blood

Table 6.5
IgM and IgC Concentrations in Umbilical Cord Serums, by Number and Percentage of
250 Cases, 1964-1971

IgM		IgG	
mg/ml	Number of cases (percentage)	mg/ml	Number of cases (percentage)
< 0.20	149 (59.6)	< 9	36 (14.4)
0.20-0.39	76 (30.4)	10-14	148 (59.2)
0.40-0.59	16 (6.4)	15-19	46 (18.4)
0.60-0.79	7 (2 8)	20-24	16 (6.4)
0.80-0.99	2 (0.8)	25-29	4 (1 6)

Table 6.6
Mean Concentration of Immunoglobulins IgM and IgG, by Birth Weight, 250 Cases,
1964-1972

Birth weight, g	Number of cases	IgM Mean ± S.E.	IgG Mean ± S.E.
< 2,001	18	0.192 ± 0.042	11.12 ± 0.98
2,001-2,500	82	0.218 ± 0.017	13.48 ± 0.37
2,501-3,000	123	0.217 ± 0.012	14.20 ± 0.38
3,001-3,500	27	0.232 ± 0.027	14.02 ± 0.86
F		0.279	3.234
d.f.		3,246	3,246
P		> .05	< .05

from the infant drawn shortly after birth. The most likely explanation is synthesis of fetal IgM in response to antigens or antibodies produced during maternal infection and released into the fetal circulation; evidence for this possibility has been obtained in American women (Stiehm and Fudenberg, 1966). A second possibility is antibody response to microbial replication in fetal tissues and membranes, a situation that sometimes occurs in village cases, although infrequently. A third possibility is that IgM passes the placental barrier more often than traditionally accepted (Gitlin et al., 1964), especially in the presence of placental abnormalities resulting from deficient maternal health and malnutrition, a common finding in various studies (Laga et al., 1972).

In view of the elevated levels of IgC and IgM among village infants, the mean concentrations of IgM and IgG versus birth weight and gestational age were then compared to determine any relationships. Although IgM showed a

Table 6.7
Mean Concentration of Immunoglobulins IgM and IgG, by Gestational Age, 244 Cases,
1964–1972

Gestational age, weeks	Number of cases	IgM Mean ± S.E.	IgG Mean ± S.E.
31–32	2	0.240 ± 0.047	7.33 ± 0.48
33–34	5	0.125 ± 0.031	11.37 ± 1.41
35–36	11	0.316 ± 0.067	11.73 ± 1.37
37–38	31	0.228 ± 0.031	12.51 ± 0.50
39–40	154	0.215 ± 0.011	13.91 ± 0.32
41–42	41	0.211 ± 0.022	14.64 ± 0.68
F		1.442	3.016
d.f.		5,238	5,238
P		> .05	< .01

poor correlation with these child variables, that of IgG was pronounced. This immunoglobulin gradually passes from the maternal to the fetal circulation; for full-term fetuses IgG reaches a level comparable to that of the mother by the end of pregnancy. An analysis of variance of concentrations of IgG versus birth weight and gestational age revealed a significant positive correlation with birth weight and even better with gestational age (tables 6.6 and 6.7). Mean IgG concentrations increased with birth weight up to 3,000 grams and with gestational age with increasing values, up to 42 weeks of gestation. With cases with 0.10 mg/ml IgA or more excluded, the correlation coefficient for IgG improved from 0.07 to 0.19 with birth weight and from 0.13 to 0.21 with gestational age.

For IgM the analysis showed no association, although the highest values of IgM were noted in infants born at 35 to 36 weeks of gestation.

If the concentration of IgG, and to a lesser extent that of IgM, is related to gestational age and birth weight, differences should be encountered among the various categories of newborn infants. Table 6.8 shows the computed averages of IgM and IgG for five groups of infants. The mean and the range of values of IgM were similar in all groups. But the three infants classed as pre-term, moderate LBW, exhibited high concentrations of this immunoglobulin. For IgG, a definite trend was noted in its mean concentration with the lowest values those of preterm, severe LBW infants, and the greatest values in the term newborns.

Thus, for IgG, gestational age is a variable with greater predictive value than birth weight. One practical derivation is that preterm infants, having a lower level of maternal antibody, will have a shorter passive immunity. As the proportion of preterm babies is greater in developing countries than in industrial nations, more infants are thereby handicapped.

Table 6.8
Mean Concentration of Immunoglobulin, by Fetal Maturity, 243 Cases, 1964–1972

Class	Number of infants	Birth weight, g	Gestational age, weeks	IgM mg/ml	IgG mg/ml
Preterm, severe LBW	14	1,640 (240)[a] (1,194–1,930)	34.0 (1.5) (31–36)	0.218 (0.195) (0.025–0.850)	10.83 (4.53) (6.30–23.00)
Preterm, moderate LBW	3	2,187 (42) (2,141–2,223)	36.0 (0)	0.446 (0.097) (0.340–0.530)	12.90 (0.81) (12.20–13.80)
Term, small-for-gestational age	81	2,305 (144) (1,900–2,490)	39.3 (1.1) (37–42)	0.207 (0.150) (0.025–0.840)	13.39 (3.36) (7.36–25.00)
Term, moderate bw	118	2,724 (135) (2,504–2,992)	40.0 (0.9) (38–42)	0.218 (0.139) (0.025–0.800)	14.13 (4.24) (7.40–28.80)
Term, high bw	27	3,144 (109) (3,003–3,374)	39.9 (0.8) (38–42)	0.232 (0.143) (0.025–0.660)	14.02 (4.48) (9.30–26.00)

[a]Mean (S.D.); below, (minimum-maximum values).

The great frequency of fetal antigenic stimulation is good reason to suspect that congenital infections may occur at a greater frequency among village newborns than in industrial societies. To explore this possibility, all cord serums with an IgM/IgA ratio greater than 1.5 were tested for antibodies to syphilis, cytomegaloviruses, and *Toxoplasma* (table 6.9). The proportion of infants with IgM antibodies to herpesviruses and *Toxoplasma* was high. The infants positive to *Toxoplasma* had specific IgM at serum dilutions of 1:2 or 1:4. No infants with reagin were detected due in large part to the fact that incidence of syphilis among Indians in highland villages is remarkably low.

Isolation of viruses from feces collected within the first two days of life provided further evidence of congenital infection (table 6.10). The agents isolated were primarily echoviruses and were present in meconium or feces in concentrations as high as 10^5 $TCID_{50}$ per gram, in itself evidence that they might have replicated in the host. Based on the shortest incubation periods for a congenital infection, agents recovered within 48 hours after birth most probably are acquired before birth (Monif, 1969). (It should be noted, however, that poliovirus shedding has been recorded 24 hours after administration of live virus [Gelfand et al., 1959].) One infant infected with echovirus 6 died of acute respiratory infection 20 days after birth.

Concentrations of immunoglobulin in cord blood of infants with suspected intrauterine infection are also indicated in table 6.10. Six of the 12 patients had IgA above the stipulated threshold level ($\geqslant 0.10$ mg/ml). The IgM/IgA ratio, however, was always greater than 1.5, suggesting that these cases truly represented antenatal infections. The estimated rate of presumed congenital infection was at least 4 percent, and diagnosed infections all involved different infants. This figure, moreover, is probably an underestimate of the actual occurrence of intrauterine infection for the following reasons:

Table 6.9
Serological Evidence of Antigenic Fetal Stimulation with Certain Infectious Agents, 303 Infants, 1964–1971

Agent	Serologic test	Number positive (percentage)
Herpesviruses	IgM-IFA[a]	5 (1.7)
Treponema pallidum	FTA-ABS[b]	0
Toxoplasma gondii	IgM-IFA	4 (1.3)
Total		9 (3.0)

[a]Indirect fluorescent antibody in IgM. The antigen used was cytomegalovirus AD169.
[b]Fluorescent treponemal antibody, absorbed.

(a) not all infants could be examined for congenital infection; (b) only cord serum and feces were examined; sampling of throat and urine conceivably could have revealed more agents; (c) collection of meconium and feces from small newborns is difficult and could not be accomplished in many cases; and (d) testing of umbilical cord serum serologically is restricted to a few selected agents, although at least 14 viruses, 30 bacteria, and several parasites and mycoplasmas have the capacity to invade, replicate, and elicit the fetal immune response (Monif, 1969; Davies, 1971; Eichenwald, 1966; Ciba Fnd., 1973; Mata et al., 1974a).

Low Birth Weight and Premature Delivery
While low birth weight is a worldwide problem affecting the lower socio-economic classes, it has a much greater impact in developing nations, which is not yet adequately recognized.* The implications, however, are important for public health in view of the well-recognized association of low birth weight with neonatal death (Corsa et al., 1952; Erhardt et al., 1964; Alden et al., 1972; Susser et al., 1972); impaired physical growth (Ounsted and Taylor, 1971; Lubchenco et al., 1972a); immune competence (Chandra, 1975); and intellectual performance (Lubchenco et al., 1963; Wiener et al., 1968; Goldstein 1971; Fitzhardinge and Steven, 1972; Hardy, 1973). One of the most significant contributions of the Cauqué study relates to the characterization of the newborn by birth weight and gestational age. In fact, mean birth weights in Santa María Cauqué were among the lowest recorded anywhere, considerably below those reported for industrial nations (Lin and Emanuel, 1972; Bjerkedal et al., 1973; Rosa and Turshen, 1970; Lechtig et al., 1971; Emanuel, 1972); for populations at similarly high altitudes (e.g., Denver,

* A high incidence of low birth weight infants has been reported—even for typical hospital populations—whenever a proper study has been made in developing nations (Salber, 1955; Jansen, 1962; Sarram and Saadatnejadi, 1967; Banerjee, 1969; Legg et al., 1969). In Latin America the incidence of low birth weights is exceptionally high even in the capitals of several nations (Coronel et al., 1968; Luna-Jaspe et al., 1969; Jurado-García et al., 1970).

Table 6.10
Cord Serum Immunoglobulins (mg/ml) in Infants with Presumed Congenital Infection, 1964–1972

Child	Specimen	Infectious agent identified	IgM[a]	IgA	IgG	IgM/IgA[b]
66	feces, 01[c]	echovirus 6, 10^3 [d]	0.56	0.04	25.00	14.0[e]
70	feces, 01	echovirus 6, 10^3	0.26	0.04	16.00	6.5
81	feces, 01	ev[f] 10^5	0.14	0.11	9.75	
82	feces, 01	echovirus 6, 10^3	0.13	0.04	10.60	3.3
166	feces, 01	poliovirus 1, 10^5	0.03	0.04	12.70	
171	feces, 01	echovirus 11, 10^4	0.03	0.04	12.20	
264	feces, 00	echovirus 7, 10^2	0.34	0.19	14.40	1.8
26	cord serum	herpesvirus[g]	0.18	0.03	13.30	6.0
117	cord serum	*Toxoplasma*	0.65	0.18	16.00	3.6
220	cord serum	*Toxoplasma*	2.30	1.10	10.70	2.1
231	cord serum	*Toxoplasma*	3.20	0.87	12.40	3.7
300	cord serum	*Toxoplasma*	2.80	1.70	12.80	1.7

[a]Values assumed elevated are (in mg/ml): IgM $\geqslant$ 0.20; IgA $\geqslant$ 0.10; IgG $\geqslant$ 15.00.
[b]IgM/IgA ratios less than 1.5 were not tabulated.
[c]00 = collected on day of birth; 01 = collected on second day of life.
[d]Virus titer, $\log_{10}$ $TCID_{50}$ per gram of feces or meconium.
[e]Died at 20 days of age. The remaining survived the first year of life.
[f]ev = enterovirus, not identified.
[g]Antigen used was CMV AD169.

Table 6.11
416 Liveborn Singletons, by Birth Weight and Gestational Age, 1964–1972

Birth Weight, g	Gestational age in weeks					
	31–32	33–34	35–36	37–38	39–40	41–42
1,001–1,500	1[a] .24	1 .24	3 .72	0	0	0
1,501–2,000	2 .48	7 1.68	10 2.40	1 .24	6 1.44	1 .24
2,001–2,500	0	0	6 1.44	31 7.45	86 20.68	18 4.32
2,501–3,000	0	0	1 .24	12 2.88	139 33.42	48 11.54
3,001–3,500	0	0	0	3 .72	29 6.97	9 2.16
$\geqslant$ 3,501	0	0	0	0	1 .24	1 .24

[a]Number of infants; below, percentage of total sample.

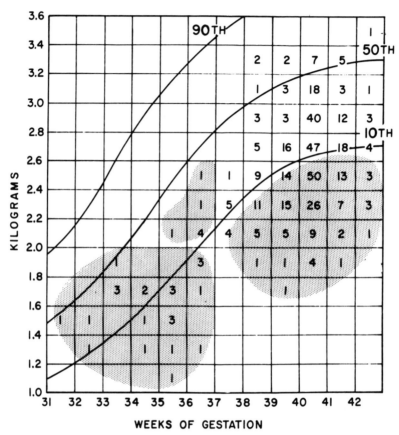

Figure 6.1
Distribution of birth weight values, 430 single live births. Numbers represent cases within each compartment.

Table 6.12
Birth Weight and Gestational Age, 415 Liveborn Singleton Infants, 1964–1972

	Abbreviation	Number of infants (percentage)	Birth weight range, g	Gestational age range, weeks
Term-high bw	Th	43 (10.3)	> 3,000	37–42
Term-moderate bw	Tm	199 (47.8)	2,501–3,000	37–42
Term-small-for-gestational age	TSGA	143 (34.4)	< 2,501	37–42
Preterm-moderate LBW	Pm	6 (1.4)	2,001–2,500	35–36
Preterm-severe LBW	Ps	24 (5.8)	< 2,001	31–36

Colorado [Lubchenco et al., 1966]), or for those with similar ethnic and genetic characteristics (e.g., North American Indians [Adams and Niswander, 1973]). Likewise, rates for premature delivery were higher than the usual levels in industrial countries. Indeed, Cauqué infants were born preterm and at low birth weights at rates comparable to those of the most stressful environmental conditions, for example, those prevalent during the siege of Leningrad (Antonov, 1947).

The distribution of 416 Cauqué infants for whom information was complete by birth weight and gestational age is seen in figure 6.1 and in table 6.11. The grouping of newborns in table 6.11 was obtained by computer. The curves in figure 6.1 correspond to the 10th, 50th, and 90th percentiles of Denver infants (Lubchenco et al., 1966), a comparison that is important in view of the biological significance of characterizing infants by criteria of birth weight and gestational age (Yerushalmy, 1967; Lubchenco, 1970). The Denver data were chosen for comparison with those of the Cauqué population because the two areas are at a similar altitude, differing only by about 1,000 feet. Data in table 6.11 show that the two variables are well correlated, with a significant number of infants with adequate gestational age exhibiting marked deficits in weight, and thus having experienced fetal growth retardation. For instance, 19 infants with 41 weeks of gestation weighed less than 2,501 grams. Only 243 (58.4 percent) newborns weighed more than 2,500 grams, of whom 1 (0.24 percent) had less than 37 weeks of gestation.

Most of the babies with adequate birth weight and gestational age fell within the 10th and 50th percentiles of the Denver grid; they will be referred to as term-with-adequate-weight for their gestational age (TAGA). Among them, 43 (10.3 percent) had birth weights of 3,001 grams or more and were arbitrarily designated term-high birth weight (Th), while 199 (47.8 percent), whose birth weights were 2,501 to 3,000 grams, were designated term-moderate birth weight (Tm) (table 6.12). No post-term infants were observed; only 16 (3.9 percent) of the total had 42 weeks gestational age, the heaviest of whom weighed 3,562 grams. There also were 143 (34.3 percent) term

Table 6.13
Incidence of Low-Birth-Weight Infants, Live Single Births, by Year, 1964–1972

	Total infants		Infants < 2,501 g[a]	Infants < 37 weeks
	with known birth weight	with known gestational age		
1964	37	36	13 (35)[b]	4 (11)
1965	45	42	19 (42)	4 (10)
1966	46	44	21 (46)	1 (3)
1967	59	55	24 (41)	4 (7)
1968	57	56	25 (44)	5 (9)
1969	53	53	20 (38)	5 (9)
1970	67	66	24 (36)	5 (8)
1971	60	58	29 (48)	3 (5)
Total	424	410	175 (41.3)	31 (7.5)

[a]All except one infant was of less than 37 weeks of gestation.
[b]Number of cases (percentage).

infants with low birth weight, here referred to as term-small-for-gestational age (TSGA).

Among the preterm infants with low birth weight, six (1.44 percent) had moderately low birth weight (2,001 to 2,500 grams) adequate for their gestational age (35 to 36 weeks gestation); they were arbitrarily designated preterm moderate birth weight (Pm). Twenty-four infants (5.8 percent) had exceptionally low (severe) birth weight (Ps). Incidence of low birth weight infants was strongly consistent throughout the study (table 6.13); that of preterm babies was less so, mainly because of the relatively small numbers involved, although a diverse causality with cyclic manifestation cannot be ignored.

Chapter 7
Maternal Factors and Fetal Growth

Although the Cauqué study did not specifically define the investigation of factors related to fetal growth in the Indian village as a primary objective, accumulated data permitted the exploration of a number of these influences. While a variety of indices have been employed to measure the adequacy of fetal growth, gestational age and birth weight were found to be the most useful indicators. Birth weight and gestational age are more readily assessed than rates of abortion, stillbirth, and congenital defects. They permit a useful characterization of the newborn. As a whole, and regardless of any particularly abnormal behavior related to congenital infection, an inborn error of metabolism, or other type of defect, a birth weight of 2,501 grams or more is considered adequate, provided gestation is between 37 and 42 weeks.

This chapter correlates maternal environment with fetal growth and development as assessed by birth weight and gestational age. The definitions are those of chapters 5 and 6. Maternal health is used throughout the text to imply a state of health in the mother that leads to optimal fetal growth and development. While most workers usually employ the expression "maternal nutritional status" or "maternal nutrition" to mean that state resulting from consumption of an adequate diet, the term "maternal health" possesses a broader biological meaning, especially for developing societies where many factors other than diet affect maternal nutritional status and fetal growth.

Data were analyzed by parametric or nonparametric methods, both when indicated. Correlations between maternal and infant variables were calculated to illustrate significant associations between birth weight and maternal variables (table 7.1).

Table 7.1
Correlation Matrix for Selected Maternal and Newborn Variables, 325 Mother-Infant Pairs, 1964–1972

	Sex of newborn	Maternal height	Maternal weight	Maternal age	Birth interval	Birth order	Duration of pregnancy	Socioeconomic index
Birth weight	-0.120[a]	0.230[b]	0.260[b]	0.117[a]	0.163[b]	0.177[b]	0.567[b]	0.150[a]
Birth length	-0.318[b]	0.166[b]	0.224[b]	-0.161[b]	-0.194[b]	-0.053	0.706[b]	0.127[a]
Birth head circumference	-0.384[b]	0.100	0.210[b]	-0.141[a]	-0.238[b]	-0.025	0.634[b]	0.160[b]
Sex of newborn		0.052	-0.037	0.045	0.014	0.045	0.004	0.031
Maternal height			0.520[b]	-0.034	0.056	0.033	0.086	0.084
Maternal weight				0.138[a]	0.115[a]	0.040	0.152[b]	0.071
Maternal age					0.527[b]	0.900[b]	0.114[a]	0.139[a]
Birth interval						0.470[b]	0.104	0.055
Birth order							0.119[a]	0.164[b]
Duration of pregnancy								0.121[a]

[a] $p < 0.05$.
[b] $p < 0.01$.

Maternal Size

To test a relation between size of the mother and that of the infant, four groups of maternal and infant values were constituted according to distribution of the variables around the mean. The mean plus and minus one standard deviation defined two intermediate groups; the other two groups included individuals falling outside those values or the largest and smallest subjects, respectively.

Maternal and infant weight proved positively correlated, that is to say, the greater the midpregnancy weight the larger the weight of the newborn (table 7.2). Since maternal midpregnancy weight is assumed to be influenced by background health and nutrition of the mother and her capacity to gain weight during pregnancy, a further comparison of infant's weight was made with maternal height, a wholly stable variable during pregnancy (table 7.2). Maternal height correlated with birth weight; as a group, taller women delivered heavier infants. This leads to an expectation that rates for low birth weight infants should be less among women of large size. Table 7.3 clearly

Table 7.2
Comparisons Between Maternal Height and Weight and Infant Weight, by Number and Percentage, 1964-1972

Birth weight, g	Maternal weight, kg[a]				
	< 47.01	47.01–52.82	52.83–58.64	> 58.64	Total
$< 2,166$	9[b] (2.6)	18 (5.2)	9 (2.6)	2 (0.6)	38 (11.0)
2,166–2,548	24 (7.0)	50 (14.5)	32 (9.3)	15 (4.4)	121 (35.2)
2,549–2,932	16 (4.7)	53 (15.4)	43 (12.5)	23 (6.7)	135 (39.2)
$> 2,932$	1 (0.3)	20 (5.8)	12 (3.5)	17 (4.9)	50 (14.5)
Total	50 (14.5)	141 (41.0)	96 (27.9)	57 (16.6)	344 (100)

Birth weight, g	Maternal height, cm[c]				
	< 138	138–142	143–147	>147	Total
$< 2,166$	9[d] (2.2)	13 (3.2)	21 (5.2)	8 (2.0)	51 (12.7)
2,166–2,548	13 (3.2)	62 (15.4)	52 (12.9)	12 (3.0)	139 (34.6)
2,549–2,932	12 (3.0)	48 (11.9)	76 (18.9)	19 (4.7)	155 (38.6)
$> 2,932$	2 (0.5)	12 (3.0)	27 (6.7)	16 (4.0)	57 (14.2)
Total	36 (9.0)	135 (33.6)	176 (43.8)	55 (13.7)	402 (100)

[a]Chi square (9 d.f.) = 25.842; P < 0.005.
[b]Number in 344 pairs (percentage).
[c]Chi square (9 d.f.) = 29.578; P < 0.001.
[d]Number in 402 pairs (percentage).

shows this to be so; only 21 percent of infants born to women weighing more than 59 kilograms (130 pounds) were of low birth weight, whereas the proportion for women of less than 47 kilograms (104 pounds) was 56 percent, a significant difference. Likewise, the frequency of low birth weight infants differed with maternal height in that taller women, as a group, delivered fewer low birth weight babies.

Table 7.4 shows the frequency of preterm infants as a function of maternal weight and height. Mothers were grouped according to their distribution around the mean, as described earlier. While 14 percent of infants born to women of less than 47 kilograms were preterm, only 2 percent were preterm among those born to women who weighed 59 kilograms or more, a significant difference. Although the combination of maternal height and inci-

Table 7.3
Incidence of Low Birth Weight Infants by Maternal Weight and Height, by Number and
Percentage of Total Cases, 1964–1972

| Birth weight, g | Maternal weight, kg[a] | | | | |
	< 47.01	47.01– 52.82	52.83– 58.64	> 58.64	Total
< 2,501	28[b] (56.0)	63 (44.7)	36 (37.5)	12 (21.1)	139 (40.4)
≥ 2,501	22 (44.0)	78 (55.3)	60 (62.5)	45 (78.9)	205 (59.6)
Total	50	141	96	57	344

| Birth weight, g | Maternal height, cm[c] | | | | |
	< 138	138– 142	143– 147	> 147	Total
< 2,501	21[b] (58.3)	66 (48.9)	64 (36.4)	15 (27.3)	166 (41.3)
≥ 2,501	15 (41.7)	69 (51.1)	112 (63.6)	40 (72.7)	236 (58.7)
Total	36	135	176	55	402

[a]Chi square (3 d.f.) = 15.32; $P < 0.005$.
[b]Number of cases (percentage).
[c]Chi square (3 d.f.) = 13.7; $P < 0.005$.

Table 7.4
Incidence of Preterm Infants by Maternal Weight and Height, by Number and Percentage
of Total Cases, 1964–1972

| Gestational age, weeks | Maternal weight, kg[a] | | | | |
	< 47.01	47.01– 52.82	52.83– 58.64	>58.64	Total
< 37	7[b] (14.0)	13 (9.2)	3 (3.1)	1 (1.8)	24 (7.0)
≥ 37	43 (86.0)	128 (90.8)	93 (96.9)	55 (98.2)	319 (93.0)
Total	50	141	96	56	343

| Gestational age, weeks | Maternal height, cm[c] | | | | |
	< 138	138– 142	143– 147	> 147	Total
< 37	6[b] (16.7)	6 (4.4)	14 (8.2)	3 (5.6)	29 (7.3)
≥ 37	30 (83.3)	129 (95.6)	156 (91.8)	51 (94.4)	366 (92.7)
Total	36	135	170	54	395

[a]Chi square (3 d.f.) = 9.38; $P < 0.025$.
[b]Number of cases (percentage).
[c]Chi square (3 d.f.) = 6.72; $P < 0.1$

Table 7.5
Incidence of Low Birth Weight Infants by Birth Order, 1964-1972

Birth order	Number of infants	Birth weight, g	
		< 2,501	≥ 2,501
0-2	129	53[a]	47[a]
3-5	140	43	57
6-8	105	32	68
9-11	49	33	67
≥ 12	7	0	100
Total	430	42	58

Note: Chi square (4 d.f.) = 17.86; $P < 0.005$.
[a]Percentage.

Table 7.6
Birth Weight, Gestational Age, and
Spontaneous Rupture of Membranes,
1964-1972

Time, hours	Birth weight, g	Gestational age, weeks
< 4	2,558 ± 18[a] (395)	39.49 ± .08 (382)
≥ 4	2,353 ± 79 (27)	38.46 ± .56 (26)
F	7.566	8.826
d.f.	1,420	1,406
P	< 0.01	< 0.01

[a]Mean ± S.E.; below, (number of cases).

dence of premature delivery showed a similar trend, the association lacked significance. The variability of gestational age across maternal weight and height, however, was more striking than that of birth weight. The above analysis suggests that the health and nutritional status of the mother, as expressed by her height and weight, influences gestational age and birth weight of the infant.

Obstetrical Characteristics and Maternal Experience
Although the extent of previous obstetrical experience is a factor in the outcome of a pregnancy, how the various factors operate and, particularly, how they influence birth weight and premature delivery nevertheless remain unclear. Rates for low birth weight infants decreased with increasing parity or the number of preceding pregnancies terminating in delivery ($P < 0.01$) and even more according to birth order, as shown in table 7.5. Obstetrical experience also appears to decrease the risk of low birth weight; while 53 per-

Table 7.7
Infant Characteristics by Birth Interval, 1964–1972

Birth interval, months	Birth weight, g	Birth length, cm	Gestational age, weeks
9–17	2,376 ± 87[a] (34)	45.0 ± 0.5 (31)	38.5 ± 0.4 (32)
18–26	2,561 ± 32 (120)	45.8 ± 0.2 (119)	39.6 ± 0.1 (117)
27–35	2,623 ± 34 (123)	45.9 ± 0.2 (123)	39.6 ± 0.1 (117)
36–44	2,593 ± 43 (51)	46.0 ± 0.3 (50)	39.8 ± 0.2 (49)
⩾ 45	2,629 ± 68 (32)	46.0 ± 0.4 (32)	39.4 ± 0.3 (32)
F	3.150	1.230	3.312
d.f.	4,355	4,350	4,342
P	< 0.05	> 0.05	< 0.05

[a]Mean ± S.E.; below, (number of cases).

cent of infants born to women of parity 2 or less were of low birth weight, only 32 percent were of low birth weight when parity was 6 to 11, and none when parity was 12 or more.

One variable definitely related to the outcome of pregnancy is the time at which the membranes rupture, relative to time of birth. As indicated in chapter 5, neither village midwives nor mothers acted to induce or precipitate membrane rupture. An analysis of variance in test of variability of birth weight and gestational age according to time of rupture of membranes showed that birth weight is less and gestational age shorter with prolonged rupture ($P < 0.01$). As would be expected, premature delivery was significantly more frequent ($P < 0.02$) in childbirth when membrane rupture occurred after 4 hours or more (table 7.6). Another obstetrical factor relating to outcome of pregnancy is the presentation of the fetus at delivery. Breech presentation and congenital malformations, both known to be associated with increased neonatal mortality, were not particularly prominent in the village and indeed were less frequent than in many industrialized nations. The reasons for the low frequency of breech presentations among the Indian population are unknown.

Birth Interval
A prolonged interval between deliveries should favor the outcome of a pregnancy on the assumption that the mother is then in a better state of health due to the added time available to replenish her nutrient stores for the new pregnancy. Birth intervals, arbitrarily subdivided into periods of nine months,

Table 7.8
Incidence of Preterm Infants, by Length of Birth Interval and Number and Percentage of Cases, 1964–1972

Gestational age, weeks	Number of cases	Birth interval, months		Chi Square	P
		9–17	18+		
< 37	24	8 (25)[a]	16 (5)		
⩾ 37	323	24 (75)	299 (95)	17.90	< 0.001
Total	347	32	315		

[a]Number of cases (percentage).

correlated directly with birth weight and gestational age (table 7.7). Birth length apparently is little affected, this variable being dependent more on maternal height than on maternal weight gain.

Shorter intervals between births consistently correlated with poor fetal growth, suggesting a deteriorated health and nutritional status of the mother as a consequence of closely spaced pregnancies and the added drain of continued breast-feeding. A birth interval of 9 to 17 months was associated with the lowest values for birth weight and length. Longer birth intervals, on the average, correlated with both higher birth weight and longer gestational age. Likewise, with birth intervals of 9 to 17 months the frequency of preterm and low birth weight infants was greater than with intervals of 18 months or more (table 7.8). Again, the shorter the interval, the more severe was the expected deterioration in nutritional status. The situation was aggravated by poor diet, frequent infection during pregnancy, and particularly by the background of poor health consistently prevalent in this population and dating from early childhood (Mata et al., 1971c).

The association of fetal growth with birth interval is not independent of maternal age since birth interval and maternal age, in turn, are highly correlated (r = 0.3719, 361 d.f., P < 0.001). In other words, longer spacing between deliveries increases with maternal age, an observation that has implications for family planning.

Diet during Pregnancy
In recent years the role of diet during pregnancy has received increasing attention (Rosa and Turshen, 1970; NAS, 1970; Bergner and Susser, 1970; Lechtig et al., 1971), largely because findings are by no means conclusive. Recent field interventions providing an improved diet in pregnancy have, for example, demonstrated a beneficial effect on fetal growth (Lechtig et al., 1972a; Blackwell et al., 1973), but such studies were conducted among populations where mean birth weights were already substantially satisfactory before the intervention began, averaging 3,000 grams, a consideration of note

Table 7.9
Newborn Size as a Function of Daily Consumption of Calories and Total Protein During
Pregnancy, 1964–1972

	Calories		Total Protein, g	
	< 2,400	2,400+	< 60	60+
Birth weight, g	2,521 ± 46[a] (37)	2,632 ± 116 (11)	2,536 ± 53 (23)	2,556 ± 71 (25)
	F = 2.213 P > 0.05		F = 0.053 P > 0.05	
Birth length, cm	45.6 ± 0.2 (37)	46.8 ± 0.4 (11)	45.5 ± 0.3 (23)	46.2 ± 0.3 (25)
	F = 6.038 P < 0.05		F = 2.213 P > 0.05	

[a]Mean ± S.E.; below, (number of cases).

in view of the relatively short stature of the women concerned in those studies. What needs demonstration is that an adequate diet during pregnancy definitely improves fetal growth in an area like Santa María Cauqué, where 40 percent of infants are of consistently low birth weight and are born to mothers of short stature.

With 47 women in the Cauqué study whose diet was investigated in pregnancy, significant correlation coefficients were observed between birth weight and the mother's consumption of animal protein ($r = 0.280$); and between birth length and intake of calories ($r = 0.299$), fat ($r = 0.296$), riboflavin ($r = 0.280$), and niacin ($r = 0.317$). Thus, when women were grouped according to whether they consumed the recommended levels of calories and protein, the mean birth length of the newborn was greater for those mothers who met the recommendations for calories (table 7.9). No differences that were statistically significant were noted in mean birth weight but a trend was observed toward a lesser frequency of low birth weight infants among mothers on higher dietary protein and caloric regimens.

Maternal Age

While the concept that exceptionally young mothers have less capacity for successful childbearing than older ones has general acceptance, much is unknown about operative mechanisms. During the study the relation of maternal age to fetal growth was explored by analysis of variance after subdividing ages into five-year subgroups (table 7.10). Birth weight, head circumference, thorax circumference, and gestational age were increasingly greater with advancing maternal age. Birth length, however, did not show a similar result, probably due to the good correlation between newborn length and maternal height, which is independent of maternal age.

Table 7.10
Newborn Variables as a Function of Maternal Age, 1964–1972

Maternal age, years	Birth weight, g	Birth length, cm	Head circumference, cm	Thorax circumference, cm	Gestational age, weeks
< 20	2,426 ± 43[a] (89)	45.3 ± 0.3 (87)	31.7 ± 0.2 (87)	29.4 ± 0.2 (87)	38.8 ± 0.3 (86)
20–24	2,521 ± 33 (118)	45.6 ± 0.2 (117)	31.9 ± 0.1 (117)	29.8 ± 0.2 (117)	39.5 ± 0.1 (116)
25–29	2,599 ± 37 (66)	45.8 ± 0.2 (66)	32.2 ± 0.1 (66)	30.2 ± 0.2 (66)	39.7 ± 0.2 (64)
30–34	2,614 ± 40 (81)	46.1 ± 0.2 (80)	32.5 ± 0.1 (80)	30.2 ± 0.2 (80)	39.6 ± 0.2 (76)
35–39	2,605 ± 52 (53)	45.7 ± 0.3 (52)	32.4 ± 0.3 (52)	29.9 ± 0.2 (52)	39.8 ± 0.2 (52)
⩾ 40	2,631 ± 102 (23)	46.1 ± 0.5 (23)	32.2 ± 0.4 (23)	30.2 ± 0.4 (23)	39.5 ± 0.3 (22)
F	3.2528	1.3608	3.1874	2.5672	3.0306
d.f.	5,424	5,419	5,419	5,419	5,410
P	< 0.01	> 0.05	< 0.01	< 0.05	< 0.05

[a]Mean ± S.E.; below, (number of cases).

Maternal Socioeconomic Status
Women lack differentiation in height and weight according to the socio-economic index. Only maternal age correlated with the SECI, an observation interpreted as indicative of an increase in relative wealth with age. All newborn variables were greater with increasing maternal SECI, but the correlation was significant only for head and thorax circumferences (table 7.11).

Since maternal age and SECI were associated, an analysis of infant characteristics against SECI was made within each maternal age category, showing an upward trend in birth weight, birth length, and gestational age with increasing maternal socioeconomic level.

Maternal Morbidity
The relation of maternal morbidity to outcome of pregnancy was investigated by establishing the association of maternal infection with serum immunoglobulins in umbilical cord blood and with fetal size or physiological maturity. Tabulating only cases where cord serums showed low or undetectable IgA (< 0.1 mg/ml), IgM was found associated with morbidity during pregnancy (table 7.12). Although a considerable proportion of infants showed elevated IgM in the absence of maternal morbidity, those born of mothers experiencing an infectious disease during pregnancy frequently showed high IgM levels (P < 0.05).

Table 7.11
Newborn Variables as a Function of Maternal Socioeconomic Index, 1964–1972

SEC Index[a]	Birth weight, g	Birth length, cm	Head circumference, cm	Thorax circumference, cm	Gestational age, weeks
15–20	2,428 ± 66[b] (37)	45.0 ± 0.4 (37)	31.6 ± 0.3 (37)	29.2 ± 0.3 (37)	39.3 ± 0.3 (36)
21–25	2,528 ± 35 (131)	45.7 ± 0.2 (131)	32.0 ± 0.1 (131)	29.7 ± 0.2 (131)	39.2 ± 0.2 (128)
26–30	2,573 ± 26 (204)	45.8 ± 0.1 (200)	32.1 ± 0.9 (200)	30.0 ± 0.1 (200)	39.5 ± 0.1 (196)
31–35	2,622 ± 80 (29)	46.1 ± 0.4 (38)	32.6 ± 0.3 (28)	30.3 ± 0.3 (28)	39.8 ± 0.3 (27)
F	1.951	1.453	2.796	3.519	1.066
d.f.	3,397	3,392	3,392	3,392	3,383
P	> 0.05	> 0.05	< 0.05	< 0.05	> 0.05

[a]Possible minimum and maximum values are 12 and 36.
[b]Mean ± S.E.; below, (number of cases).

Table 7.12
Concentration of IgM and IgG in Cord Serum in Relation to Morbidity during Pregnancy, by Number and Percentage of 201 Live Births, 1964–1972

Morbidity	IgM, mg/ml		IgG, mg/ml	
	< 0.19	≥ 0.19	< 12	≥ 12
No illness	85 (81.0)[a]	63 (65.6)	48 (69.6)	100 (75.8)
One illness or more	20 (19.1)	33 (34.4)	21 (30.4)	32 (24.2)
Chi square		6.068		0.894
P		< 0.05		> 0.05

Note: Specimens with 0.1 mg/ml (or more) IgA were not included. Morbidity included diarrheal disease, lower respiratory tract disease, cellulitis, urinary tract infection, otitis, herpes simplex, hepatitis, nonspecific fever, tenosynovitis.
[a]Number of cases (percentage).

Table 7.13
Variables Analyzed in Single and Multiple Correlations, Newborn vs. Maternal Variables

Variable	Abbreviation
Newborn	
Sex: 1, male; 2, female	ISEX
Weight, g	BWT
Length, cm	BHT
Head circumference, cm	BHEAD
Thorax circumference, cm	BTHCIR
Mother	
Age, yr	MAGE
Number of deliveries	DELIV
Birth order	BORDER
Birth interval, months	BINTER
Duration of pregnancy, weeks[a]	DPREG
Midpregnancy weight, kg	MWT
Height, cm	MHT
Tricipital skinfold thickness, mm	SKIN
Arm circumference, cm	ARM
Leg circumference, cm	LEG
Illnesses in first trimester	ILL1
Illnesses in second trimester	ILL2
Illnesses in third trimester	ILL3
Total illnesses in pregnancy	ILLT

[a]Also, gestational age (GAGE), a newborn variable.

Infectious disease of the mother correlated with a greater probability of fetal synthesis of immunoglobulin M, in agreement with the concept that the greater the incidence of maternal infection the greater the probability for fetal infection and antigenic stimulation (Mata et al., 1974a; Mata, 1974). The opposite was noted regarding IgG, but the association did not achieve statistical significance.

Mothers with the greatest morbidity showed no tendency to deliver small infants, except when illnesses included a clinical infection of the urinary tract. The lack of association of morbidity during pregnancy with fetal growth must be interpreted with caution, however, since the Cauqué study was not designed to discover all diseases or abnormalities of pregnancy. Clinical responses of mother and fetus expectedly have great variability, making it difficult to sort out those illnesses with no effect on fetal growth in order to test for statistically pertinent associations.

Table 7.14
Step-Wise Regression Analysis for Infant Variables, 325 Cases, 1964–1972

Variable in order of entry[a]	Regression coefficient (B)	Standard error of B	F value[b]	Percentage RSQ	Δ percentage RSQ
Birth weight[c]					
(Constant = -2723.24)					
DPREG	123.17	10.33	142.09	30.7	30.7
MWT	11.51	2.87	16.11	33.9	3.2
ISEX	-95.86	32.97	8.45	35.4	1.5
ILL3	-80.81	29.04	7.74	37.0	1.6
Birth length[c]					
(Constant = 60.56)					
DPREG	7.07	0.58	146.74	29.8	29.8
ISEX	-10.41	1.87	30.89	35.6	5.8
MHT	0.93	0.21	18.14	39.0	3.4
Birth head circumference[c]					
(Constant = 113.93)					
DPREG	5.06	0.38	175.39	34.5	34.5
ISEX	-7.41	1.21	37.25	41.1	6.6
MWT	0.31	0.10	8.75	43.1	2.0
DELIV	0.56	0.20	7.21	44.4	1.3
Birth thorax circumference[c]					
(Constant = -9.13)					
DPREG	5.40	0.52	107.16	25.8	25.8
MHT	0.65	0.19	11.33	28.6	2.8
ILL3	-3.89	1.46	7.01	30.2	1.6
BINTER	0.14	0.05	6.52	31.6	1.4

[a]The other variables did not add significantly to the regression (tested at the 1 percent level).
[b]$P < 0.01$.
[c]Dependent variable.

Table 7.15
Step-Wise Regression Analysis for Infant Variables, Duration of Pregnancy Excluded,
325 Cases, 1964-1972

Variable in order of entry[a]	Regression coefficient (B)	Standard error of B	F value[b]	Percentage RSQ	Δ percentage RSQ
Birth weight[c]					
MWT	0.16	0.03	22.37	6.5	6.5
BINTER	3.46	1.31	6.98	8.5	2.0
Birth length[c]					
BORDER	3.26	0.37	77.78	9.9	9.9
MAGE	-0.08	0.01	35.05	18.4	8.4
ISEX	-9.35	2.25	17.30	22.3	3.9
MHT	1.06	0.26	16.40	26.1	3.7
Birth head circumference[c]					
ISEX	-6.90	1.51	20.81	8.0	8.0
MAGE	-0.02	0.02	2.09	12.6	4.5
MWT	0	0	13.37	15.8	3.2
BORDER	-4.02	0.59	47.18	19.5	3.6
DELIV	5.42	0.95	32.60	26.9	7.4
Birth thorax circumference[c]					
BORDER	-7.60	0.59	167.49	5.7	5.7
DELIV	8.25	0.70	136.90	33.0	27.3
MHT	0.91	0.23	16.20	36.2	3.2

[a]The other variables did not add significantly to the regression (tested at the 1 percent level).
[b]$P < 0.01$.
[c]Dependent variable.

Step-Wise Regression Analysis

Correlations were prepared for 325 pairs of mothers and infants for whom data were complete, as illustrated in table 7.1. Significant correlations coefficients were obtained when birth weight, birth length, and other variables were compared with maternal characteristics, namely, height, midpregnancy weight, leg circumference, and parity. These variables were studied in multiple step-wise regression analyses (SWRAs). Each of four infant variables (weight, length, and circumferences of head and thorax) were treated as dependent variables; SWRAs were calculated using sex of the infant and 14 maternal variables treated in turn as independent variables. Tables 7.14 and 7.15 present the results.

Among maternal variables, duration of pregnancy (gestational age), a variable highly interrelated and confounded with such other factors as maternal size, obstetric experience, maternal age, and socioeconomic status, was the best predictor of the size of newborns. As expected, gestational age accounted for most of the variability in newborn size—from 26 percent to 35 percent—depending on the particular infant dependent variable under consideration. Duration of pregnancy showed the highest predictive capacity for head circumference (34.5 percent) and the lowest for thorax circumference (25.8 percent). Other maternal variables contributing to the regression included maternal height or weight, sex of infant, illnesses in third trimester of pregnancy, birth interval, and number of previous deliveries (table 7.14). The highest percentage of the total sum of squares (percentage RSQ) explained by these regressions was 44 (for head circumference) and the lowest, 32 (for thorax circumference).

With removal of duration of pregnancy from the equation, however, maternal age, weight, and height and the obstetrical experience of the mother, as expressed by birth order and number of previous deliveries, were the most important variables (table 7.15).

The present analysis agrees with the findings of other investigators on the importance of the maternal environment in fetal growth (Giroud, 1970; Tanner and Thomson, 1970; Love and Kinch, 1965; Weiss and Jackson, 1972). Size of the mother is the major determinant, a fact repeatedly confirmed by field studies (Thomson et al., 1968). The Cauqué study demonstrated that the factors most clearly associated with fetal size are those reflecting the background health of the mother, as expressed in maternal weight and height, in bodily reserves, and in a capacity to initiate pregnancy and carry a fetus through an adequate period of gestation.

In this regard laboratory studies showed a negative intergenerational effect of deficient nutrition on the offspring of animals; successive generations of malnourished rats delivered litters of small-for-dates (Stewart, 1972). Epidemiological observations revealed a secular change in birth weights in Japan within one generation, presumably the result of improved nutrition, hygiene, and social conditions (Greenwald et al., 1967). In England maternal size is associated with improved fetal growth (Thomson et al., 1968); conceivably, the tall women of that population were the consequence of improved environmental conditions surrounding their childhood and adolescence. While a genetic contribution must be accepted in partial determination of the total newborn size variability, the differences observed between contrasting societies (i.e., Guatemalan Indian villages and industrial societies) appear to be mainly due to differences in backgrounds of nutrition and hygiene. While no definitive data exist on the size of newborns in Europe 200 years ago, records of infant mortalities then suggest that fetal growth probably resembled that of Santa María Cauqué at the present time.

The broad generalization to be drawn from this chapter, and one that would enhance the positive aspects of the maternal environment, is that an effect on the newborn's birth weight can be brought about within generations by improved living conditions. This is of great importance in planning public health action. Without considering details of logistics and feasibility, health measures of obvious value to the present situation have to do with encouragement of delayed marriage, breast-feeding, adequate spacing of children, the improved social and economic status of women, and the strengthening of antenatal care. For the long range, improvement of the nutritional status of infant, child, and adolescent will lead to a better maternal environment, improved fetal growth, and the associated better survival, growth, and development of infants through childhood and adolescence. The societal contribution is cumulative. Women affected in this way will deliver larger and healthier infants than did their mothers. A positive intergenerational effect conduces to a social level comparable to that of the more developed nations.

Chapter 8
Survival

The data in this chapter relate to the survival during infancy (first year of life) and early childhood (1 to 6 years) of annual cohorts of children recruited to the study. Except when death was unexpected, followed an unusually rapid course, or was accidental, the clinic staff had knowledge of most illnesses as they evolved. In many cases a staff member was in attendance when death occurred. Of the remainder, they had regular and prompt notification. As would be expected, traditions and inherent beliefs occasionally precluded a proper determination of cause of death. No autopsies were performed. Exceptionally, an external physical examination of a deceased child was made or occasionally a throat or rectal swab obtained. No blood could be collected from the dead. Any manipulation of a dying child potentially led to a charge of responsibility for the death. Various considerations of this nature explain a moderate incompleteness of recorded information on causes of death.

Antenatal Events and Survival
Birth weight and gestational age are expressions of antenatal events since independently or combined they represent the outcome of fetal growth. Survival among singletons was studied as function of those factors according to intervals of either 250 or 500 grams of birth weight, or at intervals of two weeks of gestational age. In computing survival the only children considered were those who lived within stipulated limits of the several survival periods and were village residents. One child, who emigrated from the village in the second half of the first year and did not return, was eliminated from all computations of survival after six months.

Table 8.1
Survival During Infancy, by Birth Weight, 430 Singletons, 1964–1973

Time survived	Number of infants	Birth weight, g									Total
		1,000–	1,500–	2,000–	2,250–	2,500–	2,750–	3,000–	3,250–	3,500–	
24 hours	430	4/5[a] (80)	25/28 (89)	47/47 (100)	99/99 (100)	125/125 (100)	82/82 (100)	31/31 (100)	11/11 (100)	2/2 (100)	426/430 (99)
7 days	430	4/5 (80)	23/28 (82)	47/47 (100)	99/99 (100)	125/125 (100)	82/82 (100)	31/31 (100)	11/11 (100)	2/2 (100)	424/430 (99)
28 days	429	2/5 (40)	22/28 (79)	45/47 (96)	96/99 (97)	123/125 (98)	82/82 (100)	30/30 (100)	11/11 (100)	2/2 (100)	413/429 (96)
3 months	429	2/5 (40)	18/28 (64)	44/47 (94)	96/99 (97)	123/125 (98)	82/82 (100)	30/30 (100)	11/11 (100)	2/2 (100)	408/429 (95)
6 months	429	1/5 (20)	15/28 (54)	43/47 (91)	96/99 (97)	120/125 (96)	80/82 (98)	30/30 (100)	11/11 (100)	2/2 (100)	398/429 (93)
1 year	428	1/5 (20)	13/28 (46)	41/47 (87)	95/99 (96)	117/124 (94)	78/82 (95)	30/30 (100)	10/11 (91)	2/2 (100)	387/428 (90)

[a]Number of survivors/total cases; below, (percentage surviving).

Table 8.2
Survival During Infancy, by Gestational Age, 416 Singletons, 1964–1973

Time survived	Number of infants	Gestational age, weeks						Total
		31–32	33–34	35–36	37–38	39–40	41–42	
24 hours	416	2/3[a] (67)	6/8 (75)	19/20 (95)	47/47 (100)	261/261 (100)	77/77 (100)	412/416 (99)
7 days	416	2/3 (67)	6/8 (75)	17/20 (85)	47/47 (100)	261/261 (100)	77/77 (100)	410/416 (99)
28 days	415	1/3 (33)	5/8 (63)	15/20 (75)	47/47 (100)	254/260 (98)	77/77 (100)	399/415 (96)
3 months	415	1/3 (33)	2/8 (25)	15/20 (75)	46/47 (98)	254/260 (98)	76/77 (99)	394/415 (95)
6 months	415	1/3 (33)	2/8 (25)	14/20 (70)	45/47 (96)	247/260 (95)	76/77 (99)	385/415 (93)
1 year	414	1/3 (33)	2/8 (25)	12/20 (60)	45/47 (96)	240/259 (93)	76/77 (99)	376/414 (91)

[a]Number of survivors/total cases; below, (percentage surviving).

Tables 8.1 and 8.2 illustrate survival during various life spans. The likelihood of death clearly relates to both birth weight and gestational age. In fact, the correlation between low birth weight and infant mortality was so striking in this study that birth weight ended up as the best practical index of fetal growth and development. Combined with gestational age (American Academy of Pediatrics, 1967; Yerushalmy, 1967; Tanner and Thomson, 1970; Lubchenco et al., 1972b), low birth weight is a reliable means to predict survival, particularly neonatal, and to a lesser extent is a measure of physical growth. A level of at least 2,000 grams was associated with survival to the first week of life, while 2,750 grams reliably predicted survival for the first three months. Only one death in postneonatal infancy was observed among those who weighed more than 3,000 grams at birth.

Gestational age also correlated with survival, but with an association not as clear-cut as for birth weight. An excess frequency of deaths among infants born at term, yet with low birth weight, is discussed later.

Infant Mortality

A comparison of infant mortality rates provides an alternate means to examine the relationship between birth weight, gestational age, and survival. Neonatal mortality in Santa María Cauqué was high (37 per 1,000 live births) mainly because of the high proportion of infants of less than 2,001 grams birth weight (table 8.3); the neonatal death rate of this group was 273 per 1,000. Risk of death among these smaller infants did not lessen significantly during the remainder of the first semester of life (242 per 1,000), but continued high in the second semester (61 per 1,000). Overall, more than half of the infants in this category died within the first year of life.

Higher birth weight clearly was correlated with lower mortality. No deaths occurred within the first year of life among 44 infants weighing more than 3,000 grams at birth, except in the case of one child of 3,253 grams who died at age 48 weeks of severe diarrheal disease and dehydration, a death that seemingly could have been avoided had the parents not refused medical assistance. The inverse correlation between birth weight and mortality is more clearly shown by examining birth weight at smaller intervals (table 8.3). This further emphasizes that the decline in mortality with increasing birth weight applies not only to the neonatal age but to the remainder of the first year of life, except that three deaths in the second half of the year were among infants who weighed more than 2,750 grams at birth.

The association of infant deaths and gestational age during the neonatal period is clear-cut; only 6 deaths occurred among 385 infants (16 deaths per 1,000) born at term (37 to 42 weeks) as compared with 10 deaths of 31 infants (323 per 1,000) born at 36 weeks or less (table 8.4). In postneonatal infancy the relationship is still important although less dramatic. The

Table 8.3
Infant Deaths by Birth Weight, 430 Singletons, 1964–1973

Birth weight, g	Number of infants	Survival period			
		Birth– 28 days	29d– 5 months	6–11 months	First year
< 1,501	5	3 (600)[a]	1 (200)	0	4 (800)
1,501–1,750	11	2 (182)	3 (273)	1 (91)	6 (545)
1,751–2,000	17	4 (235)	4 (235)	1 (59)	9 (529)
2,001–2,250	47	2 (43)	2 (43)	2 (43)	6 (128)
2,251–2,500	99	3 (30)	0	1 (10)	4 (40)
2,501–2,750	125	2 (16)	3 (24)	2 (16)	7 (56)
2,751–3,000	82	0	2 (24)	2 (24)	4 (49)
3,001–3,250	32	0	0	0	0
3,251–3,500	11	0	0	1 (91)	1 (91)
> 3,500	1	0	0	0	0
Total	430	16 (37)	15 (35)	10 (23)	41 (95)

[a]Deaths (deaths per 1,000 live births).

Table 8.4
Infant Deaths by Gestational Age, 416 Singletons, 1964–1973

Gestational age, weeks	Number of infants	Survival period			
		Birth– 28 days	29d– 5 months	6–11 months	First year
31–32	3	2 (667)[a]	0	0	2 (667)
33–34	8	3 (375)	3 (375)	0	6 (750)
35–36	20	5 (250)	1 (50)	2 (100)	8 (400)
37–38	47	0	2 (43)	0	2 (43)
39–40	261	6 (23)	7 (27)	8 (31)	21 (80)
41–42	77	0	1 (13)	0	1 (13)
Total	416	16 (38)	14 (34)	10 (24)	40 (96)

[a]Deaths (deaths per 1,000 live births).

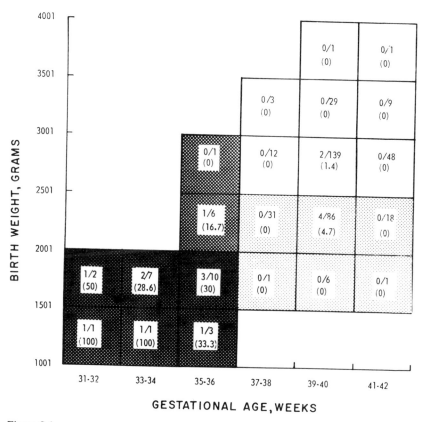

Figure 8.1
Distribution of neonates. Figures in parentheses indicate percentage of neonatal mortality.

increased deaths among infants of 39 to 40 weeks gestation were often associated with low birth weight.

Although birth weight and gestational age have individual predictive power and both are useful indices under field conditions, they are applied to best advantage when combined. The diagram in figure 8.1, for example, shows population distributions by the combined two criteria and also the corresponding neonatal mortality. That the two criteria are essential to optimal expression becomes wholly apparent. At the bottom left are the lower birth weight preterm infants with high neonatal mortality. Next upward and toward the center are preterm newborns with higher birth weight and lower neonatal mortality. Toward the right are low birth weight infants of 37 weeks or more gestation (small-for-gestational age) with neonatal death rates that are not particularly high. Term infants weighing more than 2,500 grams had negligible neonatal death rates.

Table 8.5
Infant Mortality, by Birth Weight and Gestational Age, 416 Infants, 1964–1972

Class	Birth weight, g	Gestational age, weeks	Infant mortality		
			Neonatal (< 29 days)	Post-neonatal (29 days–11 months)	Total (first year of life)
Preterm	< 2,501[a]	< 37	10 (323)[b] N = 31	6 (286) N = 21	16 (516) N = 31
Term, small-for-gestational age	< 2,501	≥ 37	4 (28) N = 143	8 (58) N = 139	12 (84) N = 143
Term	≥ 2,501	≥ 37	2 (8) N = 242	10 (42) N = 240	12 (50) N = 242
Total			16 (39) N = 416	24 (60) N = 400	40 (96) N = 416

[a]One newborn infant weighed 2,565 g.
[b]Number of deaths (deaths per 1,000 children alive at beginning of period); below, N = initial population.

Postneonatal infant mortality is summarized according to the two combined criteria in Table 8.5 along with neonatal mortality. Prematurity involves a continuing risk of death in the postneonatal period with a rate of 286 deaths per 1,000 live preterm infants. Interestingly enough, deaths among small-for-gestational age and full-term infants of adequate birth weight increased considerably during postneonatal infancy—two-fold and five-fold, respectively—a reflection of the environmental risks of malnutrition, infectious disease, and poor care that intrude after the first few months of life.

Mortality in Early Childhood

Table 8.6 presents age-specific mortality (deaths per 1,000 population) of children in the second, third, and fourth years of life. Rates continued high in these years, again a reflection of environmental stress and malnutrition. Antenatal factors still exerted an effect on mortality even at this period in life. Of special interest was the resistance of prematurely born children. Although a half had died by the end of the first year, the survivors experienced no enhanced risk during the hazardous early preschool years. Small-for-gestational age infants, judged as having experienced fetal growth retardation, performed less satisfactorily with a high age-specific mortality throughout early childhood. Children born at term and of adequate birth weight also had a high mortality, particularly in the second and third years of life (44 and 33 deaths per 1,000, respectively), but less than for corresponding small-for-gestational age children. The contrasting behavior of the two groups in the fourth year is striking; small-for-gestational age children had an age-specific mortality of 50 per 1,000, term infants only 8 per 1,000.

Table 8.6
Mortality in Infancy and Early Childhood, Children
of Known Birth Weight and Gestational Age, 1964–
1972

Class[a]	Second year	Third year	Fourth year
Preterm	0[b] N = 15	0 N = 13	0 N = 8
Term, small-for-gestational age	8 (76) N = 105	3 (39) N = 78	3 (50) N = 60
Term	9 (44) N = 204	5 (33) N = 153	1 (8) N = 122
Total	17 (52) N = 324	8 (33) N = 244	4 (21) N = 190

[a]See text and table 8.5 for criteria in classification.
[b]Number of deaths (deaths per 1,000 children alive at
beginning of period). N = initial population. Attrition
in numbers is explained because cohorts have different
ages.

Causes of Death

Neonatal deaths, including those among twins not considered previously, are
listed in table 8.7. As mentioned earlier, establishing causes of neonatal death
is difficult and requires sophisticated facilities and techniques. Accurate
diagnosis of acute respiratory disease can be established only with the aid of
chest radiography. Death in the first few days of life often is due to anoxia,
subdural hemorrhage, and other pathological manifestations that require
necropsy and whole brain sectioning (Towbin, 1970) for certain identification.

Eight of 18 deaths occurred within 48 hours of birth, all among the
smaller preterm babies. The remaining 10 deaths occurred after the ninth day
of life, again in smaller babies—but in general these latter were not as small as
the 8 who died shortly after birth: 4 were born prematurely, 4 were small-for-
gestational age, and 2 were of adequate birth weight and gestational age. The
diagnoses and certain clinical findings, also listed in table 8.7, emphasize
acute respiratory disease. Under other circumstances the cause of death might
well have been stated as prematurity. With three exceptions at least one
clinical finding in each newborn suggested a congenital abnormality of some
kind, particularly among infants who died shortly after birth. The 3 children
without detectable abnormalities died at 10, 12, and 17 days; for 2 the
certified cause of death was acute respiratory disease. No diagnosis could be
established for the child who died at 17 days; death occurred during a

Table 8.7
Classification of Neonatal Deaths by Age and Sex, Birth Weight, Gestational Age, Presumed Cause of Death, and Clinical Findings, 1964–1972

Child no.	Sex	Birth weight, g	Gestational age, weeks	Class[a]	Age at death	Presumed cause of death[b]	Membrane rupture, hours	Duration labor, hours	Skin	Respiration	Heart	Muscle tone	Cord IgM, mg/ml	Cord IgA, mg/ml
147	M	1,930	33	PT	30 min	CM	<0.5	7	Cyanotic	Poor	Abnormal	Atonic	0.14	0.04
41	F	1,687	34	PT	2 hrs	Ne	<0.5	5	Pale	Slow	*	*	0.03	0.04
285[c]	M	1,054	29	PT	4 hrs	Ne	<0.5	4	Cyanotic	Slow	*	*	0.26	0.04
286[c]	M	783	29	PT	4 hrs	Ne	<0.5	4	Cyanotic	Slow	*	*	0.26	0.04
337	M	1,225	32	PT	12 hrs	Ne	<0.5	9	Pale	Slow	*	*	0.29	0.04
33	M	1,863	36	PT	12 hrs	Ne	<0.5	4	Pale	Slow	Murmur	Hypotonic	0.10	0.04
174	F	1,761	35	PT	1 day[d]	Ne, HCNS (?)	36	4	Cyanotic	Normal	Normal	Hypotonic	*	*
426	M	1,820	35	PT	2 days	P, CM	<0.5	4	Pale	Normal	Normal	Hypotonic	0.17	0.04
184	M	2,633	40	T	10 days	P	<0.5	3	Pink	Normal	Normal	Normal	0.16	0.04
211	F	1,357	34	PT	11 days	P	<0.5	7	Pink	Normal	Normal	Hypotonic	0.03	0.13
405	F	2,109	41	SGA	12 days	P	<0.5	11	Pink	Normal	Normal	*	0.10	0.04
196	F	2,376	35	PT	16 days	Ne, HCNS (?)	<0.5	5	Pink	Normal	Normal	Normal	0.31	0.21
301	F	1,194	35	PT	17 days	P	<0.5	5	Pink	Normal	Murmur	Hypotonic	0.85	0.04
36	M	2,675	39	T	17 days	Ne	<0.5	2	Pink	Normal	Normal	Normal	0.14	0.04
396	F	2,066	40	SGA	18 days	P	<0.5	4	Pink	Normal	Normal	Normal	0.23	0.04
355	F	1,521	31	PT	19 days	P	36	6	Cyanotic	Normal	Normal	Hypotonic	0.19	0.04
66	M	2,447	40	SGA	20 days	P	<0.5	2	Pink	Normal	Normal	Normal	0.56	0.04
142	F	2,348	40	SGA	26 days	P	<0.5	11	Pink	Normal	Normal	Normal	0.61	0.41

aClassification: T = term; PT = preterm; SGA = small-for-gestational age.   bPresumed causes of death were: P = pneumonia; CM = congenital malformation; HCNS (?) = intracranial hemorrhage, central nervous system damage; Ne = not established.   cTwins.   dFracture of hip.   *Not determined.

weekend and the parents buried the child after refusing examination by a physician.

Nine deaths were classed as due to acute respiratory disease (pneumonia?), 2 of which presumably were associated with intracranial hemorrhage and central nervous system damage (HCNS) and 1 with congenital defect (club foot). Two had at least one obvious congenital malformation (absence of ears; club foot). There were 2 additional probable cases of HCNS. Cord serum IgM or IgA were appreciably elevated in half of infants dying in the neonatal period.

Causes of death in the postneonatal period differed significantly from those of the first 28 days of life (table 8.8). Although acute respiratory disease (bronchopneumonia, pneumonia) accounted for more than a third of all postneonatal deaths, a word of caution is necessary regarding this diagnosis under field conditions. Other causes of death were whooping cough, measles, and acute diarrheal disease, essentially with an underlying protein-calorie malnutrition (PCM). This condition is defined as underweight with edema or as weight deficit for age by at least 40 percent with or without edema.

Two sudden and unexpected crib deaths occurred, one an infant born prematurely (1,809 grams; 36 weeks) who died at age 14 weeks, and the other a small-for-gestational age (1,842 grams; 40 weeks) with death at 16 weeks. No pathological studies were made. Both infants had been exclusively breast-fed, which makes food aspiration an unlikely cause of death; no prior illnesses had been observed. These deaths give a rate of 4.65 sudden infant deaths per 1,000 live births in the first semester of life, a rate in excess of observations elsewhere although clearly to be appraised in relation to the small numbers in the present study.

The common communicable diseases—measles, diarrheal disease, and whooping cough—were the outstanding causes of death in the second year of life, together accounting for 79 percent of fatalities, the remainder being attributed to bronchopneumonia. Moderate protein-calorie malnutrition (PCM) and the much less frequent severe forms of marasmus and kwashiorkor were associated causes in about a fourth of deaths; retarded physical growth was evident in almost all.

Infectious diseases continued to account for significant numbers of deaths in the third and fourth years of life, particularly with a history of fetal growth retardation. The contribution of measles, whooping cough, and acute diarrheal disease to mortality in infancy and early childhood is summarized, by age, in table 8.9. The two specifically preventable diseases accounted for most deaths among children one to three years old. Even in the first year 36 percent of deaths were ascribed to measles and whooping cough. These data do not correspond to the normal distribution of causes of deaths in this population because, after an absence of more than ten years, whooping cough invaded the village in 1968 in a highly lethal epidemic.

Table 8.8
Causes of Postneonatal Death, by Age, 1964–1972

	Age				
Primary cause	29 days– 11 months	1 year	2 years	3 years	4–6 years
Pneumonia, broncho- pneumonia	9[a]	1	3	1	0
With PCM	0	1	0	0	0
With PCM and diarrhea	0	0	1	0	0
Whooping cough	5	5	1	0	0
With bronchopneumonia	0	4	2	2	0
Measles	2	0	0	1	0
With bronchopneumonia	1	4	0	0	0
With diarrhea	1	0	0	0	0
Diarrheal disease	4	2	0	1	0
With PCM	0	1	1	0	0
Meningoencephalitis	0	0	1	0	0
With bronchopneumonia	0	1	0	0	0
Sudden infant death	2	0	0	0	0
Other	1	0	0	0	0
Total	25	19	9	5	0

[a]Number of deaths in age group.

Table 8.9
Mortality of Common Infectious Diseases in Early Childhood, by Number and Relative Percentage of Deaths, 1964–1972

Age, years	Population	Total	Measles and whooping cough	Acute diarrheal disease	Measles, whooping cough, and diarrheal disease
< 1	458	41	9 (21.9)[a]	4 (9.8)	13 (31.7)
1	400	19	13 (68.4)	3 (15.8)	16 (84.2)
2	323	8	3 (37.5)	2 (25)	5 (62.5)
3	258	4	3 (75)	1 (25)	4 (100)
4	198	0			
5	148	0			
6	110	0			

[a]Number of deaths (relative percentage).

Table 8.10
Infant Survival as a Function of Birth Interval, by Number and Percentage of Cases, 1964–1972

	Birth interval, months[a]				
	9–17	18–26	27–35	36–44	45+
First 4 weeks of life $\chi^2 = 13.9; P < 0.01$					
Died	5 (14)[b]	4 (3)	1 (1)	3 (6)	1 (3)
Survived	30 (86)	116 (97)	122 (99)	48 (94)	31 (97)
First 6 months of life $\chi^2 = 19.7; P < 0.001$					
Died	8 (23)	5 (4)	4 (3)	3 (6)	2 (6)
Survived	27 (77)	115 (96)	119 (97)	48 (94)	30 (94)

[a]Interval between the birth of the present infant and that of the preceding sibling.
[b]Number of cases (percentage).

Diarrheal disease traditionally has been recognized as an important cause of death in this and other developing regions (Gordon et al., 1963; Gordon et al., 1967). That holds true in the present instance, although the relative importance is not directly apparent in table 8.8 because the tabulation was by primary causes. Diarrheal disease stands not only as the cause of 12 percent of deaths but was also associated with one death each from measles and bronchopneumonia. If these cases are included, diarrheal disease ranks with measles and is second to lower repiratory disease and whooping cough. Furthermore, diarrhea almost always is associated with PCM in the first two years of life. Judging from the profile of deaths described earlier, diarrheal disease would be second to respiratory disease as a cause of death, particularly in infancy and early childhood.

The important consideration is that postneonatal deaths and those of early childhood can be reduced by effective vaccination against measles and whooping cough. It may be argued, however, that in view of the retarded growth and poor nutritional status detailed in the rest of this study, any reduced mortality as a result of immunization probably would be of lesser magnitude than expected because of deaths from intercurrent acute diarrheal disease, respiratory infections, and growth failure.

Malnutrition and Survival
Protein-calorie malnutrition (PCM) was associated with most infectious diseases, and it had a dominant role in bronchopneumonia and such acute communicable diseases as whooping cough, measles, and diarrheal disease. Field epidemiological studies suggested that PCM had a more important place than ordinarily recognized, sufficient to induce an individual behavior among many diseases of infants and toddlers in developing nations (Béhar, 1964). The concept that malnutrition significantly contributes to morbidity and

Table 8.11
Infant Deaths per 1,000 Live Births, Santa María Cauqué and the United States, by
Birth Weight

Birth weight, g	Neonatal			Postneonatal			Infant		
	SMC	US	R	SMC	US	R	SMC	US	R
1,501–2,000	273	210	1.3	303	26	11.7	576	199	2.9
2,001–2,500	34	45	0.8	34	13	2.6	68	54	1.3
2,501–3,000	10	10	1.0	43	7	6.1	53	17	3.1
3,001–3,500	0	5	0	23	5	4.6	23	10	2.3

Note: For Santa María Cauqué, 1964–1972; for the United States, Chase (1962). Figures
rounded to the nearest integer. R = ratio SMC/US.

mortality of weanlings was inferred from such epidemiological scrutiny
(Gordon et al., 1963; Gordon et al., 1967).

Observations in Santa María Cauqué revealed significant differences in
physical growth between children dying of endemic diseases, such as diarrhea
and bronchopneumonia, and control children from the same village who
survived these diseases. The relationship of malnutrition to the outcome of
infectious disease will be further discussed in chapter 12.

A direct indication of the influence of nutrition on survival is obtained by
examining its behavior as a function of birth interval. The assumption is that
short intervals between births are likely to result in nutritional depletion and
deterioration of maternal health with a resulting negative effect on the quality and quantity of breast milk and on the mother's abilities to care for the
child. Table 8.10 presents infant survival as a function of birth interval, showing that neonatal survival was significantly less when birth intervals were short
(9 to 17 months). These findings can be attributed to deficient fetal growth
with short birth intervals.

Comparison of Infant Mortality in Developing and Industrialized Nations, by Birth Weight

Comprisons of mortality according to birth weight are necessarily limited to
infant mortality because of a lack of information in the world literature on
mortality at ages one to four years, considered as a function of birth weight,
gestational age, or newborn maturity. Even for infancy the information is
limited to certain populations of industrial nations and often for the neonatal period only, such as the studies relating low birth weight and poor survival from urban industrial settings (McKeown and Gibson, 1951; NCHS,
1967; Wegman, 1971; US DHEW, 1972c). Some information is available from
the Pan American Health Organization (PAHO) International Investigation of
Childhood Mortality (Puffer and Serrano, 1973) and from the present data of
the Cauqué study. The data provided by the PAHO investigation cannot be
projected to the general population because denominators were not available.

Other comparisons are possible using the data from Santa María Cauqué and from a study done in the United States by Chase (1962). The comparison is revealing (table 8.11) in that neonatal mortality rates in the two populations, on the basis of birth weights, are remarkably similar: the Santa María Cauqué/United States ratios were close to equality (1.0) for birth weights of 1,501 to 3,000 grams. The evidence suggests that neonatal mortality is related to antenatal events and is relatively independent of the extrauterine environment. In general, low birth weight infants receive exceptional care in the United States through special intensive care units (Klaus and Fanaroff, 1974). Under village conditions this advantage apparently is matched, for infants above 1,500 grams, by maternal-infant interactions that favor early and effective breast-feeding and probably by other desirable biological and psychological variables. While the great differences in overall neonatal mortality between developing and industrial societies obviously are associated with the greater incidence of low birth weight infants in developing areas (20 to 42 percent), there is little doubt that intensive care of high risk neonates, particularly with birth weight under 1,000 grams, results in better survival rates as revealed, for instance, by the statistics of The Royal Victoria Hospital, Quebec, Canada (Usher, 1974).

Significant differences in postneonatal mortality according to variations in birth weight are noted in table 8.11, where the larger mortality rates are among infants of lower birth weight. Two things are apparent: first, that the adverse environment, mainly through diet and infection, accounts for most of the greater risk of death for village infants as compared to those of wealthier populations; and second, that better fetal growth alone is apparently able to reduce postneonatal infant mortality to a significant degree.

The collective evidence from this study adds further proof to the concept that birth weight and gestational age correlate with survival, not only in infancy but also in later childhood. Low birth weight in particular was associated with practically all neonatal deaths and with most of those in postneonatal infancy. The present data imply that in similar regions, if infant mortality is about 100 deaths per 1,000 live births, 30 to 40 percent of infants will be of low birth weight. The generalization would not hold, however, if tetanus neonatorum was prevalent, or if infants were weaned at early ages without proper food supplementation (Plank and Milanesi, 1973), situations that result in high infant mortality independent of birth weight. A large-scale cooperative investigation of childhood mortality in Latin America (Puffer and Serrano, 1973) has further demonstrated that an interaction of poverty, low birth weight, improper weaning, and infection accounts for most infant deaths.

The long-lasting high infant mortality in Santa María Cauqué was not dramatically modified by the medical care provided during the study, a combination of simple medical services with limited provision of immunization and other preventive measures. A well-trained pediatrician, supported by a staff of auxiliary public health nurses, closely supervised almost all ill children, providing antimicrobials, rehydration, and other simple management as indicated. These measures were well beyond usual facilities available in the surrounding region, yet notably short of optimal medical care. They failed to have an impact on the well-established high neonatal and infant mortality that had prevailed in the village for the decade preceding the Cauqué study. Even if effective immunization had been employed, with the anticipated reduction in mortality, infant death rates still would have been excessive because of a hazardous environment interacting with a child population of whom a third were already malnourished at birth.

A better medical care system could be instituted, at high cost, to include a complex of sophisticated apparatus, instruments and drugs, the availability of a goodly supply of foods and special formulas, and a qualified neonatologist assisted by paramedical personnel, all with access to a complex laboratory. This undoubtedly would result in improved survival rates, yet such measures are impractical for two reasons. One is that no economic structure could bear the costs even in a relatively limited region, much less on a national basis. The other consideration is of human values, addressed to the question of what kind of survival can be expected from infants who are born after fetal growth retardation and who subsequently suffer further malnutrition along with the impact of recurrent acute infections. Accumulated evidence shows that infants born under the conditions described have physical, immunological, neurological, and behavioral abnormalities (Bengoa, 1969; Hardy, 1973; Chandra, 1975). Recognizing the medical obligation to save lives, the quality of the survivor remains a pertinent question. The stern reality is that remedy of the existing malnutrition is at best partial and the quality of survival, expectedly, is no more than relative. If nothing else, human values concerning the quality of life should act on the moral and social conscience of society to create a change in the order of priorities, substituting prevention for incomplete efforts at repairing damage already done.

What becomes evident is that a significant reduction in infant mortality, if it is to be accomplished in relatively immediate years, is directly dependent on a reduction in premature and low birth weight infants and on improved fetal and postnatal growth, especially in the early childhood years. Improvement in fetal growth alone could result in lesser mortality in infancy and early childhood, even if contemporary local and external surroundings remained unaltered. Public health action, therefore, finds its central target in the maternal environment, preferably in combination with social and humanitarian activities. Moreover, a better maternal environment inevitably produces a more favorable milieu for the growing child.

Chapter 9
Growth and Development in Infancy and Early Childhood

Most visitors from industrial societies, who come to a Guatemalan Indian village for the first time, remark on the short stature of the residents. INCAP field workers have the general impression that size is of no special concern to the villagers and that adults are little interested or preoccupied about stature, weight, or processes of growth and development. No consultations on growth were requested at the village clinic, and among both children and elders consultations on nutrition related most often to complaints of anorexia. Adults might indicate a desire for greater physical strength because of their hard work in the fields, the long distances they walk, and the huge loads they carry on their heads or backs. To this end villagers requested medicines and vitamins, especially if they were injectable, which conceivably would stimulate appetite or invigorate the body. Women were not interested in having large babies, and when asked why the usual answer was that they carried their children on their backs until 18 to 24 months of age. Possible difficulties in the delivery of large babies were not an apparent worry.

Physical size, however, is important in any society as an index of health. At the individual level, height and weight at a particular time may reveal little about general health, because individual variations are large (figure 9.1). When the data constitute the mean for a whole population, however, they attain significance since a general deficit at a particular age is likely to indicate interference with the growth potential of that population. Furthermore, measurements of body size are important because they often correlate with other

This chapter was written jointly with Juan J. Urrutia and Carlos E. Beteta.

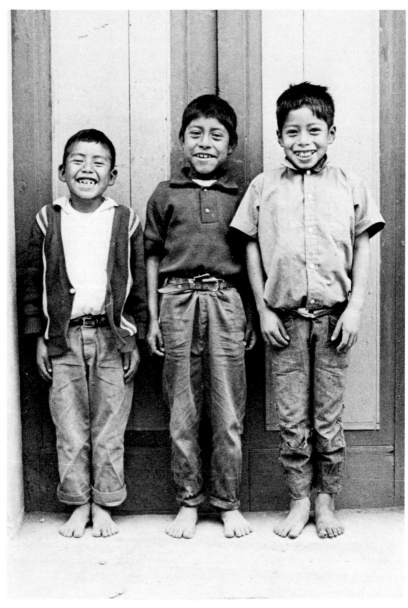

Figure 9.1
First three children of the Cauqué study at ten years of age. *From left to right*, dates of
birth and birth weights: 11 February 1964, 3,313g; 25 February 1964, 2,369g; 11 March
1964, 2,949g. By US standards the heights of all three are approximately those of seven
year olds.

functional parameters of greater relevance, such as psychomotor development, again with the important provision that judgment is at the level of
whole populations. These considerations are valid if the normal growth
pattern of a population under scrutiny has been well established, which is not
always true of developing societies.

Previous studies on the growth of Guatemalan Mayan-descent Indians have
been of a cross-sectional (prevalence) nature; they revealed large differences
in weight and height compared with industrial societies (Méndez and
Behrhorst, 1963; INCAP-CDC, 1972). A study of children in semilongitudinal
(incidence) fashion for four years came to similar conclusions through fitting
the pooled information by simple regression lines on the total data (Guzmán
et al., 1968).

The Cauqué study approached the problem differently, namely, by analysis of individual growth curves using a good fitting and by pooling information after individual children had been categorized according to birth weight,
gestational age, or both. The study had the added advantage of prospective
observation of eight annual cohorts and virtually complete data collected
under natural conditions with neither benefit nor detriment of experimental
or other programmed intervention.*

The prospective observations now presented relate to infants born during
the Cauqué study, from 1964 through 1972. Virtually all were recruited into
annual cohorts whose eventual losses were negligible other than by death and
occasional migration. Infants born after 1972 are still being studied, along
with the surviving children of the original cohorts, in a continuing investigation that assesses the effect of food fortification on health and growth
(Mata et al., 1972e). Those studies will contribute still more information to
the data archive.

Growth has been analyzed for 430 single infants and for four sets of twins,
all with known birth weights. Gestational age also was established for 416
singletons and for the twins. Seven children were lost to the study at various
ages by emigration. Occasionally a child may have escaped measurement at a
particular age because of visits to neighboring villages or cities. This was

---

* The relationship between birth weight and postnatal physical growth has been
explored by retrospective analysis by many workers with demonstration of positive
correlations (Miller et al., 1972), but all too infrequently by prospective study. Two
investigations have shown that preterm babies and small-for-dates grow abnormally
(Babson, 1970; Fitzhardinge and Steven, 1972a) despite life in adequate environments
theoretically more favorable than those of rural villages in a developing region. The
prospective study of the 1958 cohort of British children showed that birth weight and
gestational age are related to postnatal growth and development (Davie et al., 1972).

Relatively little information is available for populations of less developed countries.
Among these few studies, Nigerian infants with birth weights below the tenth percentile
for the region concerned showed a poorer weight gain than did children with greater
birth weight (Morley et al., 1968). A similar observation was recorded for Gambian newborns followed prospectively in their rural environment (McGregor et al., 1968).

uncommon and the required measurements usually were made as soon as the child returned.

Further attrition in observed numbers occurred because cohorts were recruited at a rate of approximately 50 infants per year. When data were pooled for analysis the latest cohorts expectedly were not represented in the older age groups. Thus, numbers in cohorts became fewer with advancing age (appendix E, Table E.1). An attrition of considerable magnitude was due to deaths in infancy and in the second and third years of life, as the preceding chapter demonstrated.

The eight annual cohorts were studied for weight and, less completely, for height. Head and thorax circumferences were obtained only for children of the 1964 and 1965 cohorts. The data were handled in several ways: (a) the growth of individual children was examined by graphically displaying the data points; (b) for definition of growth in the total population or in groups by birth weight or gestational age, or the two criteria combined, averages, standard deviations, and standard errors were calculated for each anthropo- metric variable at fixed intervals; (c) individual curves were fitted by a regres- sion equation with a logarithmic function to be explained later; and (d) the statistics of these equations of individual curves were used in multivariate and other types of analyses.

Physical Growth

Average curves of weight and height were computed for all children of the study, excluding the twins, by yearly cohort and by age; the data are sum- marized in tables E.2, E.3, and E.4 of appendix E. Mean curves were com- pared with those for Iowa children (Jackson and Kelly, 1945), a standard adopted by INCAP more than 15 years ago (INCAP, 1956). The Iowa curves, first released in 1945, are still applicable because no significant secular change has been noted in 20 years of observation (Jackson, 1969).

There are good reasons to believe that these standards are adequate for infants and preschool children. Growth in the first three to four months of life approximates the standard. Many INCAP studies during the last 20 years, including the comprehensive survey of Central America, have proved that growth of children of high socioeconomic strata parallels that of the Iowa curves. Furthermore, infants of Santa María Cauqué, with a birth weight of at least 3,000 grams, grow and remain in the 50th percentile of the standards for height and weight during the first three months of life. This and similar observations (Béhar, 1968; Guzmán et al., 1968; Mata et al., 1972c; Habicht et al., 1974) are reasons to believe that village children have an optimal growth potential equal to that of infants of more advanced societies.

Comparison of INCAP standard curves and those of the children of Santa María Cauqué reveals a marked deficit in weight and height. In figures 9.2a and b means and standard deviations around the mean—which approximate

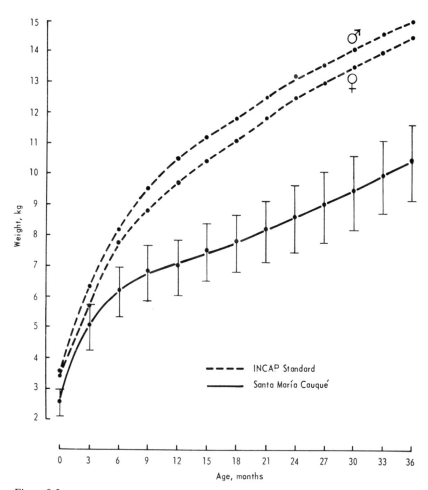

Figure 9.2a
Mean values and standard deviations for weight, all cohort children, 1964–1972

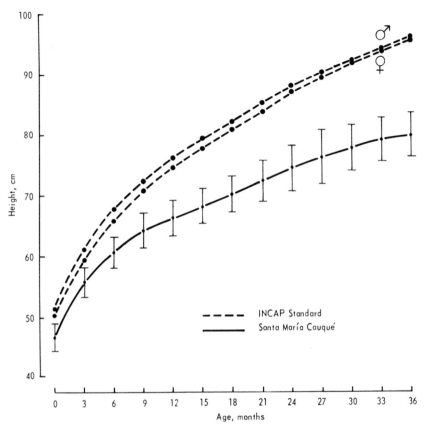

Figure 9.2b
Mean values and standard deviations for height, all cohort children, 1964–1972

the 16th and 84th percentiles in a normal distribution—are plotted. Guatemalan children of higher socioeconomic strata fall within the 30th percentile of the Harvard School of Public Health standards (Stuart and Meredith, 1946) but nearer the 50th percentile of the Denver charts (Hansman, 1970; Duncan et al., 1974). While most of the present analyses had been completed when the Denver standards became available, the Denver data do serve ideally for comparison with data from Santa María Cauqué in view of the similar altitudes of the two locations. They were processed for calculation of percentiles of weight and height in the description of growth retardation in chapter 14.

The assumption has been made that the growth potential of village children is similar to that implicit in the standards used. In fact, mean growth rates in the first three months of life are wholly comparable. Departure from the standard occurs at four to five months, and by one year of age is most

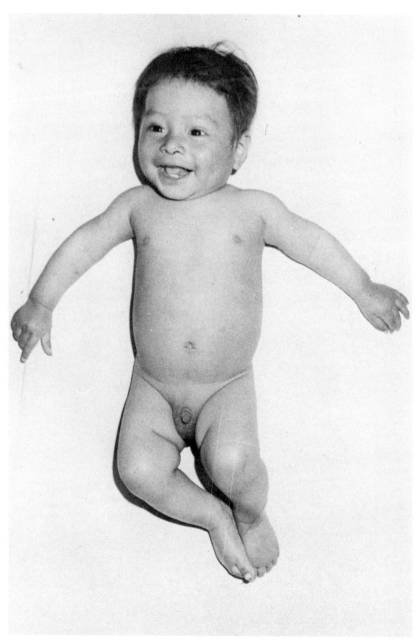

Figure 9.3
Child 3 at age six months. Weight at six months = 6,715g; birth weight = 2,949g.

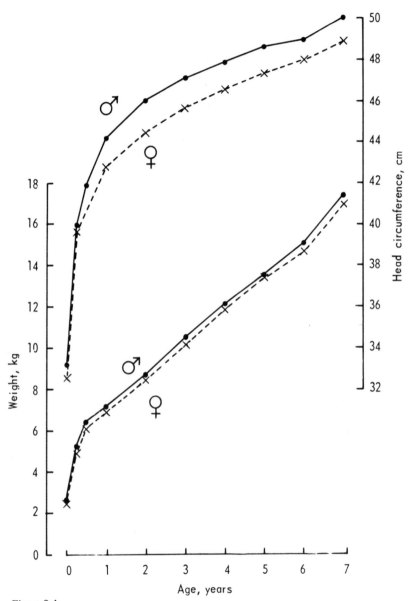

Figure 9.4
Mean weights and head circumferences, from birth to age seven years, 1964–1972

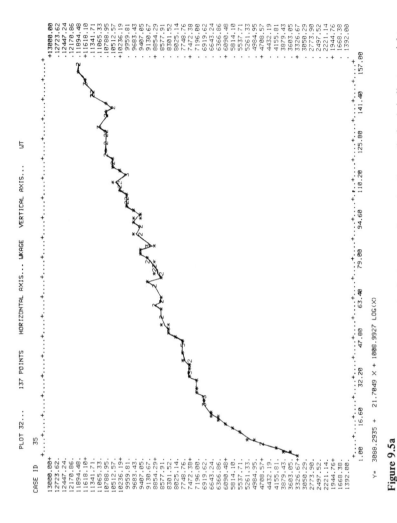

Figure 9.5a
Weight curve of Child 35. The horizontal axis shows age in weeks; the vertical axis indicates weight in grams. Equation for curve fitting: $y = a + bx + c\log x$. Numbers in curve denote number of data points.

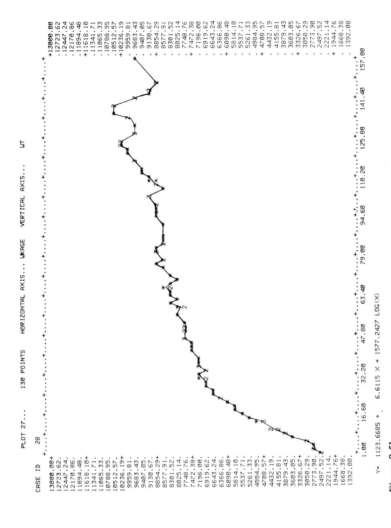

Figure 9.5b

Weight curve of Child 28. The horizontal axis shows age in weeks; the vertical axis indicates weight in grams. Equation for curve fitting: $y = a + bx + c\log x$. Numbers in curve denote number of data points.

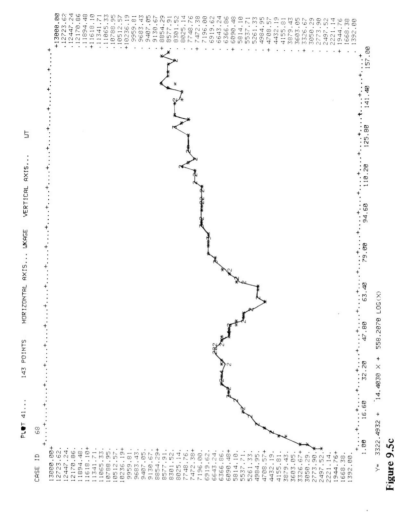

Figure 9.5c
Weight curve of Child 68. The horizontal axis shows age in weeks; the vertical axis indicates weight in grams. Equation for curve fitting: $y = a + bx + c\log x$. Numbers in curve denote number of data points.

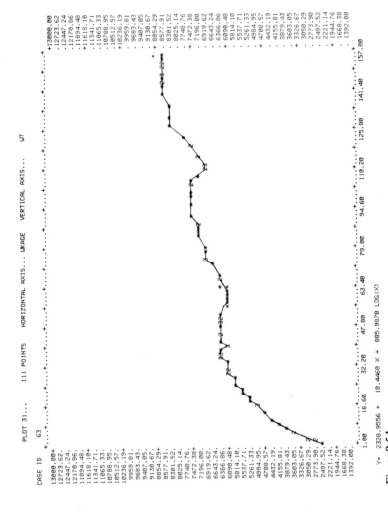

Figure 9.5d
Weight curve of Child 63. The horizontal axis shows age in weeks; the vertical axis indicates weight in grams. Equation for curve fitting: $y = a + bx + c\log x$. Numbers in curve denote number of data points.

marked, at which time infants are below the 16th percentile. Although
growth deficits begin to appear before six months, infants appear healthy and
are well developed at that age even though 40 percent originally were low
birth weight infants (figure 9.3). The slowed average growth tends to quicken
during the second and third years of life, paralleling the standard curves, yet
not reaching their level; the separation is progressive and leads to larger absolute differences with age. The short stature of adult women is evidence of
this.

Males attained greater weight and height than females at all ages, a difference established early and usually well marked by six months of age (figure
9.4). Sex differences in growth continued throughout the seven years of
observation; this is contrary to the United States where, among school
children of equivalent ages, girls are taller than boys (Johnston et al., 1973).

Growth Curves of Individual Children
Individual children exhibited great variability in growth. Differences seemed
to be determined early in life, a generalization not always applicable because
of marked differences in existing environmental influences, for instance,
degree of exposure to infectious agents and variations in response to those
agents. Figures 9.5a, b, c, and d reproduce weight curves of four children in
their first 157 weeks (three years) of life. Child 35, with a birth weight of
2,960 grams, grew better than most children; the growth curve was relatively
smooth, although with recurring periods of weight loss, particularly in the
second and third years of life. A deficit in weight and stature became marked
by the second year of age. During the first three to four months of life Child
68, with a birth weight of 2,341 grams, grew at a faster rate than expected.
An episode of marked weight loss occurred later, with protracted recuperation. The curve eventually smoothed out but with considerable periods of
slow gains and distinct growth retardation. Such growth deficits are ordinarily
associated with inadequate feeding, infections, and infectious disease, or a
combined action of these factors. Child 28, with a birth weight of 2,451
grams, had one of the better initial growth rates until 30 weeks of age. The
child experienced an acute weight loss in the second half of the third year,
along with marked deterioration of the nutritional state. Case 63 illustrates
still another growth pattern: the infant had a birth weight of 2,319 grams and
grew adequately during the first three months, after which the curve flattened
out and remained depressed for more than six months. After a short period of
growth at that time, there was a bout of acute weight loss. By the end of the
third year this child was markedly stunted. The clinical interpretation of
growth curves as a function of background health (diet, infections) has been
described elsewhere (Mata et al., 1967a; Mata et al., 1971c; Mata et al.,
1972b) and will be discussed again in chapters 11 and 12.

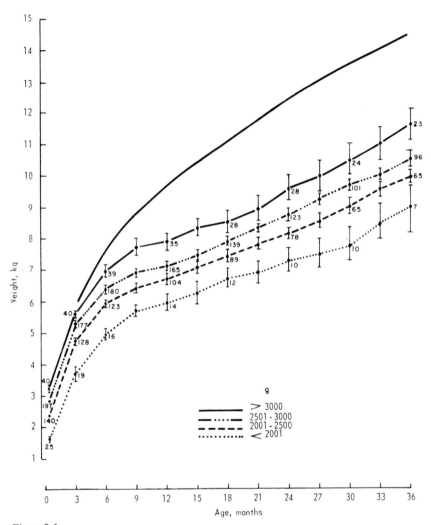

Figure 9.6a
Mean values and standard deviations of weights, cohorts of children defined by birth
weight, from birth to age three years. Figures near mean values show numbers of children
measured at each age.

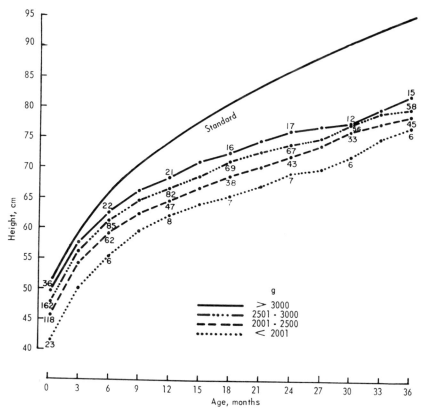

Figure 9.6b
Mean values and standard deviations of heights, cohorts of children defined by birth weight, from birth to age three years. Figures near mean values show numbers of children measured at each age.

Growth of Yearly Cohorts

The constancy of host characteristics has been a recurring theme of this book. Further support for a lack of significant change is derived from analysis of the growth attained by individual cohorts during the study period. Tables E.3 and E.4 of appendix E present mean values for weight and stature of the annual cohorts recruited from 1964 through 1971. Complete data for head and thorax circumferences are limited to the 1964 and 1965 cohorts (tables E.5 and E.6). Inspection of the rows in tables E.3 and E.4 reveals the remarkable stability of values throughout the range of one to seven years of life although differences were noted, such as those between the 1964 and 1969 cohorts. Data on mean growth of head and thorax show that these two variables behaved similarly, indeed almost identically, between the two cohorts.

Growth as a Function of Birth Weight

Observation of growth curves of individual children suggested that postnatal growth is related to birth weight. Prospective data on weight and stature were available for most newborns with recorded birth weight. This population is presented in table E.7 of appendix E.

Means, standard deviations, and standard errors were computed at various ages for subgroups of infants defined by birth weight. The mean weight and height values in tables E.8 and E.9 reveal marked differences among the four groups at prescribed ages. The differences became highly obvious when the means were plotted in figures 9.6a and b. Head and thorax circumferences also correlated with values at birth, as shown in tables E.10 and E.11 and graphically in figures 9.7a and b.

This type of analysis smoothes out differences in individual growth normally found in any population. Figure 9.8, for example, reproduces scatter diagrams of weight measurements in the first three years of life in two groups of children with contrasting birth weights. Even though some children of more than 3,000 grams birth weight exhibited a slow weight gain and eventually had a markedly deteriorated nutritional status (as indicated by the low points of one child in the figure, their postnatal weight values were better, as a whole, than those of children with a birth weight of less than 2,001 grams.

The analysis of growth patterns as a function of birth weight demonstrates a positive correlation with this isolated variable. It acquires added value when reliable information on gestational age is not available. Since weight and gestational age are two highly correlated variables, the correlations of birth weight and physical growth have implications for gestational age. Furthermore, the Cauqué study revealed, either directly or indirectly, that a high incidence of low birth weight infants characterizes Guatemala and that without knowledge of birth weights any interpretation of growth in developing countries becomes difficult.

The poorest growth curves so far presented are, as a rule, those of preterm babies of exceptionally low birth weight. The next lowest curve applies mainly to term small-for-gestational age infants, while the two upper curves are mainly those of term infants with weight adequate for gestational age.

Growth as a Function of Gestational Age

Mean values and standard deviations for weight, height, and head circumference, calculated as a function of gestational age, are presented in Tables E.12 through E.14 of appendix E. Gestational age also is a good predictor of physical growth. Two groups of children appear distinctly differentiated by their average growth curves: preterm (less than 37 weeks of gestational age) and term (figure 9.9). Head circumference also correlated with gestational

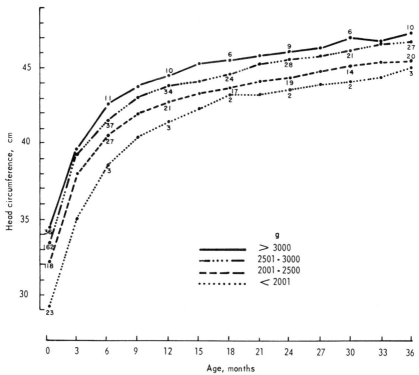

Figure 9.7a
Mean values of head circumferences, cohorts of children defined by birth weight and
INCAP standard, birth to age three years. Figures near the mean values show number of
children measured at each age.

age, particularly in the early months of life, although differences were less
marked by 15 months and even smaller thereafter (figure 9.10).

Caution should be exercised in relation to the predictive value, for groups
of infants, of either birth weight or gestational age, or of the two variables in
combination. The analyses showed that as a group children tend to remain
within a track defined by birth weight and gestational age, that is to say, by
the antenatal events. The postnatal environment, however, has an important
part in determining the growth potential of the individual. This is supported
by evidence from pediatric practice, namely, that even smaller preterm
infants can grow adequately if they are nursed and cared for under well-
defined and adequate conditions.

Newborn Maturity and Postnatal Growth
Birth weight or gestational age are often used independently of each other to
predict postnatal physical growth because of the difficulty of obtaining

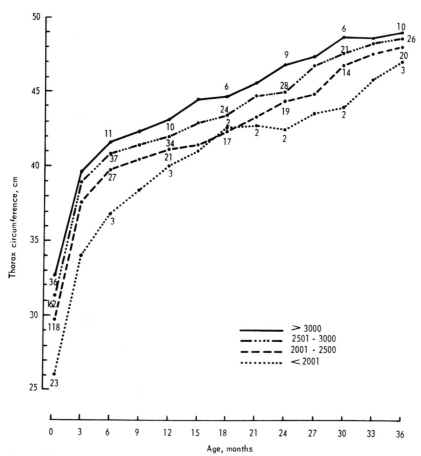

Figure 9.7b
Mean values of thorax circumferences, cohorts of children defined by birth weight and
INCAP standard, birth to age three years. Figures near the mean values show number of
children measured at each age.

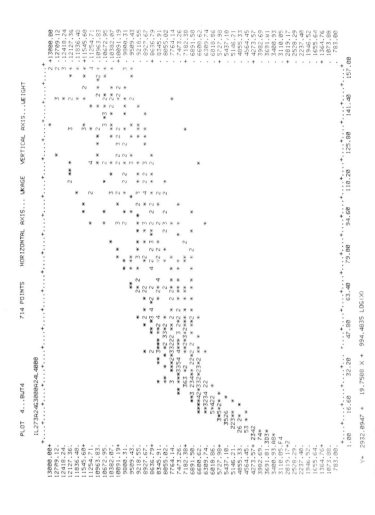

Figure 9.8
All weight points, all cohort children with birth weights greater than 3,000g, from birth to age three years. The horizontal axis shows age in weeks; the vertical axis indicates weight in grams. Numbers *2* to *9* show observations at that level; letters *A* to *G* correspond to data points *10* to *16*.

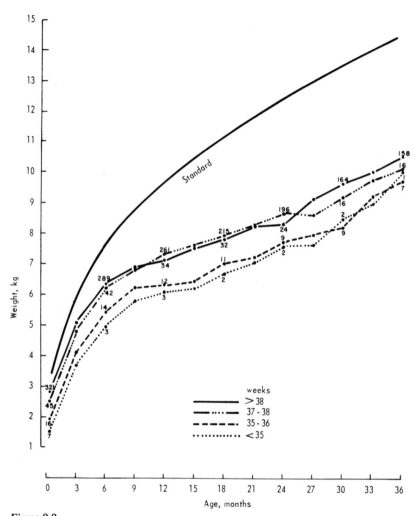

Figure 9.9
Mean weight curves, cohorts of children defined by gestational age, birth to age three years. Figures near the mean values show numbers of children measured at each age.

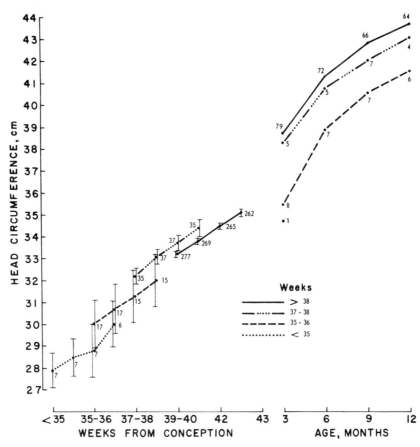

Figure 9.10
Mean values and standard deviations of head circumferences, cohorts of children defined by gestational age. Figures near the mean values represent the number of children measured at each age. Only one child of less than 35 weeks of gestation could be measured at three months of age.

Table 9.1
Weights, First Eight Days of Life, 229 Infants with Daily Records, by Fetal Maturity, 1964–1972

Age, days	Preterm (N = 9)	Small-for-gestational age (N = 86)	Term < 3,001 g (N = 112)	≥ 3,001 g (N = 22)
0	1,954 (322)[a]	2,302 (134)	2,716 (140)	3,140 (98)
1	1,897 (299)	2,261 (135)	2,664 (143)	3,064 (120)
2	1,867 (317)	2,229 (140)	2,645 (149)	3,027 (135)
3	1,861 (352)	2,236 (147)	2,660 (151)	3,031 (129)
4	1,869 (375)	2,266 (158)	2,687 (162)	3,056 (135)
5	1,904 (400)	2,297 (160)	2,720 (173)	3,081 (143)
6	1,928 (418)	2,328 (168)	2,756 (182)	3,114 (142)
7	1,960 (445)	2,367 (182)	2,797 (196)	3,140 (156)

[a]Mean weight in grams (S.D.).

combined data for the two variables in developing societies and under field conditions. The combination of data, however, describes the newborn best. Five groups of infants were recognized: preterm with severe low birth weight (Ps); preterm with moderate low birth weight (Pm); term small-for-gestational age (TSGA); term with moderate birth weight (Tm); and term with high birth weight (T). Occasionally the two groups of preterm infants were combined (table 6.12).

The average weights during the first eight days of life were computed from the daily weight measurements available for 229 infants (table 9.1). Before discussing the data it is worth emphasizing that all infants were given the breast shortly after birth. Two aspects contrast with the usual information from pediatric practice in industrial nations: first, the relatively small postnatal initial weight loss, averaging no more than 90 grams (3 ounces); and second, regain of that loss or even added weight by the end of the first week of life.

This behavior is evidenced in figure 9.11 where average weight values are expressed as a percentage of birth weight. The degree of maturity or retardation present at birth affected the way infants reacted with initial weight loss. As a group preterm infants lost most weight, yet began to recover it by the fourth day; by the end of the first week they had returned to the original level. Weight curves of term infants with fetal growth retardation (term-small-for-gestational age, or small-for-dates) and those of term infants with birth weight of 2,501 to 3,000 grams were impressive in that weight loss was the smallest and recuperation more rapid than for other newborns; within five days these babies had recovered the weight loss and two days later were showing a weight gain, as a group, of more than 2 percent of the initial weight. Term infants with the largest birth weight proportionally lost more.

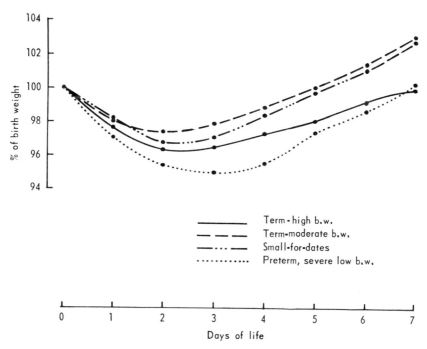

Figure 9.11
Weight loss of infants of different degrees of maturity, first seven days of life

In industrial societies mature bottle-fed babies lose about 3 to 4 percent of their weight, ordinarily recovered within seven days; breast-fed infants lose more (4 to 5 percent) and recovery requires seven to ten days (Smith, 1974).

A varying behavior of infants according to their degree of maturity was more noticeable in curves based on the first six years of life. The mean values for weight, height, and head circumference are shown in tables E.15 through E.17 of appendix E. Figure 9.12 shows mean weight curves for four groups of infants. They differ one from another. Growth was better for newborns of adequate gestational age and high birth weight. Conversely, preterm infants with birth weight below 2,001 grams had the lowest weight curve.

A group of three surviving preterm infants with moderately low birth weight was not included in figure 9.12 in order to promote clarity of the graph. These infants, who could be classed as preterm with adequate weight for their gestational age, showed a rapid growth rate in the first months of life, catching up with the term infants with moderate weight represented by the second curve from the top.

The curve for height for these four groups behaved similarly, as did that of head circumference (figure 9.13). Regarding head circumference, differences in growth rate are not striking in the first four weeks of life, provided proper

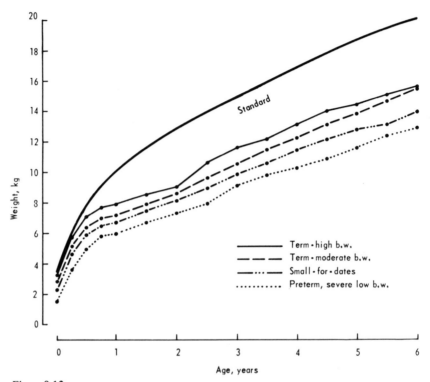

Figure 9.12
Mean values of weight, cohorts of children defined by maturity at birth, from birth to age six years

correction is made for gestational age. By so doing it became evident also that absolute differences are not marked between the two groups of term infants, but differences do exist between them and the preterm and small-for-gestational age children. Furthermore, the smaller preterm infants showed a tendency to more rapid growth in head circumference than did the other categories. At least throughout the first six years of life children classified according to fetal maturity maintained the differences in head circumference evident at birth. The group of three preterm infants with moderately low birth weight (2,001 to 2,500 grams) grew rapidly to attain a curve paralleling that of term infants of moderate birth weight.

This analysis extends the preceding analyses of growth as a function of birth weight and gestational age, but it has more biological meaning because the two variables have been combined to express the degree of fetal maturity. The result is that growth correlates with antenatal events and that discrepancies in size among the various groups of newborns, in the case of weight and height, are accentuated with time.

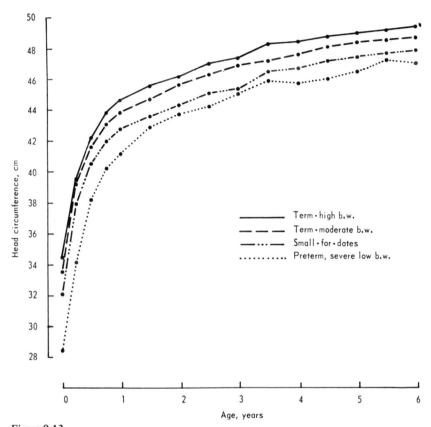

Figure 9.13
Mean values of head circumferences, cohorts of children defined by maturity at birth, from birth to age six years

A subsample of collected data will serve here to emphasize existing deficits in physical growth. The right hand-wrist radiographs of 26 boys and 24 girls, taken at six-month intervals from six months to five years of age, were assessed by the method of Greulich and Pyle (1959). Using this standard, interpolations were made to the closest month; results were recorded as arithmetic means of all bone skeletal ages.

The means and standard deviations of area skeletal ages for boys and girls are shown in table 9.2. Mean skeletal age was lower than the corresponding chronological age after six months, a deficit particularly noticeable at age 18 months and thereafter. In five year olds the mean difference between chronological and skeletal age was close to two years.

Boys showed a greater deficit in bone maturation than girls during the first three years, but at later ages the situation was reversed (table 9.2). The present observations among representative children of Santa María Cauqué

Table 9.2
Skeletal Age (Greulich-Pyle) and Bone Maturation, 26 Boys and 24 Girls Observed
Prospectively from Six Months to Five Years of Age, 1964–1971

Chronological age, years	Skeletal age, decimals of years		Difference in mean skeletal age (boys – girls)
	Boys	Girls	
0.5	0.53 (0.23)[a]	0.60 (0.30)	–0.07
1.0	0.79 (0.28)	0.94 (0.23)	–0.15
1.5	1.09 (0.37)	1.19 (0.18)	–0.10
2.0	1.31 (0.37)	1.41 (0.21)	–0.10
2.5	1.58 (0.37)	1.67 (0.25)	–0.09
3.0	1.86 (0.43)	1.88 (0.30)	–0.02
3.5	2.14 (0.51)	2.13 (0.33)	+0.01
4.0	2.52 (0.54)	2.39 (0.38)	+0.13
4.5	2.90 (0.53)	2.70 (0.41)	+0.20
5.0	3.25 (0.56)	3.03 (0.42)	+0.22

[a]Mean (S.D.).

complement transversal studies of Guatemalan children of low socioeconomic
levels (Garn and Rohmann, 1959; Blanco et al., 1972), demonstrating that
malnutrition is reflected in poor development of many organs and systems,
including the skeletal one.

Growth of Twins
It is difficult, if not impossible, to obtain a definitive answer to the relationship between independent newborn variables, such as birth weight and
gestational age, and physical growth. Further evidence, however, can be
obtained from the study of twins reared in the same environment. Ten twins
were born in the Cauqué study, two of whom died shortly after birth. Six of
those surviving were considered to be monozygotic on the basis of a single
placenta, the same sex, similar physical appearance (judged by prospective
observation), and identical ABO Rh configurations. Two pairs of twins had
known birth weights; one pair (males) was observed for five years and the
other (females) for one year. No birth weight was obtained for the other pair
of monozygotic twins (females) but measurements were made at three weeks
of age and for the next two years.
    Differences in initial size between twins of individual pairs, expressed as
absolute values and as percentage of values of the larger twin, are presented in
table 9.3. Variation in weight between twins of individual pairs were not
particularly great; they ranged from 2 percent to 10 percent for the larger
twin. Differences in length and head circumference were even less, from 0.2
percent to 4.9 percent. These differences in weight, height, and head

Table 9.3
Growth Differences Between Presumably Monozygotic Twins, 1964–1972

Pair	Child number	Sex	Birth order	Length of study, years	Birth weight, g	Δ, g[a]	Percentage[b]	Birth length, cm	Δ, cm	Percentage	Birth head circumference, cm	Δ, cm	Percentage
1	124	M	1	5	2,657			47.4			33.0		
	125	M	2	5	2,711	54	1.9	47.3	0.1	0.2	32.8	0.2	0.6
2	302	F	1	1	1,749			40.1			29.0		
	303	F	2	1	1,942	193	9.9	41.3	1.2	2.9	30.5	1.5	4.9
4[c]	498	F	1	2	3,459			49.0			35.7		
	499	F	2	2	3,106	353	10.2	48.5	0.5	1.0	34.9	0.8	2.2

[a]Difference between twins.
[b]Percentage difference from value of larger twin.
[c]Measurements are those of the third week of life.

Table 9.4
Physical Growth of Presumably Monozygotic Twins, 1964–1972

	Pair 1			Pair 3			Pair 4		
	Twin 125	Twin 124	Percentage[a]	Twin 303	Twin 302	Percentage[a]	Twin 498	Twin 499	Percentage[a]
Weight, g									
Birth	2,711	2,657	98.0	1,942	1,749	90.1	3,459[b]	3,106[b]	89.8
3 months	5,329	5,162	96.9	3,747	3,163	84.4	5,358	4,773	89.1
6 months	6,684	6,109	91.4	4,816	4,446	92.3	6,794	6,241	91.9
1 year	6,882	6,562	95.4	5,336	5,073	95.1	7,727	7,193	93.1
2 years	8,678	8,058	92.9				10,170	9,751	95.9
3 years	10,413	9,380	90.1						
4 years	12,882	10,074	78.2						
5 years	14,553	12,893	88.6						
Height, cm									
Birth	47.3	47.4	100.2	41.3	40.1	97.1	49.0[b]	48.5[b]	98.9
3 months	54.5	56.7	104.4	50.4	48.7	96.6	55.4	54.8	98.9
6 months	59.9	61.0	101.8	54.6	54.3	99.5	60.3	59.6	98.8
1 year	66.8	67.0	100.3	60.2	60.2	100.0	65.7	66.7	101.5
2 years	75.4	75.2	99.7				74.6	74.5	99.9
3 years	82.1	80.0	97.4						
4 years	87.5	84.3	96.3						
5 years	94.0	90.8	96.6						

[a]Percentage of observed value for larger twin, at birth.
[b]These measurements were taken at 3 weeks of age.

Table 9.5
Physical Growth of Pair 5 Twins, First Two Years of Life, 1964-1972

Age	Twin	Weight, g	Height, cm	Head circumference, cm
Birth	F	1,749	40.3	28.9
	M	1,600 (91.5)[a]	41.0 (101.7)	29.4 (101.7)
2 weeks	F	1,728	40.3	29.5
	M	1,603 (92.8)	40.3 (100.0)	30.2 (102.4)
4 weeks	F	1,621	40.7	29.7
	M	1,731 (106.8)	41.3 (101.5)	31.4 (105.7)
3 months	F	3,135	48.0	34.5
	M	3,078 (98.2)	49.3 (102.7)	36.3 (105.2)
6 months	F	4,275	54.3	38.5
	M	4,564 (106.8)	55.3 (101.8)	40.6 (105.5)
9 months	F	5,643	59.7	40.8
	M	5,671 (100.5)	61.5 (103.0)	42.6 (104.4)
1 year	F	5,832	61.6	41.8
	M	6,594 (113.1)	65.7 (106.7)	43.8 (104.8)
1 year 3 months	F	6,636	64.2	42.3
	M	7,392 (113.4)	69.3 (107.9)	45.0 (106.4)
1 year 9 months	F	7,930	71.5	43.8
	M	8,561 (107.9)	76.2 (106.6)	45.7 (104.3)
2 years	F	8,312	71.6	44.1
	M	9.006 (108.3)	78.2 (109.2)	45.9 (104.1)

[a](Percentage of measurement of female twin).

circumference at birth persisted in postnatal life for as long as the children were observed, adding evidence to other similar observations (Falkner, 1966; Babson and Phillips, 1973).

Anthropometric measurements at specified age intervals are presented for monozygotic twins in table 9.4. The twins of Pair 1 were born with a difference in weight of only 2 percent and no perceptible difference in length. With age the relative difference in weight became larger and more significant to the extent that by four years of age the twin born smaller had a relative weight deficit of 11.4 percent. Although lengths were comparable at birth and through the first year, after one year the smaller twin at birth lagged behind in height to reach a difference of more than 4 percent at age five years. A similar behavior was noted for the other two twins, with the differentiation less for height and head circumference than for weight.

Twin Pairs 3 and 4 showed more marked differences at birth than did Pair 1. The relative distinction at one year of age, however, was not proportionately larger than for Pair 1. Thus, postnatal physical growth correlated with birth weight independently of gestational age, but the magnitude of the phenotypic differences attained at various ages undoubtedly was influenced by environmental factors, such as infection.

Of the pair of nonidentical twins the female (Case 327) weighed significantly more at birth than the male (Case 328) but was of comparable length and head circumference (table 9.5). Measurements at two weeks showed that the male had outgrown his twin in weight and head circumference. Differences in the three variables persisted through the second year of life, as shown for height and head circumference. In this particular instance, differences in weight at birth conceivably could have been due to variations in placental function, and therefore in blood supply, or they could have been genetically determined. The first possibility seems the more likely; the male twin showed a better growth potential in postnatal life. The better growth of the male also could have been the result of greater maternal concern in nursing. In two instances the differences in weight between the twins became smaller at ages three and nine months, both cases incident to an episode of infectious disease. The growth curves of twins thus illustrate a correlation of birth weight and sex with postnatal growth, independent of gestational age.

Fitting of Growth Curves
Weight and height curves of individual children were fitted by computing regression equations according to the formula $y = a + bx + c \log x$ (Tanner, 1962) where a is an estimate of the parameter at age 0 (departing point); b is a "linear" parameter, a measure of rate of growth reflecting most of the growth trend after the period of faster growth; and c is the parameter of growth deceleration, reflecting growth in the first months of life. This treatment has been used for prevalence data (Malcolm, 1970) and has proved superior to the simple regression for prospective data when sufficient measurements are available as in the present study. Figure 9.14 illustrates the fitting of the weight curve of one child using the values collected in the first five years of life; actual or real measurements are shown for comparison. Visual inspection of the curve reveals an excellent fit as reflected in the high R^2, a value of 0.99. Irregularities in the curve decrease the R^2; for instance, the R^2 for Case 68, depicted in figure 9.5c, was 0.87, one of the lowest, although still a good fit.

The fitting of growth curves for 208 children having complete data for the first three years of life gave R^2 values in excess of 0.90 for all except three; these had values between 0.75 and 0.875. The histogram of values of R^2 is shown in figure 9.15a; most values were greater than 0.95. The distributions of parameters of the equation (a, b, and c) were bell-shaped as illustrated in figure 9.15b for b. The values of a and c were less distinctly distributed and the histograms had a wide base, particularly that of the logarithmic component of the curve (c). The excellence of fit of individual growth curves (high R^2 values) is to the advantage of the analysis because it offers a way to summarize growth data for comparison with other information, namely diet, infection, and disease.

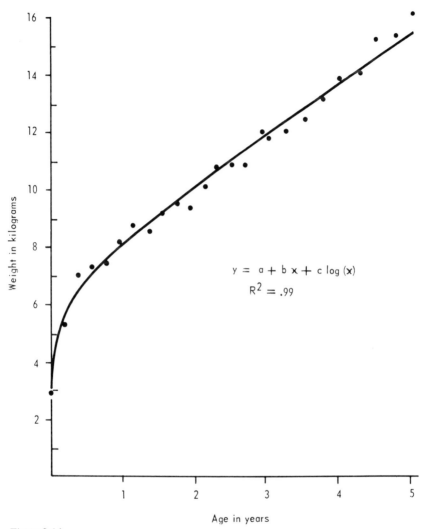

$$y = a + b\,x + c\,\log(x)$$
$$R^2 = .99$$

Age in years

Figure 9.14
Weight fitting curve of Child 35. Actual weights at three-month intervals are plotted along with the fitted line obtained from values produced by the equation.

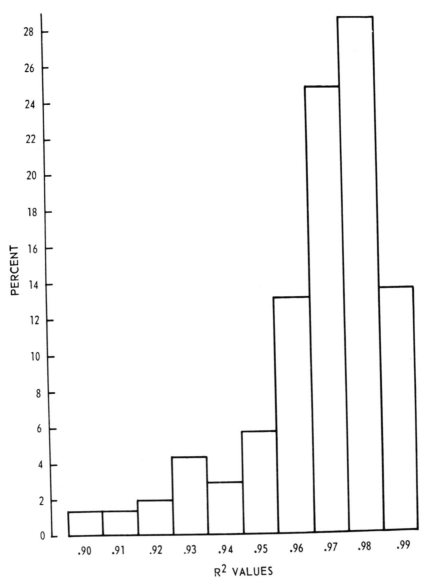

Figure 9.15a
Frequency distribution of R^2 values, 200 children, birth to age three years. The majority of fitted curves had R^2 values greater than 0.95.

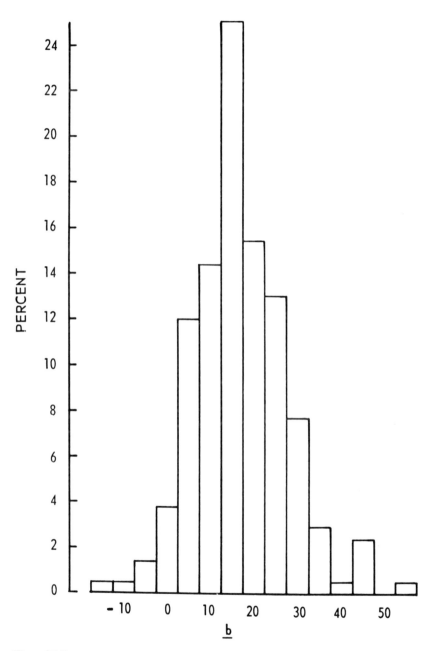

Figure 9.15b
Frequency distribution of parameter b, 200 children, from birth to age three years

Table 9.6
Correlation Coefficients for Parameters of the Weight Curve and Infant and Maternal
Variables, 1964–1972

Variable[a]	c	b
BWT	−0.02	0.14[b]
BHT	0.01	0.10
HDCIRC	−0.04	0.17[c]
THCIRC	−0.02	0.12
GAGE (DPREG)	−0.14[b]	0.11
MAGE	−0.29[c]	0.15[b]
MWT	−0.02	0.07
MHT	0.02	0.21[c]

[a]192 cases with infant variables; 174 cases with maternal variables. For codes of variables see table 7.13.
[b]$P < 0.05$.
[c]$P < 0.01$.

Parameter b was larger for term infants. The lowest b values were noted, as a group, in the term-small-for-gestational age. A comparison of the means of b for the two groups (term and small-for-dates) by Student's t test was significant ($t = 2.16$; d.f. $= 184$; $P \approx 0.03$). Thus, the overall growth rate of term small-for-gestational age infants was poorer than for term infants.

Regression Analysis with Parameters of the Fitted Growth Curve
Step-wise regression analyses (SWRAs) were computed using either parameter b or c of the fitted weight curve as the dependent variable, with several infant and maternal factors treated as independent variables. Infant variables were birth weight, birth length, head circumference, and gestational age; those of the mother were age, midpregnancy weight, and height. Gestational age could be considered a maternal variable, namely, duration of pregnancy.

Significant coefficients were observed among the three parameters, highest between b and c ($r = 0.65$), and lowest between a and b ($r = 0.24$). Correlations were calculated for the parameters of equations for individual children (table 9.6). Significant correlations also were observed between the parameters and certain maternal and newborn characteristics. Gestational age (GAGE) correlated with parameter c because the child is decelerating but not with b, which mainly reflects growth after the first few months of life. Although birth weight and head circumference correlated with parameter b, only the latter entered into the regression equation, to account for 3 percent of the variability of b (table 9.7). Gestational age (duration of pregnancy) accounted for only 2 percent of the variability of c.

Maternal variables were better correlated than those of the infant. Parameter b correlated well with maternal height and maternal age, with 6.9 percent

Table 9.7
Step-Wise Regression Analysis for Parameters of the Fitted Weight Curve, 191 Children, 1964–1972

Independent variable in order of entry	Regression coefficient (B)	Standard error of B	F value	Percentage RSQ
Birth head circumference (Dependent variable = b)	0.13	0.06	5.75[a]	2.94
Gestational age (Dependent variable = c)	-32.02	15.87	4.07[a]	2.10

[a]$P < 0.05$.

Table 9.8
Step-Wise Regression Analysis for Parameters of the Fitted Growth Curve, 173 Children, 1964–1972

Independent variable in order of entry	Regression coefficient (B)	Standard error of B	F value	Percentage RSQ	Δ percentage RSQ
Maternal height (Dependent variable = b)	0.49	0.17	8.06[a]	4.47	
Maternal age (Dependent variable = b)	0.22	0.10	6.31[a]	6.87	2.40
Maternal age (Dependent variable = c)	-11.66	2.93	15.84[a]	8.43	

[a]$P < 0.005$.

of its variability accounted for by these variables; c was inversely correlated with maternal age, with 8.4 percent of its variability explained (table 9.8).

Although the total variability accounted for was small, this association of maternal and newborn variables with physical growth is important. Maternal factors such as height and age are influenced by socioeconomic status and by health and care of the mother from childhood onward; they correlate better with the parameters of the infant's growth curve than do variables of the infant that are assessed at birth.

While the postnatal environment appears to be the logical target for intervention, particularly in early life, an improvement in fetal growth evidently will lead to a marked effect on physical growth despite the small amount of the variance explained by the regression equations. Nevertheless, the data in chapter 7 suggest that improved fetal growth will result from better nutrition and health of girls from infancy to motherhood.

Chapter 10
Feeding Practices

Feeding practices are an intimate feature of the culture of any society. The feeding of infants and children in relatively isolated and traditional societies like Santa María Cauqué customarily follows practices transmitted from one generation to the next. In Santa María Cauqué initial nutriture of the child is wholly by breast-feeding, a practice that continues for months until introduction of liquid and solid supplementary foods marks the start of a long weaning process.

Breast-Feeding and Weaning Practices
As practiced by village women breast-feeding is highly successful. Virtually no failure to nurse was recorded during the eight years of the study. All 448 live-born infants who survived 48 hours were nursed as soon as the mothers, in folk tradition, considered the milk to have "matured," a time normally two days after puerperium. Women view nursing as a wholly natural function, the only way to feed a baby, and they know little about the possibilities or methods of bottle feeding. The economic status of most families, the few cattle in the village, and the minimal influence of urbanization and education are all factors conducive to breast-feeding.

Breast-feeding begins shortly after birth. Mothers also gave sugar-water through the first week to approximately half the newborn infants by putting a piece of cloth soaked in solution in the child's mouth. Approximately half of the mothers secreted milk during some part of pregnancy and 10 percent

This chapter was written jointly with Richard A. Kronmal and Bertha García.

through delivery. In such cases the mother nursed her newborn infant without delay.

Approximately a third of the women not lactating during gestation provided their infants with colostrum while the rest offered the breast as the milk matured. Infants of women who were not lactating at the time of delivery often were nursed from birth and for two or three days by other women of the village, usually relatives who at the time were nursing their own young infants. The emphasis on foster mothers with young infants is in accord with local belief that milk output is greatest during the first months of lactation. In a few instances a grandmother, nursing her own infant, nursed her grandchild as well. The village pattern was that all babies eventually received breast milk, and some had colostrum as soon as they were born.

It is also worth recalling that steam baths are taken by the mother partly in the belief that the heat applied to the back benefits breast-feeding and that warm milk prevents colic. Most mothers drank hot chocolate during the first week postpartum, an ancient custom thought to increase milk output.

Aside from sugar-water from the first day of life, infants received no fluids or foods except breast milk on the immediately succeeding days, nor for the next several weeks or even months. Both first-born and successive children ordinarily were nursed without difficulty. To nurse the young mother usually kneels and sits on her heels on the floor in a quiet, relaxed atmosphere (figure 10.1). Mothers ordinarily nursed for as many times and as long as judged necessary by signs or other demands of the baby. Massage to the breasts is customary before beginning to feed; the child is not allowed to empty a breast completely, with the result that both breasts are offered at each nursing. Since the mother and newborn sleep together, the child has ready access to the nipple and, indeed, often holds it in the mouth while asleep. Under these conditions collection of information on the number of feedings and the output of milk is close to impossible. It does appear, however, that milk secretion by village women is efficient, although volume expectedly is often suboptimal and nutritional properties may be altered. Efficient milk secretion is substantiated not only by the commonly prolonged breast-feeding, but also by the fact that mothers often nurse during pregnancy and occasionally feed the new baby along with the preceding sibling.

Systematic interviews with village mothers in connection with feeding practices revealed that generally they favored prolonged lactation because of a well-implanted belief that breast-feeding is good for the child, even during pregnancy. Breast feeding, in fact, extends into the second, third, and even the fourth year of life. The calm, relaxed, but formal disposition observed with the first baby or in the early months of lactation eventually turns into a more casual and informal relation as the child grows older. Thus mothers are found nursing their children while attending church, in cofradía or clinic, or

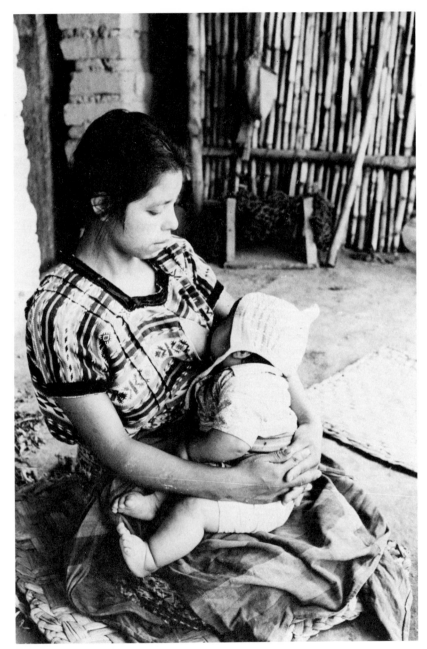

Figure 10.1
Young mother nursing her firstborn. The traditional qüipil is modernized with a zipper
to facilitate access to the breast.

Table 10.1
Intake of Supplemental Foods, Mean Grams per Day, Cohort of 45 Breast-Fed Infants, by Age, 1964–1967

	Age, months			
	2	3	4	5
Dairy products[a]	2[b]	2	2	1
	(132)	(162)	(50)	(80)
Gruels[c]	1	3	4	5
	(9)	(3)	(4)	(5)
Sugar	9	11	14	14
	(19)	(12)	(10)	(17)

[a]Equivalent to whole cow's milk.
[b]Number of infants; below, (mean grams of food consumed per day).
[c]Incaparina (see text), oatmeal, or maicena gruel.

even while walking in the village street. Breast-feeding is so much a part of the culture that the *qüipil* (blouse) is fashioned to permit easy access to the breast.

Prospective observations on all annual cohorts of infants permitted the generalization that in this culture weaning begins at about six months of age, extends in protracted fashion into early childhood, and occasionally into later preschool years. The general account of weaning that follows is based on 250 children who were fully weaned within the study period. Excluded from the analysis are 59 children who died while still being nursed, 3 who migrated from the village, and 8 for whom no adequate data were obtainable because of poor cooperation by the mother. Supplementary feeding practices refer to observations on the group of 45 cohort children. A few infants were completely weaned in the first year and a slightly larger number in the third and fourth years, but the average time was around 23 to 24 months of lactation. Girls tended to be completely weaned at earlier ages than boys, perhaps because of a preferential treatment to males or differences in rates of growth.

Recent years have seen a tendency toward introduction of other foods than breast milk at an earlier age. While modes were basically similar, more children were weaned at 15 to 20 months in the last half of the study, a finding apparently unrelated to sex differences. Further observations likely will provide additional information on similar changes in breast-feeding as rural areas are increasingly influenced by western culture.

The weaning process itself begins when supplemental foods, fluids, and *atoles* (gruels) are given to the child for the first time on a regular basis. For most infants of Santa María Cauqué this occurs at age 2 to 5 months. The most common supplementary foods were sugar-water made with either brown or refined sucrose, gruels, and cow's milk (table 10.1). Gruels were either of oatmeal, corn, flour, starch, or a high-protein vegetable mixture,

Table 10.2
Intake of Supplemental Foods, Mean Grams per Day, Cohort of 45 Breast-Fed Infants, by Age, 1964–1967

	Age, months					
	6	7	8	9	10	11
Dairy products[a]	2 (178)[b]	2 (55)	2 (32)	2 (32)	1 (36)	1 (8)
Eggs		1 (2)	2 na[c]	9 (2)	14 (4)	16 (5)
Meats				4 na	11 na	24 na
Beans						2 na
Vegetables		4 (12)	11 (15)	21 (13)	25 (12)	35 (16)
Fruits	1 (1)	3 (3)	10 (6)	11 (10)	18 (7)	18 (7)
Bananas, plantains		5 (5)	17 (7)	26 (9)	36 (10)	36 (16)
Tubers, roots			5 (4)	6 (3)	10 (4)	10 (4)
Tortilla	4 (4)	14 (6)	35 (9)	42 (16)	41 (19)	45 (23)
Bread	10 (2)	23 (8)	37 (7)	42 (9)	44 (9)	43 (11)
Rice and noodles		3 (5)	15 (5)	22 (10)	29 (6)	42 (93)
Sugar	21 (16)	38 (25)	45 (13)	45 (19)	45 (22)	45 (23)
Broths[d]	1 (5)	9 (12)	27 (12)	44 (21)	45 (29)	45 (30)
Coffee	11 na	23 na	36 na	44 na	43 (1)	44 (1)

[a]Equivalent to whole cow's milk.
[b]Number of infants (mean grams of food consumed per day).
[c]na = negligible amounts.
[d]Beef, beans.

Incaparina, marketed and sold throughout Guatemala by private industry (Bressani and Scrimshaw, 1961). Only a few infants received supplementary foods within the first six months and the amounts were so small that they contributed little to the diet. Table 10.2 illustrates the greater variety of fluids, gruels, and solid foods, the increasing number who received added food, and the larger amounts given as the children grew. Tortillas, rice and noodles, bread, broths, and some fruits were the main items by amounts consumed as well as numbers of children participating. Other foods were given to fewer children and in small amounts. The transition from a childhood to an adult diet was increasingly evident by the end of the first year, and by three years of age the two were definitely similar. The intake of dairy products, meat and eggs, and even beans was generally low, as in the general village diet (table 10.3).

The second and third years of life marked the time when tortillas began to occupy the dominant position they have in the everyday diet of the Cauqué villager; by two years of age all children were eating relatively more tortillas than any other food, as much as 40 percent of the total diet. Exceptions were the few children whose families owned a cow and had milk.

Table 10.3
Intake of Foods Other than Breast Milk, Mean Grams per Day, 45 Cohort Children, by Age, 1964–1970

	Age, months		
	12	24	36[a]
Dairy products	2 (28)[b]	8 (129)	33 (3)
Eggs	15 (4)	29 (7)	16 (8)
Meats	29 (3)	45 (5)	42 (6)
Beans	7 (2)	37 (27)	42 (27)
Vegetables	40 (18)	45 (19)	42 (41)
Fruits	25 (7)	26 (13)	41 (14)
Bananas, plantains	39 (13)	43 (16)	41 (17)
Tubers, roots	11 (20)	22 (4)	25 (1)
Maize (tortilla)	45 (28)	45 (105)	42 (226)
Bread	45 (15)	44 (13)	42 (14)
Rice and noodles	37 (3)	42 (7)	42 (7)
Sugar	45 (17)	45 (29)	42 (29)
Broths	49 (43)	45 (2)	42 (36)
Coffee	44 (1)	45 (2)	42 (2)

[a]Only 42 children remained in the cohort at age 3 years.
[b]Number of children (mean grams of food consumed per day).

As with breast milk, the child is offered food on demand. Tortillas, for instance, are kept within reach of children and can be taken freely and eaten. There is no emphasis or particular judgment by the mother regarding the amount of food a child must consume or presumably needs. The whole atmosphere surrounding maternal-infant interactions during supplementary feeding is relaxed, with a dependence on habit and custom.

The reasons advanced by mothers for completing the weaning procedure were investigated for all children of the study. Some of the stated reasons for instituting definitive weaning were wholly obvious and susceptible to direct measurement, such as failure of milk production or birth of a new child. Others were subjective reasons, their significance impossible to assess properly, such as the "milk was not good," the "child was too bothersome," or the "child was unwilling." The commonest reasons given for ending breast-feeding related to age of the child. The data suggest that underlying factors may exist other than the reasons advanced by the mothers. In order to explore the possibility of more logical causes, events such as pregnancy, abortion, and delivery of a live-born were tabulated as a function of weaning age. Among 309 histories, breast-feeding ended in 59 instances because of death of the child; for the remaining cases a tangible related event—a pregnancy, the birth of a new sibling, or an abortion—could be recorded for 186

Table 10.4
Frequency and Percentage of Events Associated with Termination of Breast-Feeding,
250 Cases, 1964–1972

Event	Frequency (percentage)
Pregnancy	150 (60.0)
Birth of sibling	32 (12.8)
Abortion	4 (1.6)
Other	
Child refused breast	24 (9.6)
Child too large	10 (4.0)
Milk scarce	7 (2.8)
Child eating well	5 (2.0)
Illness of mother	4 (1.6)
Child hospitalized	4 (1.6)
Child bothersome	4 (1.6)
Death of mother	1 (0.4)
Other reasons	5 (2.0)

Note: 59 children died and were excluded.

(74.4 percent); for the remaining 64, a variety of other reasons were noted (table 10.4).

Although the effect of breast-feeding on fertility is well noted, the concept that prolonged breast-feeding inhibits pregnancy is as yet not well established among most villagers. Despite the fact that no village woman was known to use modern methods of contraception, pregnancy rarely occurred within the first 12 months after a delivery and continued to be uncommon in the subsequent 6 months. Pregnancy became more frequent 18 to 35 months after delivery of a liveborn who survived and remained at the breast throughout that period. This fact relates well to the observed birth intervals described in chapter 5. Arrest of breast-feeding did not occur during the first month of a subsequent pregnancy, but was frequent at 3 to 6 months of gestation.

No pregnancy was recorded among 64 lactating mothers who weaned their children during the study. While illness of mother or child accounted for eight weanings (3.2 percent), most weanings in this group related to the age of the child or its appreciable size. Two children lost their mothers while still being breast-fed, one from tuberculosis and the other from acute diarrheal disease. One child was 33 months old and adapted readily to solid food. The other was 7 months old when the mother died. His sisters, 9 and 12 years old, carried him from house to house for 6 months where he had the benefit of several foster mothers, including one ladino woman. He survived the weaning period as successfully as did other children.

No differences were noted in distributions of expressed causes of weaning by age or sex of the child, nor by birth weight or gestational age. Also, no differences were observed in weaning age according to rainy or dry season despite its clear influence on crops and food availability.

Nutritional and Immune Properties of Breast Milk

No information was collected in the Cauqué study itself on volume of breast milk. Observations in Tezonteópan, a village in the Mexican highlands, similar in size, socioeconomic level, and cultural traits to Santa María Cauqué, indicated a decreased production of milk by chronically malnourished women after two months of lactation; it became markedly evident at six months (Martínez and Chávez, 1971). Similar observations have been recorded in India (Gopalan, 1956; Rao et al., 1959) and Indonesia (Bailey, 1965).

The quality of breast milk in the region was investigated from 1958 to 1959 by examination of 138 specimens from 69 mothers of Santa María Cauqué at various stages of lactation (Contreras et al., 1962). Results were compared with a similar sample from women of high socioeconomic level in Guatemala City. Maternal milk from the village had an adequate concentration of total calories, proteins, vitamin A, and riboflavin during the first three months of lactation. The concentration of free riboflavin, however, was significantly less than in milk from urban women. During the second quarter the concentration of vitamin A and total riboflavin was less than values for women of a higher socioeconomic level although proteins and calories remained comparable. No determinations were made of volume of milk; the cited information from India, New Guinea, and Mexico thus continues to be the most satisfactory base for interpreting effects of breast-feeding on growth and health of village children in developing regions.

As to the immune properties of breast milk, a significantly enhanced resistance to enteric infection has been observed among breast-fed babies not only when the environment is favorable, but also when environmental sanitation was at less than acceptable levels (Mata et al., 1969c; Mata and Wyatt, 1971). While the mechanisms are poorly understood, some resistance seemingly is engendered by the indigenous microflora characterizing the breast-fed child (Mata and Urrutia, 1971) by constituting a protective barrier against pathogenic infectious agents. This flora is predominantly of gram positive anaerobic bacilli (*Bifidobacterium, Eubacterium*) and probably develops from the combined stimulus of bifidus factor(s), lysozyme, lactoferrin, secretory IgA, and other antibodies. It is known that secretory IgA and the other immunoglobulins have anti-infectious properties and that specific antibodies to enteroviruses and enterobacteriaceae are present, especially in samples of colostrum (Mata and Wyatt, 1971; Wyatt et al., 1972; Goldman and Smith,

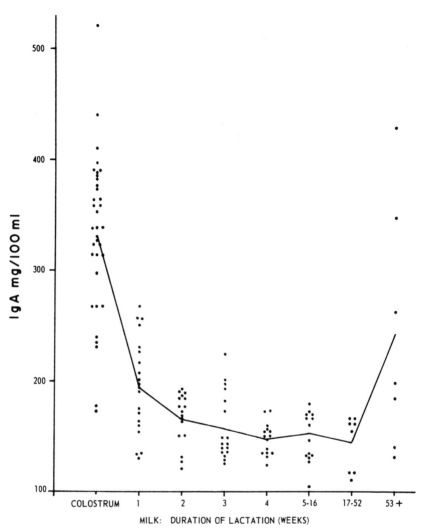

Figure 10.2
Concentrations of secretory IgA in colostrum and milk, 133 specimens from 43 women,
1968

Table 10.5
Mean Daily Nutrient Intake, 45 Cohort Children, Birth to Age Three Years, by Age, 1964–1970

	Age, months					INCAP Recommendation for 3-Year-Olds
	12	24		36		
	45 b-f[a]	31 b-f	14 w[b]	11 b-f	31 w	
Calories	214 (101)[c]	530 (236)	619 (176)	754 (261)	992 (272)	1,550
Total protein, g	4.8 (2.5)	14.3 (6.5)	17.4 (4.9)	21.4 (7.3)	26.9 (6.6)	30
Animal protein, g	0.4 (0.7)	2.7 (3.2)	3.1 (2.5)	5.9 (3.0)	9.7 (7.3)	
Iron, mg	1.6 (0.9)	4.7 (2.0)	5.9 (1.8)	7.5 (2.4)	9.6 (3.6)	10
Total retinol, μg	15 (18)	71 (88)	90 (95)	53 (35)	111 (77)	250
Thiamin, mg	0.12 (0.06)	0.30 (0.15)	0.37 (0.17)	0.44 (0.16)	0.55 (0.13)	0.6
Riboflavin, mg	0.07 (0.05)	0.26 (0.24)	0.29 (0.14)	0.24 (0.07)	0.36 (0.15)	0.9
Niacin, mg	1.31 (0.07)	3.06 (1.25)	3.42 (1.06)	4.29 (1.41)	5.81 (1.49)	10.2
Ascorbic acid, mg	7.2 (6.0)	15.9 (9.2)	16.2 (8.3)	18.6 (7.1)	24.3 (10.2)	20

[a] b-f = breast-fed. The contribution of breast milk was not assessed. None of the 45 children was weaned at 12 months of age. One was weaned at 18 months, because he had diarrhea at that time; his diet is not included in the table.
[b] w = wholly weaned.
[c] Mean (S.D.).

1973). Macrophages. lymphocytes, and other factors also are present in breast milk (Mata and Wyatt, 1971; Goldman and Smith, 1973).

Maternal milk from Santa María Cauqué revealed significant concentrations of secretory IgA, IgM, complement (C3), and specific antibodies, values which dropped considerably after the first week of lactation but persisted in significant amounts if the volume of milk secreted is taken into account (Wyatt et al., 1972). Figure 10.2 shows the values for secretory IgA in milk at various stages of lactation; an active secretion of this immunoglobulin is evident. Greater concentrations after one year of lactation have been interpreted as an indication that milk secretion has decreased, giving a higher relative concentration of IgA. The possibility, however, that this immunoglobulin is synthesized at a greater rate in late stages of lactation as a result of antigenic stimulation is not to be discarded.

Nutritive Value of Foods Other than Breast Milk   The nutrient intake of supplemental foods was measured for the 45 cohort children. The value of supplemental foods for breast-fed children compared with those weaned at selected ages are shown in table 10.5.

With no equivocation, weaned children had a decidedly lower intake of calories and nutrients, except for ascorbic acid, iron, and thiamin, as judged by the recommendations for well-nourished children of comparable age presented earlier in table 4.7. This is particularly true for children weaned before two years of age. Such comparisons at later dates, however, may not be wholly justifiable because village children are born smaller and they grow less, so that by age three years their mean weight and standard deviation are 10.4 (1.2) kilograms, no more than two-thirds of the weight of the well-nourished three year old children for whom the recommendations were formulated. There is no doubt that Cauqué children in general consume less than the amounts recommended as necessary to promote growth and adequate resistance to infection.

Assessment of dietary adequacy of this population of children will be made first, according to the ages for which the recommendations were projected, and second, according to the observed weight of the children studied. The first analysis assumes that the child needs certain prescribed amounts of calories and nutrients according to chronological age regardless of deficits in weight and height. The second analysis assumes that the child has adapted to a state of nutritional deprivation and therefore the needs are those of his actual weight under existing conditions.

Table 10.6 shows the first comparison. Of 14 fully weaned two year old children, only one consumed the recommended amounts of retinol and thiamin. More than a half received less than 50 percent of the calories, total retinol, and riboflavin recommended for that age; all children consumed less than 50 percent of the recommended niacin. Some improvement was noted for 28 children of the cohort at three years of age, particularly in respect to

Table 10.6
Adequacy of Diet of Children Weaned at 2 and 3 Years of Age, as Percentage of
Recommendation for Age, 1964-1970

Percentage of recommendation	Cal.	Total protein	Iron	Total retinol	Thiamin	Ribo-flavin	Niacin	Ascorbic Acid
14 two year olds								
< 50	8[a]	2	2	10	2	11	14	2
50-99	6	12	12	3	11	3	0	8
⩾ 100	0	0	0	1	1	0	0	4
28 three year olds								
< 50	2[a]	2	1	19	1	25	9	1
50-99	18	18	16	7	20	3	19	8
⩾ 100	8	8	11	2	7	0	0	19

[a]Number of children.

Table 10.7
Adequacy of Diet of Children Weaned at Two and Three Years of Age, as Percentage of
Recommendation for Weight, 1964-1970

Percentage of recommendation	Calories	Total protein	Total retinol	Riboflavin
13 children weighing 11.4 kg[a]				
< 50	0[b]	0	10	3
50-99	8	2	3	8
⩾ 100	5	11	0	2
3 children weighing 13.8 kg[c]				
< 50	0[b]	0	1	0
50-99	2	0	1	3
⩾ 100	1	3	1	0

[a]Only 13 two year old children weighed 11.4 kg, the standard value for that age.
[b]Number of children.
[c]Only 3 three year old children weighed 13.8 kg, the standard value for that age.

Table 10.8
Calories from Net Dietary Protein (NDpCal), Diets of Children One to Three Years Old,
1964–1972

Age, months	Number of children	Feeding	Percentage of mean NDpCal[a]
12	45	b-f[b]	4.1
24	33	b-f	5.2
	12	w[c]	5.6
36	11	b-f	5.7
	31	w	5.5

[a]Assuming a net protein utilization of 50 percent.
[b]b-f = breast-fed. The contribution of breast milk was not assessed.
[c]w = wholly weaned.

calories, total protein, thiamin, niacin, and ascorbic acid. Iron was adequate for 11 of these children but was poorly absorbed because of its source and nature of the diet. The same can be said about quality of protein since 40 percent of the protein in the diet of preschool children was derived from maize.

Assessment of adequacy of diet on the basis of weight of the child was difficult since no weight approached the expected level and only 13 two year old children and 3 three year olds had weights corresponding to the standard weight for respectively one and two year olds. If, however, the actual weight of a child, and not his age, was the basis for comparison, adequacy appeared more favorable. The comparisons are shown in table 10.7; the diet appears adequate for most nutrients except total retinol and to a lesser extent ribo-flavin.

Calculation of the percentage of calories derived from the net dietary protein (NDpCal%) shows that the protein is not deficient (table 10.8). Considering a net protein utilization (NPU) of 50 percent, an underestimate, the values obtained are in agreement with recommendations set by FAO/WHO for children one to three years old.

Thus, although village children continuously exposed to a suboptimal environment show deficient physical growth, many are able to survive under poor dietary regimens. However small the amounts of animal protein consumed by the child, the usual result is an adequate amount of calories derived from net dietary protein, although some children showed an extreme situation of inadequate food consumption. The deficit in total calories, or better, in total food, appears to be more significant than that of protein alone, as indicated by the Cauqué study in its early phases of development (Mata et al., 1967a). The concept that calories seem to be a more limiting factor in areas of poverty was decisively advanced by workers from India (Narasinga-Rao et al., 1969). In this regard several nutrition interventions in which improvement of protein levels was the primary objective failed to show any convincing

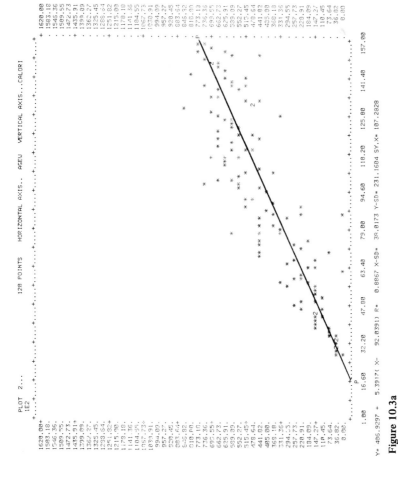

Figure 10.3a
Caloric intake of Child 2. The horizontal axis shows age in weeks; the vertical axis represents calories.

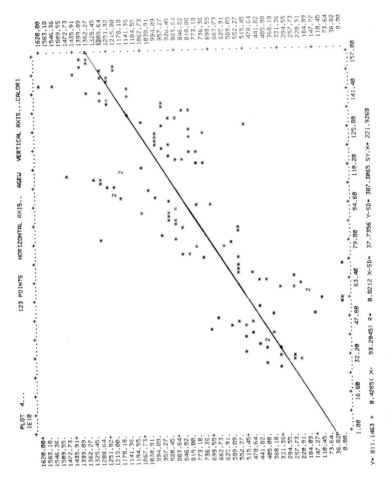

Figure 10.3b
Caloric intake of Child 10. The horizontal axis shows age in weeks; the vertical axis represents calories.

effect on growth; calorie supplementation had a more dramatic impact on the nutrition of children in India (Gopalan et al., 1973). Furthermore, recent observations in rural Costa Rica revealed a childhood population with significant deficit in growth yet consuming adequate amounts of animal protein (Valverde et al., 1975); the amount of calories consumed was low, however, a finding difficult to reconcile with the availability of calorie sources in the fertile and rainy region where the study was conducted.

The INCAP formulation of adequate diets at minimal cost for rural Guatemala (Flores et al., 1969) required a minimum of 0.15 quetzales per day (US $0.15) to feed a preschool child with local foods. This amount cannot be met by many families within the stringent budget of the rural farmer (see cost of labor, food, and clothing in table 2.10), a fact further complicated by current inflation and the energy crisis. Thus, poverty and deficient nutrition education constitute important factors that further limit amounts of calories and quality of the protein available to village children.

Supplemental Foods and Physical Growth   Food intake and growth were examined in two ways: first, through correlation of parameters of growth curves versus those of food curves; and second, through an analysis of the parameters of growth curves in relation to weaning age and child characteristics at weaning age.

In order to examine correlations between growth and food intake the nutrient value of all foods except breast milk was first measured for each child at weekly intervals during the first three years of life. Using the data obtained, curves were fitted by simple regression ($y = a + bx$) for calories and nutrients and for individual children, revealing a series of good fits. Correlation coefficients were of the order of 0.4 or more (P < 0.001) for calories, protein, and certain nutrients, and to a lesser extent for ascorbic acid and total retinol. Figures 10.3a through 10.5 indicate considerable scatter due to within-child and method variability, although the more accentuated differences can be traced generally to reduction of intake in connection with infectious disease or increased intake with recuperation. Figure 10.3a represents the caloric curve of Child 2 observed during the first three years, giving an R value of 0.89 with a range of ± 107 cal. Most of the calories are derived from maize, bread, noodles, and sugar. The diet of Child 10 (figure 10.3b) showed a coefficient of 0.82 (P < 0.001) and a greater variability (± 221 cal). Fittings for other nutrients such as niacin also were good as revealed by correlation against total protein (figure 10.4). While nutrients such as retinol and calcium varied more markedly with age than did calories, protein, and niacin, the correlation coefficients ordinarily were significant (figure 10.5). Total protein and calories were highly correlated, as were calories and niacin and thiamin because maize and a few other foods, regularly consumed, constitute a substantial portion of the total intake. Fittings

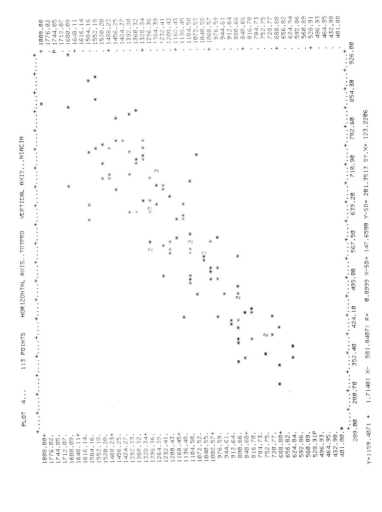

Figure 10.4
Correlation of niacin and total protein. The horizontal axis shows total protein in decigrams; the vertical axis represents niacin in mg × 10⁻³ .

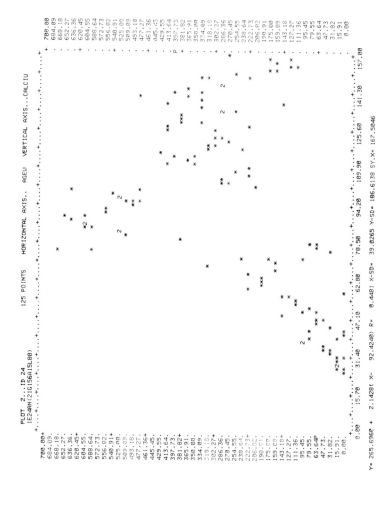

Figure 10.5
Calcium intake of Child 24. The horizontal axis shows age in weeks; the vertical axis represents calcium in decigrams.

for riboflavin, vitamin A, and ascorbic acid were not as good due to greater variability in intake of the foods contributing those nutrients, namely animal protein, fruits, and vegetables.

Figure 10.6a shows the distribution of R^2 values to illustrate the adequacy of fit. Three-fourths of the R^2 values were above 0.50 for thiamin, while 82 percent of the R^2 for calories were greater than 0.60. Low R^2 values correspond to a greater variability in dietary intake, mainly due to periods of anorexia incident to infectious disease. The slopes (b) of the fittings had a wide range of variation as shown in figure 10.6b, but in general they maintained a symmetrical bell-shaped distribution for calories and most nutrients, indicating differences in nutrient consumption among cohort children. The histogram of intercepts (a) showed a much wider base, because a values are influenced strongly by the time at which supplemental feeding begins.

The pattern of intake of supplemental foods, adequately reflected by fitting regression lines, by the distribution of slopes, and to a lesser extent by the intercepts just described, offers an opportunity to look for correlations with weaning age and physical growth.

Calories were chosen for the analysis because most R^2 values were high and because calories correlate strongly with most other nutrients. The analysis was made on the cohort children for whom the value of supplemental foods had been determined and fitted by regression analysis. Comparisons were between the parameters of diet (a and b) and those of the weight curve (a, b, and c) described in chapter 9. To emphasize, in the fitting of diet a is the intercept of the regression line with the y axis and falls quite close to the time supplemental feeding begins; b is the slope of the line and is larger for larger food intakes. The parameters of the growth curve, on the other hand, are: a, the starting point in the fitting; b the linear function of rate of growth, generally reflecting the trend over most of the curve, that is to say, after the first year of life; and c, a measure of growth deceleration, reflecting the growth trend particularly in the first months of life when growth is most rapid. Correlation coefficients obtained by regressing the parameters a and b of the calorie curve against the parameters a, b, and c of the growth curve of corresponding children are shown in table 10.9. None of the parameters of caloric intake showed a significant correlation with growth except b of the diet, which was correlated with a and to a lesser extent with b of the growth curve. Food intake summarized by regression lines did not correlate well with physical growth.

The lack of strong correlations could be accounted for by several factors. One is the great variability of caloric intake, which makes it difficult to detect correlations with the growth parameters. Another is the irregularity of growth curves of certain children, mainly the result of infectious disease. Infection, even asymptomatic, is highly prevalent at all ages with its anorexia, nutrient losses, and nutrient wastage, all of which interact with absorption of sufficient

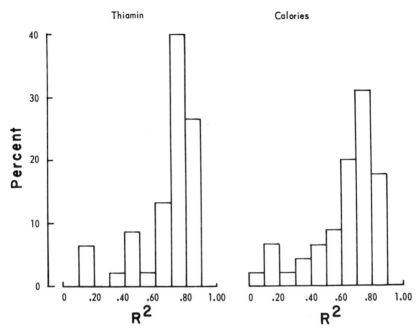

Figure 10.6a
Percentage distribution of R^2 values of the fitted curve for thiamine and calories, 45 cohort children, 1964-1972

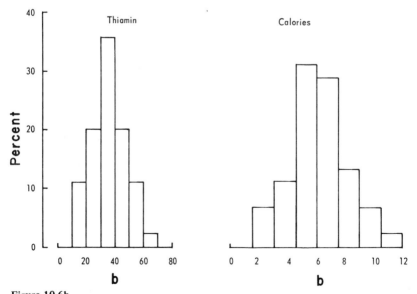

Figure 10.6b
Percentage distribution of b values of the fitted curve for thiamine and calories, 45 cohort children, 1964–1972

Table 10.9
Correlations Between Parameters of the Calorie and the Growth Curves, 44 Children, Birth to Age Three Years, 1964–1970

Parameters of calorie curve	Parameters of growth curve		
	a	b	c
a	−0.2415	−0.0302	−0.0790
b	0.2804	0.1850	0.0785
	$P \approx 0.05$		

calories and protein by the weanling and weaned child.* Finally, it should be recalled that in these studies the contribution of maternal milk to total intake was not measured.

The next step in the analysis was to remove "outliers" or cases with markedly different growth curves. On the basis of the histogram of R^2, only children with $R^2 \geqslant 0.6$ for calories and $R^2 \geqslant 0.93$ or $R^2 \geqslant 0.95$ for weight were included, which is to say that those children who showed a poor fitting of the caloric curve, the weight curve, or both, were excluded. The correlation coefficients of the comparisons are presented in table 10.10.

Only after removing the children with poor fittings did this analysis show any correlation between caloric intake and the linear term of the equation expressed in parameter b. In fact, only those curves with an $R^2 \geqslant 0.95$ were capable of revealing the association with caloric intake. The correlation with b and not with c was expected since supplemental foods are introduced after most of the period of growth deceleration has passed.

Other correlations investigated were between parameters of the caloric curve and newborn characteristics and age at weaning, shown in table 10.11. Birth weight showed some correlation with caloric intake, an observation that fits with the general concept that infants with greater birth weight tend to grow better than those with low birth weight. The other variables tested (birth length and head and thorax circumferences) yielded no significant correlation coefficients.

Breast-Feeding, Weaning, and Growth

A similar analysis was made using weaning age (in months) against the parameters of the growth curve. The correlation coefficients are given in table 10.12 and clearly show a significant association between growth and weaning (implying complete weaning) as follows: late weaning correlated with growth in the largest portion of the curve, expressed mainly in b, that is, after the rapid growth of the first months of life had ended. On the other hand, late

*In this regard, it would appear that a limited source of calories was not the primary reason for the calorie deficiency reported in the Costa Rican study (Valverde et al., 1975). Alternative explanations are cultural factors and infection with resultant reduced intakes.

Table 10.10
Correlations Between Parameters of the Calorie and the Growth Curves, Selected
Children Observed from Birth to Age Three Years, 1964-1970

Number of children	Restriction	Parameters of calorie curve	Parameters of growth curve		
			a	b	c
33	R^2 diet $\geqslant 0.6$ R^2 growth $\geqslant 0.93$	a	-0.2234	-0.1614	0.0804
		b	0.3230 $0.1 > P > 0.05$	0.3067 $0.1 > P > 0.05$	-0.0379
27	R^2 diet $\geqslant 0.6$ R^2 growth $\geqslant 0.95$	a	-0.0460	-0.1552	0.0251
		b	0.1563	0.3898 $0.05 > P > 0.02$	-0.0150

Table 10.11
Correlations Between Parameters of the Calorie and the Growth Curves, Selected
Children, Birth to Age Three Years, 1964-1970

Parameters of calorie curve	Birth weight	Gestational age	Age at weaning
a	-0.2673 $0.1 > P > 0.05$	-0.0980	-0.0791
b	0.2871 $P \approx 0.05$	0.0415	-0.0613

Table 10.12
Correlations Between Age at Weaning and the Parameters of Growth Curve, 38 Children,
Birth to Age Three Years, 1964-1970

Number of children	Restriction	Parameters		
		a	b	c
38	R^2 growth $\geqslant 0.93$	-0.3078 $0.1 > P > 0.05$	0.5369 $P < 0.001$	-0.4371 $0.01 > P > 0.005$
13	R^2 growth $\geqslant 0.93$ bw $< 2,501$ g	-0.3938 $P > 0.1$	0.6862 $0.005 > P > 0.001$	-0.5042 $0.1 > P > 0.05$
25	R^2 growth $\geqslant 0.93$ bw $\geqslant 2,501$ g	-0.2425 $P > 0.1$	0.4252 $0.05 > P > 0.02$	-0.3760 $0.1 > P > 0.05$

Table 10.13
Mean Weights of Cohorts of Children Weaned at Various Ages, 1964–1972

Age, months	Age at weaning, months						F	d.f.	P
	12-17	18-23	24-29	30-35	36-41	42-47			
0	2,682 ± 103[a]	2,665 ± 41	2,715 ± 45	2,652 ± 56	2,724 ± 170	2,617 ± 123	0.285	217	> 0.05
3	5,059 ± 154	5,197 ± 80	5,303 ± 83	4,970 ± 109	4,863 ± 256	4,520 ± 302	3.543	211	< 0.01
6	6,459 ± 141	6,398 ± 93	6,466 ± 93	6,130 ± 105	5,804 ± 361	5,766 ± 295	3.385	221	< 0.01
9	6,891 ± 213	6,969 ± 98	7,055 ± 92	6,610 ± 121	6,411 ± 394	6,444 ± 272	3.002	223	< 0.05
12	7,165 ± 281	7,241 ± 96	7,240 ± 97	6,871 ± 140	6,703 ± 332	6,656 ± 193	2.469	223	< 0.05
18	7,784 ± 291	7,901 ± 100	7,913 ± 110	7,613 ± 131	7,629 ± 227	7,347 ± 289	1.606	214	> 0.05
24	8,751 ± 444	8,617 ± 122	8,745 ± 120	8,590 ± 159	8,376 ± 256	8,194 ± 323	0.790	218	> 0.05
30	9,221 ± 500	9,489 ± 152	9,510 ± 144	9,621 ± 194	9,503 ± 339	9,277 ± 315	0.297	193	> 0.05
36	10,542 ± 467	10,278 ± 169	10,434 ± 157	10,419 ± 200	10,432 ± 152	10,370 ± 294	0.150	188	> 0.05
42	11,187 ± 427	11,189 ± 186	11,316 ± 191	11,366 ± 252	11,197 ± 239	11,059 ± 314	0.160	156	> 0.05

[a]Mean ± S.E., grams.

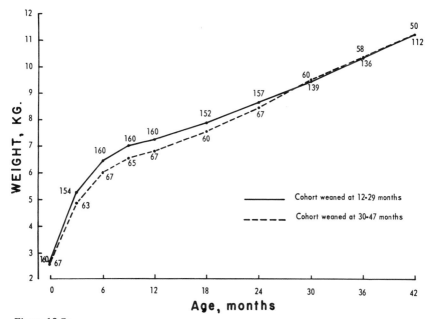

Figure 10.7a
Weight curves in the first 42 weeks, two cohorts of children defined by weaning age,
1964–1972

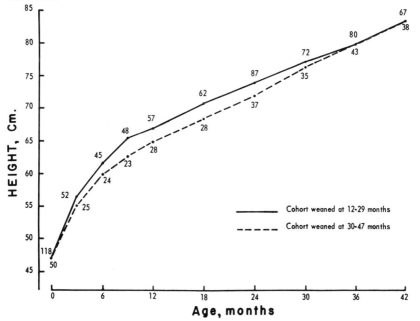

Figure 10.7b
Height curves in the first 42 weeks, two cohorts of children defined by weaning age,
1964–1972

weaning correlated inversely with parameter c, which reflects growth in the first months of life. In other words, it appears that infants growing faster in the first year of life are weaned earlier, while those growing more slowly are weaned later and tend to grow better in the late part of the breast-feeding period. This analysis was of 38 children after removing those with fittings yielding R^2 values of less than 0.93.

Further evidence supporting the observation that children growing faster in the first months are weaned earlier was obtained by computing the mean growth curves of all cohorts of the Cauqué study, defined by the age at which weaning was complete. Table 10.13 shows growth of six cohorts defined according to weaning age. Means and standard errors in grams were computed at the age intervals shown in the table. The groups had no observed differences at birth. By analysis of variance, increasing differences were detected at 3 to 12 months of age; thereafter differences were less and F values began to diminish till becoming insignificant. By 42 months of age the cohorts had the same average weight and linear growth. In view of the similarities between the first and second three cohorts, they were combined into two larger groups, as shown in figures 10.7a and b.

Analysis then revealed that children weaned earlier were indeed larger in the first year of life, while those weaned late had been smaller in the first year. Children weaned at 12 to 29 months had grown faster in the first year; once weaned, however, these children showed smaller growth velocities. Those weaned later at 30 to 47 months had a lower growth rate in the first year of life, but grew faster as weanlings. Both groups were virtually identical in weight and height at 42 months.

While weaning age is a complex maternal variable, strongly dependent on the child's growth, health, and behavior, as well as the influence of culture and behavior (Oberndorfer and Mejia, 1968; Sanjur et al., 1970), the high correlation demonstrated above between growth and weaning further suggests that biological phenomena are important in determining the length of breast-feeding. A hypothesis could also be advanced that infants growing faster in the first few months receive more maternal milk because their mothers have better health and nutrition, a situation that appears to influence fecundity because a new pregnancy occurs sooner than in women who breast-feed for longer periods. A smaller milk output, indicative of maternal malnutrition (Martínez and Chávez, 1971), could explain the slower growth rate of some children in the early months of lactation. Prolonged breast-feeding is more frequent in such cases along with an accompanying decreased fecundity, a finding also in agreement with increased fecundity of rural Mexican mal-nourished women who improved their nutrition (Chávez and Martínez, 1973).

Children weaned early were exposed to an obviously deficient solid diet, and their nutritional status deteriorated. Those still at the breast continued to receive a complement of maternal milk, which also contributed secretory IgA, lactoferrin, macrophages, and other resistance factors that constitute a defense mechanism against intestinal infection (Mata and Wyatt, 1971; Goldman and Smith, 1973). The result is faster growth of these children at later dates. As wholly weaned individuals, both groups eventually become similar in weight and height.

Although the benefits of prolonged breast-feeding on child growth and survival and as a mechanism for child-spacing are often limited by the nutrition-infection interaction exemplified by weanling diarrhea (Gordon et al., 1963; Scrimshaw et al., 1968a), breast-feeding is undoubtedly the single most important factor in assuring survival of low weight urban and village children. If sanitation and education were improved sufficiently to lower the risk of weanling diarrhea and other infectious diseases, growth and health of infants would increase without the provision of supplemental foods in addition to breast milk in the first year of life.

From the present analysis one could expect, even in the absence of proper education, a faster growth rate of infants in the first months of life through better maternal health and nutrition, abetted by earlier weaning or longer birth intervals. Education, however, is fundamental to ensure proper supplementary feeding of children weaned early and effective spacing of children through family planning measures.

An important consideration here is the extent to which biological and cultural phenomena of mother and child are interwoven in complex fashion. Modification of one factor may generate a favorable or an adverse effect on another characteristic. A multidisciplinary approach is crucial in the analysis of these problems, especially in decisions on interventions directed toward prevention and control.

Most prospective data on intestinal infection derives from the generally well-nourished infants and children of industrial nations. They have relatively low rates of infection compared to Cauqué children (Gelfand et al., 1958; Gelfand et al., 1963; Fox et al., 1966; Hall et al., 1970). Infection of Cauqué children, in fact, occurred from the moment of birth; the study discovered many neonatal infections with viruses, bacteria, and parasites. These recur throughout infancy and significantly affect the child's growth and development. This chapter will discuss colonization of the intestine, early invasion by pathogenic agents, and the various rates and significance of intestinal infections.

Colonization is defined here as the entry and replication of indigenous or autochthonous microbial species at any site of the intestinal tract. Indigenous and autochthonous microbes are generally nonpathogenic and constitute the normal microbial flora (Dubos et al., 1965). This term is applied to colonization by yeasts, bacteria, and mycoplasma, but not to protozoa, although there are some which behave similarly to indigenous microbes. Infection is the entry followed by development or replication of an infectious agent in the body. It can be inapparent (subclinical) or be associated with signs or symptoms, in which case the term infectious disease applies (APHA, 1970). An infected person is a carrier: a healthy carrier if no symptoms are manifest during the course of infection; a convalescent carrier if the individual continues to harbor the infectious agent after symptoms have disappeared.

Intestinal Colonization by Indigenous Microorganisms
Research on colonization was carried out in connection with the Cauqué study (Mata and Urrutia, 1971; Mata et al., 1971b; Mata et al., 1972a). Prospective observation of village newborns from birth until one year of age, in some instances until the second or third years, revealed that colonization with indigenous microbial species is readily accomplished and effectively maintained. It begins with exposure to fecal and skin bacteria during childbirth and is favored by defecation during parturition and by frequent skin-to-skin contact shortly after birth. Although some infectious agents have pathogenic properties, most are harmless or even beneficial to the newborn. They rapidly invade the skin, gastrointestinal tract, and other surfaces to constitute stable and persistent microflora, important as a defense mechanism (Rosebury, 1962; Dubos et al., 1963; Gorbach, 1971). Various studies have demonstrated a variety of factors in breast milk that promote certain kinds and concentrations of organisms, particularly bifidobacteria.

On the other hand, mothers living in unsanitary environments often harbor pathogenic organisms that are transferred to the infant during childbirth and thereafter in the same manner as the indigenous flora. In fact, the Cauqué study showed a high prevalence of maternal infection which likely accounts for enhanced antenatal infection in this population (Mata, 1974).

The Neonatal Period   The acquisition of bacteria by 30 breast-fed newborns was investigated during neonatal life. The plate dilution technique was used to estimate numbers of aerobic, facultative, and anaerobic bacteria detectable in concentrations of at least 10^4 per gram of wet feces. The counts were approximated to the nearest log. Bacteria occasionally were cultivated from meconium as early as 4 hours after birth; 6 of 9 samples passed 4 to 7 hours after birth contained facultative bacteria, mainly micrococci, streptococci, and enterobacteriaceae.

The pattern in which bacteria appear in the course of the first four weeks is seen in figure 11.1. The fecal flora for the first two days of life consisted of streptococci, clostridia, bifidobacteria, and facultative gram-negative bacilli. Half of the infants had *Escherichia coli* within the first 24 hours of life at concentrations of 10^8 to 10^{11} bacilli per gram of wet feces. Bifidobacteria appeared in a few infants on the first day of life, but by the second day cultures of a third showed these bacilli. By the end of the first week, bifidobacteria proliferated to outnumber all other bacteria; the feces of all infants had concentrations that ranged from 10^9 to 10^{11} per gram.

Eighty-three percent of infants showed anaerobic streptococci within the first day at concentrations of 10^6 to 10^{10} per gram. By the second day the counts were of 10^9 to 10^{11} per gram. Streptococci and *E. coli*, present in greater numbers than bifidobacteria during the early days of life, decreased

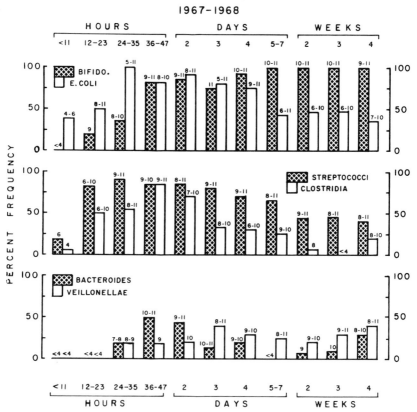

Figure 11.1
Frequency of bacterial groups in meconium and feces collected during neonatal periods, 1967–1968 (from Mata and Urrutia, 1971). Numbers above columns indicate range of bacterial counts as reciprocal of $\log_{10}$ per gram of wet meconium or feces.

by the end of the neonatal period to low frequencies. When found, however, the concentrations were from 10^7 to 10^{11} per gram. Clostridia appeared in a few infants from the first day of life; high titers were obtained on the second day, but few infants excreted bacilli thereafter.

By the end of the first week all breast-fed babies had a simple flora almost wholly of bifidobacteria in concentrations of the order of 10^{11} per gram of wet feces, while the average concentration of *E. coli* was several logs less. The flora remained in this state during exclusive breast-feeding, that is to say, from birth to about three months.

A few infants were colonized by bacteroides and veillonellae during the first weeks of life, with initial appearance usually after the second day. Bacteroides and veillonellae were not frequent in breast-fed neonates, but concentrations when demonstrated ranged from 10^8 to 10^{11}.

Table 11.1
Frequency of Bacterial Groups, 262 Fecal Samples of Healthy Infants, First Nine
Months of Life, 1967–1968

Bacterial group	Lowest concentration detected	Samples positive	
		Number	Percentage
Bifidobacteria		258	98.5
Veillonellae		157	59.9
Streptococci		152	58.0
Bacteroides	8^a	75	28.6
Lactobacilli		27	10.3
Clostridia		17	6.5
Micrococci	4^a	255	97.3
Enterobacteriaceae	4^a	233	88.9
Enterococci	6^a	184	70.2

^{a}Log$_{10}$ of bacterial concentration per gram of wet feces.

The Postneonatal Period   To gauge the changes after the first 4 weeks the frequency of bacteria in 12 breast-fed infants was studied throughout the first 9 months of life, as shown in table 11.1. Bifidobacteria were regularly the most frequent and numerous bacterial group in concentrations of 10^{10} to 10^{11} per gram. Streptococci, veillonellae, and bacteroides became prominent, increasing to concentrations of 10^8 per gram or more with age so that they were present in more than 75 percent of infants observed for one year. The relative frequency of the various bacterial groups is presented in table 11.2 for 12 infants whose feces were cultured fortnightly during the first year of life. Results apply only to periods of good health.

Enterobacteriaceae and other aerobic or facultative bacteria were normally present in each age group in concentrations two to three logs below that of bifidobacteria. The relative concentration of the facultative component increased particularly during weeks 13 to 16 and 21 to 32. Facultatives were almost exclusively enterobacteriaceae, of which *E. coli* predominated.

Concentrations of at least 10^6 *E. coli* were not common before two months, but thereafter titers of 10^6 and 10^{10} were usual and this bacterial group was present in all infants at all examinations. Other gram-negative facultative bacterial groups such as Providence and *Klebsiella-Enterobacter* were found in high titers. Lactobacilli and clostridia were relatively rare. *Proteus* was rare, and *Pseudomonas* was consistently absent. The anaerobic component of the flora, however, always outnumbered the aerobic by two to three logs, although the differences were less marked after the first year.

Similarities in flora among individuals are illustrated in table 11.3. Total bacterial counts for three pairs of twins were studied during the first two

Table 11.2
Fecal Bacterial Flora in Breast-Fed Children and in Adults, 1967–1971

Bacterial group	12 breast-fed children				12 weanlings (2 to 3 years old)	12 adults (13 to 37 years old)
	5–8 weeks	13–16 weeks	21–24 weeks	45–48 weeks		
Bifidobacteria	11.1[a] (31/31)†	11.4 (24/24)	11.6 (22/23)	11.0 (13/13)	10.6 (12/12)	9.4 (9/12)
Bacteroides	9.6 (6/31)	10.3 (6/24)	10.2 (11/23)	9.9 (10/13)	9.2 (10/12)	10.3 (12/12)
Total anaerobes	11.5	11.6	11.6	11.2	11.0	10.5
Total aerobes	8.0	8.8	9.2	9.3	9.0	8.8
Ratio $\frac{\text{anaerobes}}{\text{aerobes}}$	$\frac{3160}{1}$	$\frac{630}{1}$	$\frac{250}{1}$	$\frac{79}{1}$	$\frac{100}{1}$	$\frac{50}{1}$
% anaerobes in total	> 99.9	> 99.8	99.7	98.8	99	98

[a] Average $\log_{10}$ of bacterial counts per gram of wet feces; below, (number of cultures with 10^8 or more of the bacterial groups/total number of cultures).

years of life with specimens collected monthly except when the subjects were ill. The small standard deviations indicate the stability of bacterial populations throughout many months of observation. This was also true when microbial groups were examined individually, although differences were apparent among infants (table 11.4). Twin 327 showed veillonellae regularly during the first 32 weeks of life at concentrations of at least 10^6 per gram, whereas Twin 328, of the same pair, showed fewer of this group of anaerobes. The first twin became negative for veillonellae, but again presented as positive in the 60th and 68th weeks of life but not thereafter during the succeeding 14 weeks. The other twin, not demonstrably colonized by veillonellae during the first 75 weeks of life, excreted these bacteria in significant numbers (more than 10^6 per gram) for approximately 4 months after the initial 75 weeks of absence (Mata et al., 1972a). It should be noted that this and other bacterial groups probably are present at all times under normal conditions, but in concentrations so low as to preclude their demonstration by the usual laboratory methods.

Similar findings were observed regarding bacteroides, streptococci, *E. coli*, and enterococci in this and other pairs of twins. The ratio of concentration of anaerobes to facultatives, as well as the predominance of certain anaerobes, however, remained rather constant in each pair.

Shift of Fecal Flora of the Breast-Fed Child to an Adult Type   The indigenous flora of the breast-fed infant from birth to about three months consists virtually of the gram-positive nonpathogenic bacilli, bifidobacteria, and eubacteria, both with unique metabolic and biologic properties that act

Table 11.3
Fecal Bacterial Flora in Three Pairs of Twins, First Two Years of Life, 1967–1971

Twin	Anaerobes	Facultatives
302	10.9 ± 0.6 (21)[a]	9.6 ± 1.0 (22)
	(9–11)	(6–10)
303	10.9 ± 0.5 (21)	9.6 ± 0.7 (22)
	(10–11)	(8–10)
498	10.7 ± 0.7 (20)	9.3 ± 0.9 (20)
	(9–11)	(7–10)
499	10.8 ± 0.6 (19)	9.1 ± 1.1 (19)
	(9–11)	(6–10)
327	10.5 ± 0.5 (18)	9.7 ± 0.8 (18)
	(10–11)	(9–11)
328	10.9 ± 0.3 (18)	9.3 ± 0.8 (18)
	(10–11)	(8–10)

[a]Mean ± S.D. of $\log_{10}$ bacterial counts (number of specimens examined). Specimens corresponded to periods of health. Below, (range of bacterial counts).

against intestinal infection and other varieties of stress. Undoubtedly, the marked resistance to pathogens such as *shigellae* and *salmonellae* during this time is related to this prevailing type of flora (Mata and Urrutia, 1971) as well as to immune properties of breast milk (Mata and Wyatt, 1971; Wyatt et al., 1972).

The indigenous intestinal microbiota of the breast-fed child provides protection for several months, but the mechanism begins to fade when supplemental foods are offered and a resulting shift in flora follows. Since supplementary foods are frequently handled by dirty hands and exposed to water usually polluted with *Escherichia coli* and frequently with enteric pathogens, parasites, bacteria, and viruses also are introduced with ensuing disease. With regular and progressive food supplementation and establishment of a solid diet and eventual weaning, the anaerobic gram-negative and non-sporulated bacilli (bacteroides groups) appeared more frequently and in greater numbers, to eventually outnumber the other bacterial groups.

The flora of breast-fed infants, weaned children, and adults of the area were compared in table 11.2. Nearly 100 percent of all identifiable bacteria from breast-fed infants were bifidobacteria. During weaning there was a decrease by one log in the concentration of anaerobes and a proliferation of bacteroides. In the adult these two organisms were encountered more frequently than bifidobacteria and outnumbered all other bacterial groups. The transition from one type of flora to another is a slow and subtle process that begins with supplementation of maternal milk and continues throughout the prolonged weaning period usual in this region. Weaning is characterized by an increased frequency of diarrheal disease (Gordon et al., 1963).

Table 11.4
Fecal Bacterial Groups and Relative Frequency in Three Pairs of Twins, First Two Years of Life, 1967–1971

Group	Lowest concentration detected	Twin 302 N = 22[a]	Twin 303	Twin 498 N = 20	Twin 499	Twin 327 N = 18	Twin 328
Bifidobacteria	9	10.7 ± 0.7 (91)[b]	10.7 ± 0.7 (91)	10.4 ± 0.6 (90)	10.6 ± 0.7 (100)	10.8 ± 0.6 (83)	11.0 (94)
Bacteroides	7	10.2 ± 0.6 (77)	10.4 ± 0.5 (73)	10.2 ± 1.1 (80)	10.4 ± 0.6 (74)	10.6 ± 0.5 (94)	10.6 ± 0.5 (89)
Streptococci	8	10.1 ± 0.8 (82)	10.1 ± 0.7 (73)	9.9 ± 0.7 (80)	9.9 ± 0.5 (74)	10.0 ± 0.4 (94)	10.4 ± 0.5 (83)
Veillonellae	8	9.8 ± 0.8 (55)	9.8 ± 0.7 (50)	9.6 ± 0.7 (55)	10.1 ± 0.4 (42)	9.6 ± 0.8 (94)	10.4 ± 0.9 (28)
Enterococci	6	8.1 ± 1.0 (82)	7.6 ± 1.3 (82)	7.9 ± 1.0 (75)	7.9 ± 1.2 (74)	8.4 ± 1.3 (83)	8.7 ± 1.2 (94)
Escherichia coli	6	9.1 ± 1.0 (91)	9.3 ± 0.5 (82)	8.8 ± 1.0 (100)	9.2 ± 0.8 (89)	9.5 ± 0.8 (94)	8.7 ± 1.2 (100)

[a]N = number of specimens examined; specimens corresponded to periods of health.
[b]Mean ± S.D. of $\log_{10}$ bacterial count (percentage of specimens positive in total examined).

Table 11.5
Parasites in Meconium and Feces, First Week of Life, 1964–1966

Child number	Age, days	Parasitic form[a]
12	1	E. histolytica (c); E. nana (c)
	4	E. histolytica (c); E. nana (c)
	5[b]	E. coli (c)
23	1	E. coli (c); E. nana (c); E. hominis (t)
186	3	E. coli (c, t); E. nana (c, t); C. mensinili (t); G. lamblia (c, t)
	5	E. nana (c, t)
42	4	G. lamblia (t)
172	4	E. nana (c)
175	4	G. lamblia (c)
80	4	G. lamblia (c)
9	6	E. coli (c); E. nana (c)
49	6	I. bütschlii (c)

[a] c = cyst; t = trophozoite.
[b] This child had diarrhea in the second week of life, but the cause remains unknown. The other infants were free of gastrointestinal symptoms.

Early Invasion by Pathogens

The newborn infant is usually considered pathogen-free, a concept largely derived from hospital practice in industrialized countries despite colonization there by pathogenic *Staphylococcus aureus*. Nevertheless, considering the unsanitary environment that surrounds the Cauqué mother and infant and the frequency with which the mother is infected concurrently with pathogenic bacteria, it is not surprising that invasion of the newborn by pathogenic microorganisms occurs rather promptly.

The Cauqué study, by collection of fecal specimens on the day of birth, was able to demonstrate with much frequency early infections with parasites, bacteria, and viruses. Table 11.5 shows parasitic forms in feces in the first week of life. Nine infants among 192 (4.7 percent) excreted some form of one or more species of a variety of protozoa, two infants as early as the first day of life. In five instances the infectious agent was of recognized pathogenic properties, either *Entamoeba histolytica* or *Giardia lamblia*.

The usual course of these infections, however, was almost invariably asymptomatic. The parasitic forms detected were primarily cysts and the presence of parasites in the intestine was short-lived, although a number were detected on a single day. Furthermore, cysts generally showed signs of degeneration, despite prompt processing of fecal specimens in the field. This suggests that some infections were spurious, that is to say, they represented no more than simple transit through the gut of parasitic forms presumably ingested with feces during delivery. On the other hand, trophozoites of *Enteromonas hominis* were discovered in a child on the first day of life, a circumstance, along with shedding of trophozoites of *G. lamblia, Chilomastix mesnili, Endolimax nana*, and *E. coli* by other children, suggesting actual multiplication of the agent in the infant gut. Because such infections do not appear to establish themselves and are asymptomatic, breast milk stands out as the factor directly or indirectly responsible for the observed resistance. Indeed, when weaning begins and the maternal milk-mediated resistance weakens and eventually fades, infection tends to become firmly established with entrance of an infectious agent, as does infectious disease.

Similarly pathogenic enterobacteriaceae may invade early in life. In three cases of *Shigella* infection during the first week of life one was detected in the feces the first day of life, one on the second day, and one on the third and fifth day, although there were no clinical manifestations. Enteropathogenic *E. coli* 0119:B4 (*EEC*) was detected in another case on the third day and was also asymptomatic. The rate of *Shigella* infection in the first week of life was 1.6 per 100 infants and that of *EEC* only 0.5. While *Shigella* infection in Santa María was remarkably more frequent than in industrial societies, rates for *EEC* were negligible. This contrasting behavior seemingly relates to a village ecosystem that permits a high dosage of *Shigella* organisms, but with enteropathogenic *E. coli* (a nosocomial bacterium) a rarity. Transient excretion of these bacilli with absence of symptoms appears to relate again to the practice of breast-feeding. Clinical neonatal infections appeared when nursing was inadequate and supplemental foods were not given (Mata et al., 1969c).

With regard to viruses, table 11.6 summarizes early excretion of enteroviruses, again at a frequency greater than in industrial nations. The observed rates, however, are similar to those in Toluca, Mexico (Sabin et al., 1960) where environmental conditions also were poor and to some extent similar to Santa María Cauqué.

Because the replication cycle of enteroviruses is rapid and highly lytic, virus shedding may begin 24 hours after invasion, as has been demonstrated for live attenuated polioviruses (Gelfand et al., 1959). This may not hold for all enteroviruses, because the infecting dose of enteroviruses to which village infants are exposed in early life could be smaller than that of poliovirus vaccine. Infections of the first day, particularly those showing high titers, suggest a congenital origin, an event favored by premature delivery, recognized or unrecognized rupture of membranes, maternal illness, and prolonged labor. Enterovirus infections demonstrated 48 hours after birth are arbitrarily considered postnatal but may indeed be of antenatal origin as well as those of the third day of life. The whole area of perinatal infection in populations with low standards of living deserves further investigation to clarify the precise time when these early infections occur.

Table 11.6
Viruses in Meconium and Feces, First Three Days of Life, 1964–1966

Day of life	Number of children tested	Number positive (percentage)	Child number	Virus isolated	Viral concentration, $\log_{10}$ $TCID_{50}$ per gram
1	79	1 (1.3)	264	Echo 7	2
2	54	4 (7.4)	66	Echo 6	3
			70	Echo 6	3
			82	Echo 6	3
			166	Polio 1	5
3	61	5 (8.2)	63	Polio 1, Echo 6	4
			162	Echo 9	5
			171	Echo 11	5
			251	Echo 7	5
			296	Echo 6	5

Rates of Intestinal Infection

The Cauqué study revealed overwhelming rates for enteric bacteria, parasites, and viruses (Mata et al., 1967b; Mata, 1969). The common occurrence of infection with toxigenic *E. coli* (Gorbach, 1973), and with other varieties of infectious agents possessing specific pathogenic properties, is expected. A similar behavior occurs in respect to infectious agents of the skin, the rhino-oro-pharynx, the mucosae of the external genitalia and the respiratory tract, confirmed by prospective isolation and serological studies of populations of low socioeconomic development (Kloene et al., 1970; Ota and Bang, 1972; Monto and Johnson, 1967; Olson et al., 1973).

One way to fully appreciate the intensity of intestinal infection in this region is to examine its natural history in individual children (Mata, 1969). Figure 11.2 shows excretion of viruses in feces for 18 of the cohort children, determined by weekly cultures made during the first three years of life. Due to a faster replication cycle of enteroviruses, the isolation rate of adenoviruses was probably less than actual fact; the recovery rate likely would be greater after blocking of enteroviruses with specific sera (Parks et al., 1967). Figure 11.2 shows individual variations in the pattern of excretion, but overall, virus shedding was extremely frequent in the first year of life and even more extensive in the second and third years (Mata et al., 1972c).

Equally illustrative is the natural history of parasitic infections for two children during a part of their second year (table 11.7). The common occurrence of parasitic infection and of such multiple infections in a single person suggests that the risk of invasion from environmental sources must be extremely high, a consideration of import for public health measures directed toward community dosage and means of transmission.

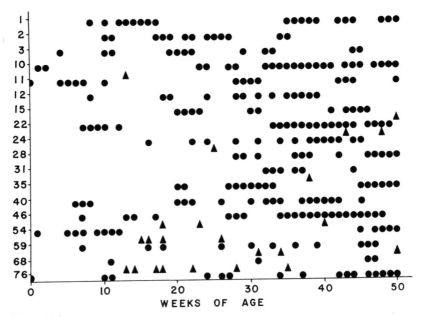

Figure 11.2
Enteroviruses and adenoviruses isolated by weekly cultures from feces of 18 infants,
1964–1967 (from Mata et al., 1972c). Circles show enteroviruses; triangles show adenoviruses.

Parasites   Percent prevalence of parasites was calculated by dividing the
number of specimens with a demonstrated parasite by the number of fecal
samples examined over a three-month period. Only one specimen per child
per week was tabulated. When more than one specimen was collected within
a week, only the first finding was entered into the tabulations; specimens of
the sixth or seventh day of life represented the first week.

Incidence rates were computed through specimen examinations made in
specific weeks during the first year of life, or alternatively, within periods of
six months. Children once demonstrated as infected were counted only once
within a particular period. Similar criteria were used to calculate prevalence
and incidence rates of bacteria and viruses.

Prevalence rates for parasites with pathogenic and presumed nonpathogenic potential are presented in table 11.8. Prevalences for the first three
months of life were comparatively low and to an extent reflected the heavy
exposure of the infant to fecal contamination during childbirth (Melvin and
Mata, 1971). Rates thereafter remained low, or even decreased, presumably
attributable to the particular intestinal milieu associated with breast-feeding.
For instance, the percentage prevalence of *E. histolytica* dropped from 1.3
percent in the second trimester of life, to 0 at the end of the first year. Other

Table 11.7
Six-Month Experience with Parasitic Infection, 2 Cohort Children, Beginning at Age
18 Months, 1965–1966

Child 3			Child 11		
Date		Parasite	Date		Parasite
Nov.	24–1965	*Giardia*	Mar.	25–1966	*Giardia*
	29–	*Giardia*		28–	*Giardia*
Dec.	16–	*Giardia*	Apr.	3–	*Giardia*
					Entamoeba coli
Jan.	12–1966	*Giardia*		20–	*Giardia*
	17–	*Giardia*			
	24–	*Endolimax*	May	5–	*Giardia*
				10–	*Giardia*
Feb.	1–	Negative		25–	Negative
	12–	*Entamoeba coli*		31–	*Giardia*
		Ascaris			*Ascaris*
	15–	*Ascaris*			
			June	6–	*Endolimax*
Mar.	1–	*Giardia*			*Iodamoeba*
		Ascaris			*Chilomastix*
	7–	*Giardia*		14–	*Giardia*
	8–	*Entamoeba coli*		22–	Negative
		Endolimax		28–	*Entamoeba hartmanni*
		Giardia			*Endolimax*
		Ascaris			*Chilomastix*
	9–	*Giardia*			
		Ascaris	July	7–	*Entamoeba coli*
	19–	*Entamoeba coli*			*Ascaris*
		Ascaris		12–	*Ascaris*
	27–	*Giardia*			*Hymenolepis nana*
		Ascaris		20–	*Entamoeba hartmanni*
	31–	*Giardia*			*Entamoeba coli*
					Endolimax
Apr.	4–	*Giardia*			*Chilomastix*
	19–	*Ascaris*			*Ascaris*
	26–	*Ascaris*			
		Giardia	Aug.	8–	*Entamoeba histolytica*
					Iodamoeba
					Trichomonas
					Giardia
					Ascaris
					Hymenolopis nana

Table 11.8
Prevalence of Pathogenic and Nonpathogenic Intestinal Parasites, by Percentage of Positive Specimens per Trimester, 45 Cohort Children, Birth to Age Three Years, 1964–1970

Years	Months	Number of specimens[a]	Intestinal parasites with pathogenic potential				Intestinal parasites with presumed nonpathogenic potential						
			Entamoeba histolytica	Giardia lamblia	Ascaris lumbricoides	Trichuris trichiura	Entamoeba hartmanni	Entamoeba coli	Endolimax nana	Iodamoeba bütschlii	Trichomonas hominis	Chilomastix mesnili	Hymenolepis nana
0	0	471	0.21[b]	0.21	0.21	0	0.21[b]	2.34	4.03	2.34	0.42	0.85	0
	3	556	1.26	2.16	0.36	0.18	0	1.98	3.06	2.16	0.54	0.72	0
	6	569	0.18	3.69	0.53	0.18	0	0.18	0.53	1.23	0	0.53	0
	9	578	0	8.13	1.21	0.17	0.17	0.87	0.52	0.52	0.52	0.35	0
1	12	549	0.73	12.57	9.29	0	0.91	1.09	1.28	0.55	1.09	1.09	0
	15	554	0.90	15.52	27.26	1.62	0.72	3.79	0.90	1.62	0.54	2.17	0
	18	573	1.57	15.53	34.55	3.49	1.75	7.85	2.97	2.44	1.57	2.79	0
	21	566	2.47	17.14	33.04	4.77	1.24	10.78	4.59	3.00	1.77	5.83	0.53
2	24	559	4.47	17.53	54.74	5.19	3.39	18.75	6.25	4.11	3.04	6.79	3.21
	27	545	7.52	19.82	26.54	6.24	4.95	24.04	11.74	8.07	4.40	10.46	4.95
	30	538	9.11	18.77	69.54	4.28	7.25	30.86	15.06	11.52	5.02	17.29	2.97
	33	525	6.86	22.10	69.71	3.81	7.81	33.90	16.38	11.43	7.62	13.14	1.71
3	36	298	10.40	19.13	77.85	3.02	6.64	35.94	20.31	17.97	10.55	11.72	2.34

[a]The study aimed at collecting weekly specimens from all children from birth to age three years.
[b]Percentage positive specimens in trimester.

Table 11.9
Frequency of Multiple Parasitic Infections, by Specific Age Intervals, 45 Cohort Children, Birth to Age Three Years, 1964-1969

Number of parasitic species	Age, weeks					
	25 (N = 45)[a]	51 (N = 45)	77 (N = 45)	103 (N = 45)	129 (N = 43)	155 (N = 42)
1	1	9	21	16	13	13
2	1	1	2	11	8	10
3				1	9	8
4			1	2	2	4
5					3	3
6				1		3
7					1	
8						
9					1	
10					1	
1+	2	10	24	31	38	41
0	43	35	21	14	5	1

[a]N = number of children.

parasites apparently were restricted during the first year of life. *Giardia* presents an exception, in that prevalence increased steadily with age to reach a ratio of 8 percent by the end of the first year.

The second year of life undoubtedly marked a greatly increased occurrence of intestinal parasitism because all rates passed those of the first year by a third and sometimes were doubled or tripled. Although rates in general were still greater in the third year, the degree of change from second to third year was less than from the first to the second.

The high prevalence suggests that most children become infected and thereby contribute to perpetuation of parasite frequency and parasite transmission in the ecosystem. Confirmatory evidence derives from incidence rates for intestinal parasites, estimated for selected weeks at regular intervals as shown in table 11.9. While only 2 cohort infants had 1 parasite at the 25th week of life, 10 were so infected by one or another species at week 51. At week 103, 31 of the cohort children were infected. The burden of infection is reflected in the number of multiple parasitic infections.

Infections with two different parasites became frequent in the second year (table 11.10). The third year, however, was characterized by still more frequent infections with multiple species: one child had 7, one 9, and another 10 different parasites at the specified week of life.

A more illustrative way to demonstrate incidence is to calculate rates for individual parasites for whole periods; for instance, table 11.10 shows

Table 11.10
Incidence of Parasitic Infections, by Six-Month Intervals, 45 Cohort Children, Birth to
Age Three Years, 1964–1969

| Parasite | Age, months | | | | | |
	0–5	6–11	12–17	18–23	24–29	30–35
E. histolytica	5[a]	0 (5)[b]	6 (11)	9 (20)	12 (32)	5 (37)
E. coli	17	2 (19)	7 (26)	8 (34)	6 (40)	2 (42)
D. fragilis	0	3 (3)	1 (4)	1 (5)	1 (6)	5 (11)
G. lamblia	8	13 (21)	14 (35)	4 (39)	1 (40)	2 (42)
A. lumbricoides	4	9 (13)	14 (27)	14 (41)	1 (42)	0 (42)
T. trichiura	2	2 (4)	4 (8)	6 (14)	3 (17)	3 (20)
H. nana	0	0	0	1	3 (4)	2 (6)

[a]Number of children with parasite.
[b](Accumulated number of children with parasite).

numbers of children who had experienced infections at various ages by six-month intervals. For example, 5 different children had acquired E. histolytica within the first six months after birth; no more children were added during the second semester, but six others became infected in the third semester, thus raising the incidence to 24.4 percent with 11 positive among 45 children. Within an initial three years all children had experienced at least one infection of Giardia and Ascaris, 80 percent had been infected by E. histolytica and 44 percent by Trichuris.

Due to altitude and other peculiarities of the village habitat there were no indigenous hookworm infections. Schistosoma and Trichinella are unknown to the region. Other parasites identified in low frequencies are shown in table 11.11. The few instances of Enterobius are merely mentioned here since examination of feces is not the preferred method to investigate this common parasite. INCAP studies in Central America have revealed that Dientamoeba is common, especially in El Salvador (Mata, 1969). In the village 8 children were infected with this parasite, more than a half in association with other protozoa; 3 had frank diarrhea in the absence of other potential pathogens (table 11.12).

Bacteria Shigellae were the preponderant enteropathogens; they appeared among village children with three to four times the frequency as did salmonellae and enteropathogenic E. coli combined (Mata et al., 1969b). They are the most important known agents of diarrheal disease. They also provide

Table 11.11
Infection with Uncommon Intestinal Parasites, 45 Cohort Children, Birth to Age Three Years, 1964–1969

Parasite	Child number	Age, weeks	Month of year	Observations
Entamoeba polecki	80	121	February	cysts
Enteromonas hominis	23	1	October	trophozoites
	22	92	July	trophozoites
	24	128	April	trophozoites
Strongyloides stercoralis	40	58	March	larvae
	69	129	February	larvae
	83	124	March	larvae
	23	147	August	larvae
	52	145	February	larvae
Taenia spp.	28	139	June	eggs
	79	146	July	eggs
	202	48	November	eggs
	197	53	November	eggs

Table 11.12
Dientamoeba Fragilis Infections, 45 Cohort Children, Birth to Age Three Years, 1964–1969

Child number	Age, weeks	Month of diagnosis	Gastrointestinal symptoms	Other parasites in specimen
50	28	October	None	None
34	31	July	None	None
22	34	June	Diarrhea	None
80	56	November	None	*E. hartmanni, E. coli, E. nana, I. bütschlii*
2	85	October	Diarrhea	None
68	123	January	None	*E. nana, I. bütschlii, Ascaris*
49	130	September	None	*E. hartmanni, T. hominis, Giardia*
45	133	September	Diarrhea	*E. hartmanni, E. coli, E. nana, I. bütschlii, Ch. mesnili, Giardia*

Table 11.13
Shigellae Isolated, by Year, 45 Cohort Children, 1964–1969

Shigella subgroup	1964	1965	1966	1967	1968	1969	Total
S. dysenteriae							
1	0	0	0	0	0	1	1
2	0	1	72	88	20	0	181
3	0	1	0	1	0	1	3
Total *S. dysenteriae*	0	2	72	89	20	2	185
S. flexneri							
1	0	7	1	0	10	0	18
2	0	3	17	21	16	90	147
3	0	4	12	6	9	25	56
4	0	0	0	233	36	7	276
5	0	0	0	8	0	0	8
6	0	0	100	56	71	5	232
Total *S. flexneri*	0	14	130	324	142	127	737
S. boydii							
1	0	6	2	1	4	0	13
2	0	0	10	0	16	1	27
3	0	0	0	4	0	0	4
4	0	0	5	0	0	7	12
5	0	0	8	0	0	0	8
Total *S. boydii*	0	6	25	5	20	8	64
S. sonnei	0	2	3	21	12	8	46
Total all *Shigella* serotypes	0	24	230	439	194	144	1,032

the best index of sanitation in any given community (Hollister et al., 1955; Van Zijl, 1966).

Because the cohort children who provide the supportive evidence of prevalence and incidence were recruited one by one as they were born, the interpretation of data necessarily is in terms of the experience of the aging cohort.

Table 11.13 shows the 15 different *Shigella* serotypes that infected the cohort during the first three years of life. As noted before (Beck et al., 1957; Mata, 1957; Gordon et al., 1962) *Shigella flexneri* was the most common with 71 percent of all isolates, followed by *S. dysenteriae* and *S. sonnei*. This epidemiological relation is neither stable nor fixed. *S. flexneri* 6 and other serotypes were more prevalent in the village in other years (Gordon et al., 1962). More shigellae were isolated in 1967 than in any other year, but the findings were those of an aging cohort; the isolations were expectedly fewer

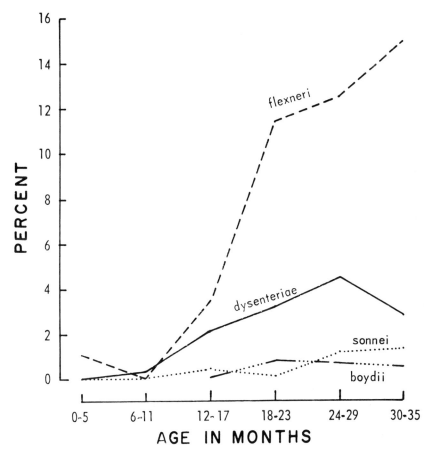

Figure 11.3
Percentage of prevalence of *Shigella* cases and carriers, by age, 45 cohort children, birth to age three years, 1964-1969

in the first year of life. Furthermore, data collected after children were three years old were not tabulated.

   The epidemiological contribution of the cohort in terms of *Shigella* infection (cases and carriers) is set forth in figure 11.3, where the most common serotypes are plotted as a function of age. The number of infections rose abruptly in the second year of life and continued at high levels in the third. The extensive contribution of the *flexneri* and *dysenteriae* subgroups is evident. Figure 11.4 illustrates the epidemic curves of the most frequent serotypes isolated from cases and carriers, with evidence of serious outbreaks of *S. flexneri* 4 in 1967, *S. flexneri* 6 in 1966 and 1967-68, *S. flexneri* 2 in 1969, and *S. dysenteriae* 2 in 1966-67.

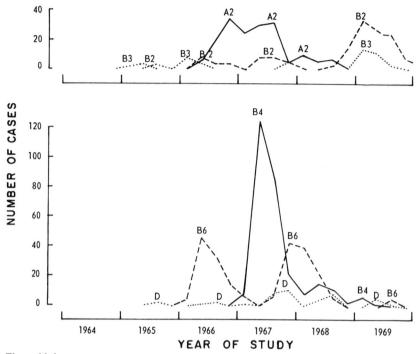

Figure 11.4
Outbreaks of *Shigella*, cases and carriers, 45 cohort children, birth to age three years, 1964-1969. Few *Shigella* were isolated during the first year of life; as the cohort aged, infections increased. Outbreaks of *S. flexneri* 4, *S. flexneri* 6, *S. dysenteriae* 2, and *S. flexneri* 2 were more prominent.

In 1969 a serious epidemic of Shiga dysentery (*S. dysenteriae* 1) began in Guatemala, involved the whole country, and spread that same year to adjoining nations to become one of the largest regional epidemics ever recorded (Mata et al., 1970; Gangarosa et al., 1970). Before this outbreak the Shiga bacillus had been found sporadically in isolated instances (Beck et al., 1957; Mata et al., 1964). A long protracted epidemic of acute diarrheal disease in Santa María Cauqué with a component of Shiga dysentery was recorded in 1960 to 1961 (Gordon et al., 1965b) but that part of the outbreak ended rather promptly, and during the subsequent eight years *S. dysenteriae* type 1 was not found despite systematic and continued study of the childhood population. The 1969 regional epidemic reached Santa María Cauqué, but only one of the 45 cohort children became ill with Shiga dysentery in the first three years of life (table 11.13).

These data show how an entire cohort of susceptibles meets the challenge of such a variety of serotypes resulting in much infection and evidently an enlarged community dosage. It must be realized, however, that cohorts of

Table 11.14
Prevalence of *Shigella* Infection, Six-Month Intervals, 45 Cohort Children, Birth to Age
Three Years, 1964–1969

Shigella subgroup	Age intervals, months					
	0–5 (N = 1,105)[a]	6–11 (N = 1,131)	12–17 (N = 1,105)	18–23 (N = 1,131)	24–29 (N = 1,090)	30–35 (N = 1,071)
Dysenteriae	1 (0.09)[b]	3 (0.27)	24 (2.17)	37 (3.27)	50 (4.59)	41 (3.83)
Flexneri	13 (1.18)	0	39 (3.53)	132 (11.67)	140 (12.84)	165 (15.41)
Boydii	0	1 (0.09)	9 (0.81)	9 (0.80)	6 (0.55)	17 (1.59)
Sonnei	1 (0.09)	0	3 (0.27)	1 (0.09)	12 (1.10)	14 (1.31)
All	15 (1.36)	4 (0.35)	75 (6.79)	179 (15.83)	208 (19.08)	237 (22.13)

[a]N = number of cultures.
[b]Number of *Shigella* strains isolated (percentage of prevalence).

children born before and after the 45 cohort children also are contributing to the total complex picture of transmission of infection and disease in the village.

Prevalence rates of *Shigella*, at age intervals of six months, are given in table 11.14. Prevalence in the first six months of life was 1.36 percent, composed mainly of neonatal infections. Prevalence dropped to 0.35 percent in the second half of the first year, a circumstance to be taken as evidence of the marked resistance to most infections possessed by breast-fed children. Such resistance appears to be effective for pathogenic enterobacteriaceae and protozoa and to a lesser extent for enteroviruses.

The highest prevalence of *Shigella* occurred at the end of the second year of life and during the third year when weaning was under way and as it neared completion. The *flexneri* and *dysenteriae* subgroups contributed the majority of isolates and behaved as described before. Arbitrarily, a second demonstration of the same serotype after an absence of at least two weeks following the initial finding was sufficient to recognize a new infection in a particular child. This permitted computation of incidence rates of infection, cases and carriers included. Incidence rates of *Shigella* and *EEC* shown in table 11.15 clearly indicate that *Shigella* has the more important role in the village epidemiology of enteric infection. Rates of *EEC* and *Salmonella* consistently were lower than those of *Shigella*. Rates clearly indicate that the second and third years of life are the most important in that they reflect the principal experience with these organisms in serious clinical manifestations. Rates decline slowly after age three years (unpublished observations) as has been noted before (Beck et al., 1957; Mata, 1957; Gordon et al., 1962; Gordon et al., 1965b).

Table 11.15
Shigella and Enteropathogenic *Escherichia coli* (*EEC*) in Children, Birth to Age Three Years, 1964–1969

Age, weeks	Number of children	Weeks at risk[a]	Shigella	EEC
0–25	81	1,783	1 (0.06)[b]	6 (0.34)[b]
26–51	65	1,546	11 (0.7)	7 (0.45)
52–77	52	1,192	20 (1.7)	7 (0.59)
78–103	46	1,096	37 (3.4)	12 (1.1)
104–129	44	1,100	39 (3.6)	3 (0.27)
130–155	43	1,075	40 (3.7)	5 (0.46)
Total		7,792	148 (1.9)	40 (0.51)

[a]Weeks in which children were examined clinically and bacteriologically.
[b]Number of new infections (rate per 100 child-weeks).

Viruses   Prevalence rates of viral infections in table 11.16 reveal that 21 percent of all specimens from infants under six months of age contained at least one enterovirus presumptively grouped as echo-like, but including coxsackie and polioviruses. The rates rose abruptly to 42 percent in the second half of the first year, to reach an eventual 61 percent at the end of the third year. As judged by figure 11.2, the conclusion is that all children shed viruses frequently, with the true rates probably higher than those recorded.

Regarding adenoviruses, prevalence rates by six-month intervals doubled among children in the course of weaning or with complete weaning (table 11.16). In view of the high rates of enteroviruses, adenovirus rates presumably are underestimates. Full typing of isolates was limited and was completed only for infections of the first week of life and for polioviruses. Incidence rates of poliovirus infection are shown in table 11.17 for the first year of life. Twenty-four percent of the 45 cohort infants excreted presumably wild poliovirus type 1 at some time during that year; the rate for type 2 was similar; and for type 3, 16 percent. Considering all types combined, at least 21 infants were infected with at least one type of poliovirus.

Chronicity and Duration of Enteric Infection
In a region where enteric infection is so common it is difficult, if not impossible, to determine duration of any specific infection unless the affected child is isolated promptly after the first demonstrated infection. While that is impossible under field conditions, the nature of the Cauqué study did permit information on the length and chronicity of certain selected infections. *Giardia, Entamoeba* and *Shigella*, in fact, virtually "colonized" the intestinal tract.

Giardia infections in general were long-lasting; they continued for weeks and sometimes months, especially if the child began to take supplementary

Table 11.16
Fecal Excretion of Enteroviruses and Adenoviruses by Six-Month Intervals, 45 Cohort Children, Birth to Age Three Years, 1964–1969

Age, months	Number of specimens	Enteroviruses	Adenoviruses
0–5	1,116	230 (20.6)[a]	34 (3.1)
6–11	1,162	483 (41.6)	46 (3.9)
12–17	917	481 (52.5)	33 (3.6)
18–23	953	438 (45.9)	60 (6.3)
24–29	908	446 (49.1)	58 (6.4)
30–35	867	530 (61.1)	48 (5.5)

[a]Number of positive specimens (percentage).

Table 11.17
Fecal Excretion of Poliovirus, First Year of Life, 45 Cohort Infants Examined Weekly, 1964–1967

Poliovirus type	Number of children positive (percentage)
1	7 (15.6)
2	5 (11.1)
3	3 (6.7)
1 and 2	2 (4.4)
1 and 3	1 (2.2)
2 and 3	2 (4.4)
1, 2, and 3	1 (2.2)
Total	21 (46.7)
Total with type 1	11 (24.4)
Total with type 2	10 (22.2)
Total with type 3	7 (15.6)

Table 11.18
Duration, Carriers, and Cases, of *Shigella* Infection, 45 Cohort Children, Birth to Age Three Years, 1964–1969

Shigella subgroup	Number of infections	Duration, weeks[a]					
		1	2–4	5–8	9–12	13–16	17–38
Dysenteriae	29	7 (24)[b]	10 (34)	4 (14)	3 (10)	2 (7)	3 (10)
Flexneri	75	18 (24)	21 (28)	18 (24)	9 (12)	5 (7)	4 (5)
Boydii	21	14 (67)	6 (28)	1 (5)			
Sonnei	7	7 (100)					
Total	132	46 (35)	37 (28)	23 (17)	12 (9)	7 (5)	7 (5)

[a]Two isolations were considered independent infections if separated by more than two weeks.
[b]Number of cases (row percentage).

foods at the time of attack. *E. histolytica* infections ordinarily were shorter although prolonged periods were observed with continued excretion of cysts. The pattern was for parasitic forms to appear and disappear at intervals, indicating the need for serial examinations to portray true incidence.

Contrary to the classical expression of acutely developing and abruptly terminating infection, chronic *Shigella* infections were frequent among village children (Mata et al., 1969b). Several problems remain to be solved before interpretation can be conclusive. In table 11.18 the reappearance of the same serotype after a demonstrated absence of more than two weeks was considered a reinfection. *Shigella* may remain submerged in the mucosa, however, with shedding delayed, to recur after prolonged intervals. How long a particular infection may persist remains unknown. One child of this study excreted *S. dysenteriae* 3 for two short periods separated by 15 weeks. A village adult presented two typical bouts of clinical dysentery due to *S. dysenteriae* 1 one year apart, with the Shiga bacillus isolated and a demonstrated rise in antibodies in each instance. While the question of duration of any single episode cannot be answered satisfactorily in all cases, most infections, clinical or asymptomatic, are characterized by well-defined episodes of bacterial shedding. Two bouts of dysentery in the same individual due to the same serotype could represent chronic infection with recurrence.

The arbitrary definition given above permits, however, an orderly estimate of duration (table 11.18). The chronicity is striking, with about 10 percent of infections lasting two to three months and 10 percent with a duration of more than three months. *Shigella* carriers of months' duration were documented in rural children (Mata et al., 1969b) and among children in a convalescent home (Mata et al., 1966). The longest recorded continuous infection was 38 weeks. During bouts of diarrhea or dysentery, organisms are excreted in concentrations of 10^6 to 10^8 viable bacilli per gram (Dale and Mata, 1968; Mata et al., 1974b). Since chronic infections are characterized by recurring forms

Table 11.19
Duration, Carriers, and Cases of *EEC* and *Salmonella* Infections, 45 Cohort Children,
Birth to Age Three Years, 1964–1969

Enteropathogenic *E. coli*			*Salmonella*		
Serotype	Number	Duration weeks[a]	Serotype	Number	Duration, weeks[a]
0111:B4	9	1–2	*derby*	3	1–6
055:B5	10	1–4	*typhimurium*	4	1
0127:B8	4	1	*infantis*	1	1
026:B6	3	1	*montevideo*	1	6
086:B7	1	1	*muenchen*	2	5–13
0124:B17	1	1	*manhattan*	1	13
0125:B15	7	1–2	*newport*	6	1–3
0216:B16	4	1	*miami*	2	1–2
0128:B12	1	1	*panama*	4	1–29
			dublin	1	1
			anatum	6	1–2
			give	4	1
			new brunswick	1	5
			senftenberg	1	1
			abaetetuba	1	1
			3:10:lv mono	1	1

[a]Two isolations were considered independent infections if separated by more than two weeks.

of diarrhea (Mata et al., 1966; Mata et al., 1969b), they probably are responsible for an effective seeding of the community environment and a consequent natural immunization of the population.

In contrast to *Shigella*, infections with *EEC* and with *Salmonella* to a lesser extent, were of shorter duration (table 11.19). Such infections ordinarily were effectively and naturally eliminated by the host with no evidence of recurrence as with *Shigella*. It is reasonable to postulate that host defense mechanisms against invading shigellae are sufficiently less operative in the presence of malnutrition to result in chronicity. The indigenous flora and B-cell immunocyte conceivably may be more important in *Salmonella* and *EEC* infections. The flora, the T-cell immunocyte, and certain factors in the amplification of the immune response may be more important in shigellosis. With malnutrition there is a more marked effect on cell-mediated immunity than on the B-cell system (Awdeh et al., 1972; Mata and Faulk, 1973; Faulk et al., 1974). Also, malnutrition reduces intestinal capacity for cell turnover. These factors could explain the persistence of shigellae in malnourished individuals, in contrast to the brief periods of a week or so, usually reported from more favored regions. Persistence of *Giardia* could be mediated by deficient

Table 11.20
Duration of Poliovirus Fecal Shedding, First Year of Life, 45 Cohort Children Cultured
Weekly from Birth, 1964–1967

Duration, weeks[a]	Poliovirus 1	Poliovirus 2	Poliovirus 3
1	7 (54)[b]	3 (28)	4 (50)
2	3 (23)	3 (28)	1 (13)
3	1 (8)	1 (9)	1 (13)
4	1 (8)	3 (28)	1 (13)
5	0	0	1 (13)
6	1 (8)	1 (9)	0
Total	13	11	8

[a]Two periods of virus shedding were considered different infections if separated by three or more weeks.
[b]Number of infectious episodes (relative percentage).

secretion of secretory IgA since this immunoglobulin interferes with attachment of antigens to the mucosal epithelium and thus exerts a mechanism for
antigen clearance (Williams and Gibbons, 1972).

With regard to viruses, information from the Cauqué study was limited
because only a few isolates were typed. Table 11.20 summarizes all attacks by
polioviruses within the first year of life. Half of the infections with types 1
and 3 were short-lived (less than eight days), while type 2 tended toward
greater chronicity. Heavier infections represented by concentrations of at
least 10^2 TCID$_{50}$ lasted six weeks.

For polioviruses, subclinical malnutrition apparently was no determinant
of persistence. Children from other rural areas of Guatemala with severe
protein-calorie malnutrition, however, show fewer enteroviruses and in lesser
concentrations in duodenum, jejunum, and colon than do well-nourished
controls from the same areas, suggesting that severe malnutrition is antagonis-
tic to viral replication. Overall, the flora of enteroviruses present in all
children almost at all times could also reflect a deficiency of the immune
mechanism that facilitates virus persistence in the gut.

The impact of repetitive and recurring infection, whether manifest or
asymptomatic, on nutrition and growth is difficult to assess under field conditions, particularly for children continuously being invaded by a variety of
agents. All too often, however, the significance of high infection rates among
poor children has been discounted by health workers and nutritionists.
Viruses and parasites are such frequent inhabitants of the intestinal tract that
sometimes they are mistakenly viewed as a part of the indigenous microbiota.
That belief has discouraged needed research on the interrelation of infection
and nutrition and has prompted the recommendation and implementation of
applied nutrition programs in total disregard of principles of sanitation and

prevention of infection. The findings of this study hopefully will counteract this trend.

The simple move from a crowded unhygienic rural environment to an urban setting offers to some the promise of improved control of infection. The urban environment, however, almost invariably leads to early weaning and a deterioration of nutritional status due to lack of proper food supplementation and the occurrence of diarrhea of similar or different etiology to that observed in the field. Furthermore, community infection commonly continues, sometimes in lesser magnitude than in the rural environment, although it can often be greater due to greater population density and poorer sanitation.

Ideally, rural environments like that of Santa María Cauqué should be improved beginning at childbirth by the control of certain infections of pregnancy, by improved measures at delivery, and by more hygienic practices of child care (diaper change, food preparation, and better personal hygiene). This has to be done, however, without necessarily discarding certain traditions such as breast-feeding which represents the most important protective mechanism against enteric infections. Emphasis should also be given to environmental sanitation and particularly to restricting contamination of supplemental foods, through measures including boiling of water, washing of hands, adequate cooking of meals, proper waste disposal, and rapid provision of medical attention when the child is ill. Such a multidisciplinary effort can be promoted through all-purpose clinics where maternal education, prenatal care, child immunization, medical care, supplementary feeding, and family planning programs are combined and coordinated with other community efforts. Much could be gained also by use of mass communication media and education programs through community development.

Chapter 12
Diseases and Disabilities

Except for the wholly apparent cases of infectious disease and injury so common in a village setting, the discovery, definition, and classification of most ailments in this context require more than the usual consideration. In part this is due to profound influences of the cultural, social, and biological qualities of host and environment. Many physicians and other health workers, however, tend to view disease solely as a biological problem. They soon come to recognize the great variations in individual response of a host to a given infectious agent. The result, exemplified by numerous studies, is an exploration of differences in resistance, hygiene, feeding practices, nutrition, and medical care, directed primarily toward better understanding of the individuality of disease manifestations. The social and behavioral determinants of morbid states, however, are not always appreciated to the extent they rightfully demand.

The contrasting and traditional characteristics of societies like that of Santa María Cauqué are so complex that to fully understand their interrelation with biological phenomena is no simple task (Fábrega, 1974).

An outstanding objective of the Cauqué study in this respect was that of pointing out the complexity and multiplicity of clinical manifestations experienced by every village child practically from birth. Table 12.1 details the history of infectious diseases experienced by a wholly ordinary pair of monozygotic twins (not belonging to the group of cohort children) who were

* This chapter was written jointly with Juan J. Urrutia and John E. Gordon.

Table 12.1
Illnesses in Pair 1 Twins, Birth to Age Three Years, 1966-1969

Age, weeks	Twin 124	Twin 125
First year		
0-12	Conj.	Conj.
	Impetigo	Impetigo
	Diarrhea	Diarrhea
	URI	URI
	Diarrhea with mucus, URI[a]	Diarrhea
13-25	Conj.	Conj.
	Conj.	URI
	URI	Conj.
	Diarrhea and vomiting	Diarrhea
26-38	URI, Conj.	URI, Conj.
	Diarrhea with mucus, URI, Conj.[a]	Bronchitis, Conj., Diarrhea[a]
	URI, Conj.[a]	
	Exanthem	
	Bronchopneumonia	
39-51	URI	Rubella
	Rubella, Bronchopneumonia[a]	URI
	Diarrhea with mucus, Exanthem[a]	Diarrhea, dehydration, URTI, URI[a]
Second year		
52-64	URI	URI
	URI	Diarrhea with mucus
	Diarrhea	
65-77	Herpes simplex oralis	URI
	URI, Conj.[a]	
	URI	
78-90	Whooping cough, Bronchopneu-	Dysentery
	monia, Stomatitis, URI, Diarrhea[a]	Whooping cough, Bronchopneu-
		monia, Diarrhea[a]
91-103	None	URI
		Vomiting
Third Year		
104-116	URI	URI, Diarrhea[a]
	Diarrhea	
	Vomiting	
117-129	Bronchitis, Impetigo, Conj.[a]	URI, Conj.[a]
		Diarrhea and Vomiting

Table 12.1 (continued)

Age, weeks	Twin 124	Twin 125
130–142	Dysentery, Conj.[a]	Impetigo
	Impetigo, URI[a]	Diarrhea
	Diarrhea	
143–155	Impetigo	Bronchitis
	Varicella	Varicella
	Bronchitis	
	Laryngotracheobronchitis	

Note: Conj. = conjunctivitis; URI = upper respiratory illness; URTI = urinary tract illness.
[a]Two or more overlapping illnesses.

observed during the first three years of life, prospectively, and who revealed a high frequency of diseases of striking similarity.* Dates of clinical attacks often coincided; beginning and termination rarely differed by more than a few days or a week. The data illustrate a home environment that provides essentially equal exposure to all siblings, a consideration to keep in mind when interpreting and evaluating applied health programs.

While morbidity rates compiled by workers using different methods cannot be compared, some idea of the magnitude of disease in Cauqué is possible by comparing the present findings with those of populations under better standards of living (Dingle et al., 1964; Tyrrell, 1965; Fox et al., 1966; Fox et al., 1972; Monto and Ullman, 1974). Rates for village children were five- to fifty-fold greater than those of children in most industrial societies. These rates and their implications are the focus of this chapter. First, however, necessary definitions and clinical considerations will be detailed.

As defined in the previous chapter, infectious disease is a morbid process having a definite set of symptoms and signs, commonly constituting the clinical picture of the disease. Illness is equivalent to disease and is used interchangeably. Recuperation is defined as the required interval for complete disappearance of symptoms of disease and recovery from any associated complications.

In this description of illness in Santa María Cauqué a relatively stereotyped response by individual children has been assumed. Signs such as fever,

* Anthropometric data on the identical twins discussed in this chapter was presented in chapters 6 and 9. The field physician who examined the children had no special awareness at the time that differences in factors such as birth weight could relate to clinical reaction. Both twins were visited weekly, thereby eliminating a possible bias due to recording events more in one case than in the other. The degree of exposure to infection can be assumed as equal, judging by similarities in intestinal flora already described and by similar excretion of pathogenic organisms. It can also be assumed that the twins had equal medical care; both were attended throughout by the same physician and nurse.

appearance of blood in the stools, vomit, or an evolving exanthem are susceptible to measurement and of decided aid in establishing a diagnosis. Symptoms such as headache, irritability, despondency, anorexia, and weakness were subjective and hard to evaluate since they were reported by the mother or attendant. They were, however, additionally assessed as far as possible by direct observation, that is, if the child did not eat well or was crying or apathetic, the symptom was accepted as real.

In the following analysis weight loss is defined as the deficit determined from onset while signs and symptoms of disease are still present, and, during subsequent recuperation, as the sum expressed as a percent of the weight at onset.

Environmental conditions of the Guatemalan highlands, such as climate and soil, eliminate many infectious diseases classically considered tropical, namely, malaria, bilharziasis, hookworm disease, Chagas' disease, and jungle fevers, which are found in the hot and humid lowlands and coastal regions of the country. In other times smallpox, yellow fever, louse-borne typhus fever, and cholera provided sporadic and sometimes widespread epidemics (Shattuck et al., 1938) but none of these diseases has been known in more than a half century. Smallpox was successfully eradicated through vaccination; no cases have been reported in Guatemala during the last 40 years. Louse-borne typhus fever disappeared from the highlands as a result of aggressive spray with DDT in the 1940s and greater availability of clothing. Impressive epidemics of cholera were recorded up to the beginning of the present century, but never since. The influenza pandemic of 1918 and the more recent ones (for instance, the Asian varieties) reached the village and contributed their share to community debility. Tuberculosis in its more severe manifestations has been a sporadic yet consuming disease of adults; its contribution to childhood morbidity and mortality has been little assessed. Syphilis is an exceptionally rare disease in highland villages. Yaws and trachoma are not present.

Specific nutritional deficiencies are not often recognized in the village despite a known marked deficiency of calories, protein, and vitamins in the local diet and an accompanying excess incidence of infection; nutritional deficiencies are multiple rather than specific (Autret and Béhar, 1955). Endemic goiter, prevalent in the past, has been controlled effectively by iodination of salt (Ascoli and Arroyave, 1970). The main nutritional problem is low-grade protein-calorie malnutrition (PCM), discernible by clinical means, by prospective observation of the child, or by biochemical studies of blood and urine. Studies of childhood growth and development, the irregular occurrence of the more severe forms of PCM, namely, marasmus and kwashiorkor, and particularly their occurrence in conjunction with outbreaks of infectious diseases are other indicators. For purposes of discussion malnutrition has been classed here as first, second, or third degree (Gómez et al., 1956), a division that expresses degrees of physical growth retardation more accurately than it does malnutrition. These distinctions will be useful, however, in the later discussion of the relation of nutritional status and the outcome of disease.

Infectious diseases, particularly of the intestinal and respiratory tracts, dominate the morbidity of the highland village child population. Most of the data in this chapter refer to the first three years of life of the 45 cohort children. The files of morbidity data for Santa María Cauqué are among the most extensive and complete of the study.* A thorough description of clinical manifestations and epidemiologic behavior is beyond the scope of this book and awaits future publication. The present emphasis is on the comparative frequency of infection and infectious disease and the relation of each to the outcome of infection and illness and to growth and development.

Diseases, illnesses, and symptoms are grouped in four subdivisions: infectious, nutritional, other manifestations, and traumatic injuries. Morbidity is expressed here as rates per 100 person-months, by six-month or longer intervals of observation. In computing rates, all diseases and illnesses separated in onset by at least 24 hours were assumed to be independent events, a premise of reasonable validity in view of the variety of infectious agents to which a child is so frequently and indeed almost continuously exposed. The procedure is strengthened by the varying pathogenic potential of viruses, bacteria, and parasites and the wide range of clinical manifestations associated with these agents.

Since the cohort children were recruited over a span of two years, and each was then observed for three years, it seems unlikely that the methods used to collect the information had any decisive influence on the results. The rates discussed later indicate that diseases, illnesses, and symptoms began to appear more frequently after the first half year, that numbers reached a peak in the second year, and that they then began to decline.

Noninfectious Diseases

Infectious syndromes were so frequent that other instances of morbidity elicited lesser interest. Table 12.2 shows cases per hundred person-years of the more severe forms of protein-calorie malnutrition (PCM), skin disorders of noninfectious origin, and traumatic injuries. The first group, severe forms of PCM, represents only the visible fraction of a general problem already evident in the patterns of physical growth and mortality already described. The rate of severe PCM was 6.8 per hundred. Marasmus is not tabulated here but will be discussed at greater length in chapter 13.

* A record of diseases, illnesses, and symptoms among the cohort children is given in appendix C. A clinical guide that served the field physician for recognition of the main items was prepared and can be requested from INCAP. The treatments employed for most of the patients are also listed in appendix C. These procedures resulted in data of consistently good quality.

Table 12.2
Noninfectious Diseases and Injuries, 45 Cohort Children, Birth to Age Three Years,
1964–1969

Disease, illness, or injury	Code	Number of cases	Rate per 100 person-years[a]
Severe protein-calorie malnutrition[b]			
Prekwashiorkor	(1202)	4	6.0
Kwashiorkor	(1203)	2[c]	1.5
Marasmic-Kwashiorkor	(1204)	3	2.3
Total PCM		9	6.8
Skin illnesses			
Eczema, intertrigo	(0916)	7	5.3
Dermatitis	(0917)	10	7.6
Urticaria, papular	(0918)	4	3.0
Total skin illnesses		21	15.9
Injuries			
Wound	(0911)	3	2.3
Burn	(0912)	3	2.3
Laceration	(0913)	1	0.8
Contusion, bruise	(01303)	3	2.3
Total injuries		10	7.6

[a]Based on 132.5 person years, accounting for attrition.
[b]Nutritional marasmus not included (see chapter 13).
[c]Hospitalized.

Noninfectious illnesses of the skin were predominantly allergies, often complicated by an infection. Intertrigo in all likelihood included a number of cases of scabies, an infectious disease commonly unrecognized because of its benign behavior, the frequency of an associated bacterial infection, and the usual dirt on the skin of village children. The demand put on the laboratory by other more important infections precluded microscopic diagnosis of many suspected cases of scabies and also of impetigo.

Injuries were surprisingly rare among children less than four years old; mainly minor wounds from agricultural tools, machetes, and knives; first- and second-degree burns by fire or hot water; and various skin lacerations and contusions.

Infectious Diseases
Rates   The clinical entities assumed to be infectious and occurring during the first three years of life are listed in table 12.3 for the cohort children as cases per hundred person-years. Diarrhea (without mucus or blood) and upper respiratory illnesses (mainly common colds) had the highest rates, respectively 483 and 372 per hundred person-years. More serious diseases such as diarrhea with mucus and bronchitis occurred less frequently, although

Table 12.3
Frequency of Infectious Disease and Illness, by Age and Number and Percentage of Cases, 45 Cohort Children, Birth to Age Three Years, 1964–1969

Disease or illness	Code[a]	Frequency Cases	Percentage all cases	Rate per 100 person-years[b]	Age, months 0-5 (N = 270)[d]	6-11 (N = 270)	12-17 (N = 270)	18-23 (N = 270)	24-29 (N = 255)	30-35 (N = 250)
Respiratory										
Upper respiratory tract infection	(0101)	493	20.14	372.1	25.2[e]	33.7	32.6	30.4	29.0	34.5
Purulent rhinitis	(0103)	1	0.04	0.8						
Tonsillo-pharyngitis, with exudate	(0102)	10	0.41	7.6	0.4	0.4	0.7	0.7	1.1	1.2
Pharyngitis	(0109)	1	0.04	0.8						
Acute laryngitis	(0111)	7	0.29	5.3	0.7	0	0	1.5	1.9	0
Acute laryngotracheobronchitis	(0113)	4	0.16	3.0						
Bronchitis	(0114)	256	10.46	193.2	12.6	18.5	20.0	18.9	17.4	10.5
Bronchiolitis	(0115)	5	0.20	3.8						
Bronchopneumonia, pneumonia	(0116)	70	2.86	52.8	2.6	4.4	3.7	7.0	5.0	3.5
Gastrointestinal										
Diarrhea	(0211)	640	26.14	483.0	18.9	41.1	47.4	50.7	47.1	35.3
Diarrhea with mucus	(0212)	313	12.79	236.2	13.0	17.8	22.6	26.3	22.4	15.5
Dysentery (diarrhea with blood and mucus)	(0213)	97	3.96	73.2	1.5	4.1	7.8	10.4	8.5	4.3
Eye										
Conjunctivitis	(0301)	213	8.70	160.8	21.5	18.5	13.0	14.1	8.5	4.7
Hordeolum	(0302)	6	0.25	4.5	0.4	0	0.7	0.4	0.4	0.4
Ear										
Otitis externa	(0401)	11	0.45	8.3	0	0.7	1.1	0	1.5	0.8
Otitis media, suppurative	(0403)	6	0.25	4.5	0.7	0.4	0.4	0.4	0.4	0

Mouth and throat										
Herpes simplex, primary	(0501)	20	0.82	15.1 }	0	1.9	3.0	1.9	2.7	1.2
Herpex simplex, recurrent	(0502, 0928)	8	0.33	6.0 }						
Stomatitis	(0503)	23	0.94	17.4	0.4	2.2	1.1	1.1	1.9	1.9
Herpangina	(0504)	7	0.29	5.3	0	0.7	1.5	0	0.4	0
Thrush	(0505)	28	1.14	21.1	8.9	0.4	0.7	0.4	0	0
Alveolar abscess	(0506)	1	0.04	0.8	0	0	0	0	0	0.4
Glossitis and cheilitis[c]	(0508, 0509)	14	0.57	10.6	0	1.1	1.9	0.7	1.9	0.4
Genitourinary										
Urinary tract infection	(0801)	1	0.04	0.8						
Balanoposthitis	(0802)	3	0.12	2.3						
Skin, scalp										
Impetigo (vesicles, pustules, crusts)	(0902, 0903, 1002)	31	1.27	23.4	0.7	1.9	1.1	3.3	1.9	3.5
Abscess, furuncle	(0904, 1003)	16	0.65	12.1	0.4	0.7	1.9	1.9	0.8	0.8
Cellulitis	(0905)	4	0.16	3.0						
Necrosis	(0910)	1	0.04	0.8						
Secondary infection	(0914, 0919)	4	0.16	3.0						
Lymphatic										
Adenitis, lymphadenitis	(601, 602)	4	0.16	3.0						

Table 12.3 (continued)

Disease or illness	Code[a]	Frequency		Rate per 100 person-years[b]	Age, months					
		Cases	Percentage all cases		0-5 (N=270)[d]	6-11 (N=270)	12-17 (N=270)	18-23 (N=270)	24-29 (N=255)	30-35 (N=250)
Common communicable diseases of childhood										
Measles	(0921)	32	1.31	24.2	0.4	4.1	1.5	3.3	0.8	1.9
Rubella	(0922)	15	0.61	11.3	0	0.4	0.7	3.0	0.8	0.8
Chickenpox	(0923)	26	1.06	19.6	0.7	1.1	3.0	3.0	1.9	1.9
Exanthem subitum	(0924)	1	0.04	0.8	0	0.4	0	0	0	0
Erythema infectiosum	(0925)	3	0.12	2.3	0	0.4	0	0.4	0.4	0
Undifferentiated febrile exanthem	(0930)	25	1.02	18.9	0.7	2.6	2.6	1.9	1.2	0.4
Undifferentiated febrile vesicles	(0931)	5	0.20		0	0.7	0.4	0	0.4	0.4
Mumps	(1103)	1	0.04	0.8	0	0.4	0	0	0	0
Scarlet fever	(0926)	1	0.04	0.8	0	0	0	0	0.4	0
Whooping cough	(0121)	10	0.41	7.6	0	0	0	0	1.9	1.9
Other										
Fever of unknown origin	(1105)	14	0.57	10.6						
Tenosynovitis	(1309)	1	0.04	0.8						
Omphalitis	(1107)	2	0.08	1.5						
Ringworm	(1004)	8	0.33	6.0						

[a]See appendix C.
[b]Based on 131.5 person-years, taking attrition into account.
[c]These have a nutritional origin and are included here because they were associated with infection and febrile episodes.
[d]N = Number of person-months.
[e]Rate per 100 person-months, by six-month intervals.

comparatively high rates, respectively 236 and 193 per hundred, were noted. This means that each child averaged from two to four attacks of such illnesses per year. Debilitating and killing diseases like bronchopneumonia and dysentery (diarrhea with blood and mucus) were relatively frequent, at rates of 53 and 73 per hundred person-years.

The percent contribution of each specific illness or disease to total morbidity is also shown in table 12.3. Diarrheal diseases as a whole were responsible for 43 percent of total recognized cases, followed in order by respiratory tract infections. Measles and whooping cough accounted for only 1.7 percent of cases, but they called for a community reaction and response greater than for any other disease. Bronchopneumonia, both primary and secondary to other infectious diseases, was often fatal and contributed 4 percent of total cases, but along with diarrheal disease was of much less family and community concern than were measles and whooping cough.

Except for whooping cough no apparent differences between sexes occurred among patients with infectious diseases. As to age-specific rates, cases per 100 person-months at intervals of six months are summarized in table 12.3 by major groups of diseases. Although rates were high during the first six months, the main import is the extent to which they increased thereafter, particularly in the critical second year. Diarrheal disease was a striking example: that rate went from 33 per hundred person-months in the first six months to 63 in the second semester and to 87 by the end of the second year after which it declined. Rates of respiratory tract disease varied less. The second half of the second year of life showed the highest rates for infectious diseases, which declined thereafter. Diseases of the eye, mainly conjunctivitis, were exceptional in that rates dropped steadily with age.

Table 12.3 also presents the observations by individual conditions of the main groups of diseases. Worthy of mention are the increased rates for bronchopneumonia and the diarrheal diseases with advancing age, reaching maximal values at the end of the second year. Herpes simplex and abscesses were among other infectious diseases which reached their greatest frequency in the second year. Thrush was virtually restricted to the first six months.

Rates of occurrence of exanthematic and other common communicable diseases of childhood for the 45 cohort children are presented in table 12.3. Because of the exceptional importance of measles and whooping cough in relation to nutritional depletion, these two diseases are described in more detail later in the chapter. Chickenpox occurred most frequently in the second year of life, although onset in the first year was not unusual and 1 case developed during the neonatal period. Rubella was rarely identified under field conditions; the 15 cases were mainly in the second and third years. Febrile exanthematic and vesicular diseases of mucosa and skin, probably of enteroviral origin, occurred mainly in the second and third semesters. Scarlet fever was an exceptionally rare condition.

Table 12.4
Infectious Diseases, Illnesses, Symptoms, and Signs, Rates per 100 Person-Months,
by Birth Weight, 45 Cohort Children from Birth to Six Months of Age, 1964–1967

	Birth weight, g	
	< 2,501 (N = 17)	2,501+ (N = 28)
Diseases and illnesses		
Upper respiratory tract illness	21.6	27.4
Tonsillo-pharyngitis	0	0.6
Laryngotracheobronchitis	0	1.2
Bronchitis	12.8	12.5
Pneumonia, bronchopneumonia	2.0	3.0
Vomiting	4.9	1.8
Diarrhea	16.7	20.2
Diarrhea with mucus	9.8	14.9
Diarrhea with blood and mucus	1.0	1.8
Conjunctivitis	28.4	17.3
Hordeolum	1.0	0
Otitis media	0	1.2
Thrush	12.8	6.5
Stomatitis	0	0.6
Abscess, furuncle	0	0.6
Secondary infection, wound	1.0	0.6
Undifferentiated febrile exanthem	1.0	0.6
Symptoms and signs		
Fever, °C		
37.5–38.4	22.6	25.6
38.5–39.4	7.8	6.6
39.5+	2.0	2.4
Diarrhea, number of stools per day		
4–6	22.6	25.6
7–9	8.8	8.9
10–12	3.9	3.0
13–15	0	0.6
Anorexia	13.7	10.7
Despondency, irritability	28.4	45.8

Birth weight had no consistent relation to susceptibility to infection or to the extent of clinical manifestations as evidenced in the summed experience of the cohort children. Table 12.4 presents rates for infectious diseases per 100 person-months during the first six months of life, according to birth weights of children above and below 2,500 grams. Although rates of upper respiratory tract illnesses and diarrhea were greater for infants with the better birth weights, those of conjunctivitis and thrush (oral candidosis) were markedly greater among low birth weight infants. No differences in overall rates of infectious diseases occurred after six months, however.

Prevalence rates for simple infection, in contrast to manifest clinical infectious disease, did vary with birth weight; infection rates of *Shigella, Entamoeba histolytica*, and *Giardia* were greater among low birth weight infants during the first six months than for infants of adequate birth weight (table 12.5). No consistent differences in virus excretion worthy of mention were noted among cohort infants distinguished by birth weight.

The excessive frequency of infections and the large dose to which the childhood population is exposed are also reflected in the precocious development of high concentrations of serum immunoglobulins (Ig's). Adult levels of IgM and IgG are attained early in life, with IgA developing more slowly (Cáceres and Mata, 1974). The rapid development of serum Ig's is illustrated in figure 12.1 for IgM and in table 12.6 for IgG. The data derive from a sample of 15 percent of the village population and reveal that by six months infants have synthesized IgM to levels comparable to those possessed by adults of the village. Indeed, adult IgG levels were demonstrable in most one year olds. The Ig values are definitely greater than ordinarily observed in humans living in industrialized nations (Rowe et al., 1968; McGregor et al., 1970; Lechtig et al., 1972d; Cáceres and Mata, 1974).

Occurrence of Symptoms   The detailed description of each clinical manifestation among village children provided data on the relative frequency of signs and symptoms usually associated with acute infectious disease (table 12.7). Diarrhea, considered here as an isolated clinical sign, was the most common, accounting for 27 percent of all observed symptoms among the cohort children during the three year study period. Fever was next, accounting for 26 percent. Despite the common occurrence of diarrhea, clinical dehydration was rare, probably because most patients continued to breast-feed while ill. Incidentally, this could be a reason why smaller children, with more diarrhea, are kept at the breast longer. Table 12.7 shows rate of occurrence of selected symptoms per hundred person-months, by age. Vomiting was comparatively infrequent during the first six months (three cases per hundred person-months), but increased to sixteen per hundred in the second half of the first year. Since the rate was considerably higher in the second year of life, it is rather clearly one of the manifestations of infection. Fever

Table 12.5
Percentage of Prevalence in Trimester of *Shigella*, *Entamoeba histolytica*, and *Giardia* Infections and of Intestinal Viruses, by Birth Weight, 45 Cohort Infants, First Year of Life, 1964–1966

Month of life	Number of specimens[a]		Shigella		E. histolytica		Giardia		Enteroviruses		Adenoviruses	
	< 2,501g	2,501g+	<2,501g	2,501g+	< 2,501g	2,501g+	< 2,501 g	2,501g+	< 2,501g	2,501g+	< 2,501g	2,501g+
0-2	286	486	2.1[b]	0.4	0	0.6	0.4	0.6	10.8	14.4	0.7	0.6
3-5	222	360	0.9	1.4	2.7	0.3	3.6	0.8	31.5	20.6	4.5	5.8
6-8	217	362	0	0	0	0.5	3.2	4.1	44.7	39.0	3.7	3.3
9-11	219	364	1.8	0.8	0	0	5.5	10.7	40.6	42.9	2.7	5.5
Total	944	1,572	1.3	0.6	0.6	0.3	3.0	3.8	30.4	28.1	2.8	3.6

[a]Collected from 18 low birth weight infants and 28 infants with adequate (≥ 2,501 g) birth weight.
[b]Percentage prevalence in trimester.

Table 12.6
Concentration of Serum Immunoglobulin G, by Age, 1970

Age, years	Number of subjects	Geometric Mean Concentration		Min-Max values, mg/100 ml	Percentage of adult concentration
		IU/ml[a]	mg/100 ml		
0–5	9	106.4	872	305–1,720	56.7
1	30	178.0	1,459	955–2,055	94.9
2	21	166.7	1,366	1,115–1,920	88.8
3	17	162.4	1,331	1,080–1,850	86.5
4	7	169.8	1,392	1,260–1,630	90.5
5–9	28	171.5	1,406	1,090–2,020	91.4
10–14	17	175.6	1,439	1,060–2,000	93.6
15–29	25	174.7	1,432	1,195–1,930	93.1
30+	68	187.6	1,538	1,195–2,100	100.0

[a]International units, WHO (Rowe et al., 1970).

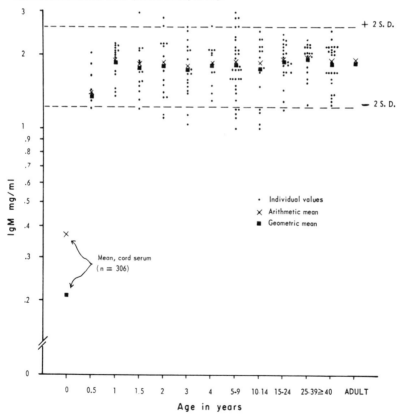

Figure 12.1
Concentrations of immunoglobulin M, mg/ml, by age, 1964–1970 (from Cáceres and Mata, 1974)

Table 12.7
Frequency of 4,462 Observed Symptoms and Selected Symptoms and Signs, by Age per 100 Person-Months, 45 Cohort Children, Birth to Age Three Years, 1964–1969

Symptom	Number observed	Percentage Frequency, all Symptoms	Rates of occurrence, by age per 100 person-months					
			0–5[a] (N = 270)[b]	6–11 (N = 270)	12–17 (N = 270)	18–23 (N = 270)	24–29 (N = 255)	30–35 (N = 250)
Vomiting	235	5.3	3.0	16.3	26.3	18.9	13.1	10.5
Fever[c]								
37.5–39.4 } 39.5+	1,148	25.7	31.5	73.3	73.0	71.5	69.9	67.1
Diarrhea[d]								
4–9			3.7	5.9	10.7	11.1	7.7	7.8
10–15 }	1,205	27.0	33.3	66.7	78.9	83.7	78.4	60.1
20+			3.7	7.8	12.2	10.0	9.7	4.7
Dehydration	32	0.7	0	1.1	1.1	0.4	0.8	0.4
Anorexia	823	18.4	0	1.9	3.7	3.3	1.9	1.2
Despondency, irritability	1,008	22.6	11.9	55.2	73.7	70.4	56.0	41.9
Other	11	0.3	39.3	71.9	80.0	75.6	63.3	48.1

[a] Age in months.
[b] N = Total number of person-months.
[c] Rectal temperature, °C. Equivalent oral temperatures = 37.0–38.9, and 39.0+.
[d] Number of stools per day.

Table 12.8
Mean Values and Standard Deviations for Duration of Respiratory Illnesses, Conjunctivitis, Bronchopneumonia, and Diarrheal Disease, by Age, 45 Cohort Children, Birth to Age Three Years, 1964–1969

Patient age, months	Upper respiratory tract illness	Bronchitis	Conjunctivitis	Broncho-pneumonia	Dysentery	Diarrhea with mucus	Diarrhea
0–5	8.6 ± 0.6 (69)[a]	12.0 ± 1.1 (34)	7.3 ± 0.6 (58)	7.6 ± 1.0 (7)	5.8 ± 1.6 (4)	4.2 ± 0.5 (35)	5.2 ± 0.6 (57)
6–11	8.1 ± 0.6 (93)	10.1 ± 0.8 (48)	7.3 ± 0.8 (50)	7.1 ± 0.7 (12)	4.7 ± 0.6 (12)	3.9 ± 0.4 (52)	4.3 ± 0.3 (123)
12–17	7.9 ± 0.5 (88)	9.2 ± 0.7 (57)	5.6 ± 0.7 (35)	8.7 ± 1.4 (12)	4.2 ± 0.8 (22)	4.0 ± 0.4 (70)	5.8 ± 0.6 (149)
18–23	6.5 ± 0.4 (82)	9.4 ± 0.8 (52)	5.4 ± 0.7 (38)	8.1 ± 0.6 (21)	4.2 ± 0.6 (39)	4.2 ± 0.3 (101)	5.2 ± 0.5 (173)
24–29	6.3 ± 0.4 (76)	7.3 ± 0.5 (43)	3.9 ± 0.4 (22)	8.4 ± 1.2 (14)	3.5 ± 0.5 (26)	4.2 ± 0.5 (75)	5.4 ± 0.5 (144)
30–35	6.9 ± 0.5 (92)	7.8 ± 0.8 (27)	5.5 ± 1.2 (12)	5.4 ± 0.7 (9)	3.5 ± 0.7 (11)	4.3 ± 0.7 (46)	6.4 ± 0.8 (115)
F	2.654	3.205	3.228				
P	< 0.05	< 0.01	< 0.01				

[a]Mean days ± S.E. (number of cases).

is important because of its relation to nutritional depletion. Rates increased significantly by the end of the first year and remained high in the second. Other symptoms such as diarrhea behaved in similar fashion.

Duration and Severity Relatively little is known about the duration of infectious diseases in populations with endemic, firmly established, and persisting chronic protein-calorie malnutrition so that global experience may not apply to village situations in developing regions (American Public Health Association, 1970). Table 12.8 presents mean duration for various illnesses. The days involved for upper and lower respiratory tract illness and for conjunctivitis are significantly shorter with progressive advances in age. The reasons are indeterminate although a relation to development of the immune system is suspect, particularly secretory IgA. Bronchopneumonia and diarrhea exhibited no such variations in duration with age, nor did impetigo, rubella, and varicella. Duration of clinical disability in measles did not differ with age, as illustrated in table 12.9; the fever of measles, however, was significantly longer when onset was after the first year of life and continued this way from age two to five years.

Except for whooping cough, differences in duration of disease by sex among patients of equivalent age were not identified. Females with whooping cough tended toward longer clinical course and greater fatality to an extent suggesting an inborn susceptibility to the disease.

The clinical severity of a disease is also measured by the nature and number of associated diseases or complications that occur. This is well illustrated by measles, a disease frequently complicated by bronchopneumonia, diarrhea, or the two combined. The origin and mechanism of these two complications are not clear. Bronchopneumonia usually is presumed to be bacterial but the possibility of giant cell pneumonia as a result of diminished cellular immunity cannot be eliminated (Mata and Faulk, 1973). The common bacterial pathogens are found in the diarrhea of measles, but there is evidence to suggest that some of these diarrheas are a true result of measles infection in a malnourished host (Gordon et al., 1965a; Urrutia and Mata, 1974).

Treatment Considerable effort was directed in the Cauqué study toward prompt treatment of patients with an illness or disability, regardless of cooperation with the study. Injuries were treated according to standard procedures at the village clinic since most were cases of first- and second-degree burns and minor wounds. More serious injuries among older children and adults occasionally required hospitalization. Of the cohort children, three were hospitalized, one at age 14 months because of severe diarrhea and dehydration, two at 26 and 34 months of age because of severe protein-calorie malnutrition. Since these two children by the best clinical judgment would have died had they remained in the village, they were excluded from

Table 12.9
Clinical Duration and Common Complications of Measles, by Age, 1965–1971

Age, years	Number of cases	Days of measles fever	Cases of fever ≥ 39.5°C	Days	Number of cases	Diarrhea[a]	Broncho-pneumonia	Diarrhea and broncho-pneumonia	Total
< 1	46	10.2 ± 2.1[b]	28	1.4 ± 1.6[b]	50	50[c]	12	28	90
1	35	11.6 ± 1.8	28	3.1 ± 2.1	37	27	8	54	89
2	34	11.1 ± 1.7	23	3.8 ± 1.7	34	29	18	41	88
3	16	11.1 ± 2.0	5	3.7 ± 1.0	16	6	19	63	88
4	14	10.3 ± 1.1	8	3.0 ± 2.0	14	43	14	43	100
5+	22	10.8 ± 1.5	8	3.0 ± 1.9	23	26	30	30	87
Total	167	10.8 ± 1.9	100	2.8 ± 2.0	174	33	16	41	90

[a]Dysentery excluded.
[b]Mean ± S.E.
[c]Percentage of cases.

Table 12.10
Number and Percentage of Treatments of 2,949 Illnesses and Injuries, 45 Cohort
Children, Birth to Age Three Years, 1964-1969

Treatment	Number (percentage)	Treatment	Number (percentage)
None	98 (3.3)	Ophthalmic ointment	119 (4.0)
Aspirin	679 (23.0)	Gentian violet	88 (3.0)
Kaolin-pectin, placebo	619 (21.0)	Antispasmodics	90 (3.1)
Expectorants	606 (20.6)	Oral fluids	75 (2.6)
Penicillin	243 (8.2)	Parenteral fluids	3 (0.1)
Sulfonamides	74 (2.5)	Hospitalization	2 (0.1)
Other antimicrobials	32 (1.1)	Other	221 (7.5)

these tabulations for those ages. The 2,949 treatments applied at home or
under clinic auspices to the cohort children during the first three years of
life included aspirin (23 percent), kaolin-pectin or placebos (21 percent), and
expectorants (21 percent). The indication for these treatments is easy to
visualize in the light of the predominating respiratory and diarrheal diseases.
Nevertheless, in 8 percent of all treatments penicillin was used, and in an
additional 3.6 percent sulfonamides or other antimicrobials were prescribed
(table 12.10).

The case fatality in measles, whooping cough, and bronchopneumonia was
less than usual in rural health centers of Guatemala, yet understandably high
because of underlying malnutrition. Simplicity of treatment was dominant
for even the most serious diseases: measles, acute diarrhea, and dysentery.
Penicillin was administered to 81 percent of patients with rales or other
evidence of lung congestion or consolidation. Thirteen percent of children
with diarrheal disease received oral fluids, a rather low proportion in the face
of the severity of the disease in underweight children, yet explainable on the
basis of the long continued breast-feeding and the usual custom of continued
nursing during illness. Of measles patients, 34 percent received kaolin-pectin
because of the commonly associated diarrhea. For dysentery or diarrhea with
bloody stools, sulfonamides were administered to 10 percent of patients;
many responded satisfactorily to symptomatic management alone. Patients
with Shiga dysentery were treated with nalidixic acid or with trimethoprim-
sulphamethoxazole (Mata et al., 1971a).

Epidemiologic Behavior of Infectious Disease *Diarrheal Disease* Observed
epidemiologic characteristics of acute diarrheal disease and related conditions
continued during the Cauqué study with no significant departure from earlier
descriptions (Gordon et al., 1963; Gordon et al., 1964; Scrimshaw et al.,
1968b). For Guatemala as a whole, however, the changes were outstanding.
At the end of 1968 and in early 1969 a series of outbreaks of dysentery

caused by the Shiga bacillus, *S. dysenteriae* type 1, struck sharply on the Western Guatemala-Mexican border and eventually extended to the whole of the country. A broader regional epidemic involved Mexico, Belize, and all other Central American republics except Panama (Mata and Castro, 1974) with repeated importation of the strain to the United States of America (CDC, 1970; Gangarosa et al., 1970). Although the epidemic included hundreds of thousands of cases of dysentery, with deaths into the thousands, the outbreak brought no serious consequences to Santa María Cauqué (Gangarosa et al., 1970; Mendizábal et al., 1971). The first attack of a cohort child involved a four-year old at the end of 1969. Another case among the 45 cohort was a child less than three years old. For the village as a whole, this organism caused the death of one child not in the cohort. Compared with the regional situation (Gangarosa et al., 1970; Mata et al., 1972d) and the past experience of the village itself with this bacillus (Gordon et al., 1965b), the dramatically smaller effect of the 1969 to 1971 epidemic on Santa María Cauqué is worth noting. Among other possible explanations than a persisting immunity from the 1965 epidemic were the awareness of the clinic staff of the nature and management of the problem; prompt epidemiologic, clinical, and bacteriologic diagnosis; and the availability of effective drugs to treat the disease (Mata et al., 1971a).

Measles   The epidemiological behavior of measles in present-day rural Guatemala (Gordon et al., 1965a) differs markedly from the outbreaks in Indian populations exposed for the first time to the virus and decimated by sweeping epidemics in times of the Spanish Conquest. Eventual endemic establishment of the disease in local communities occurred through frequent and repeated introduction of the virus, sometimes as often as every year. The result is small, localized outbreaks every one or two years, as fresh susceptibles accumulate by birth (Urrutia and Mata, 1974).

Measles outbreaks in villages are traceable in general to effective contact with an infected person, usually through a visit to one of the markets in urban cities. Better motor transportation in recent decades has prompted these changes in the epidemiology of measles. As a consequence relatively more infants and young children are exposed than in former times; the disease appears less frequently among persons more than ten years old. In fact, 19 percent of all cases of the Cauqué study occurred during the first year of life and 22 percent in the second year (table 12.11). Because the nutritional status at this time has deteriorated, the expected result is a more serious disease and higher fatality than with measles occurring at school ages, as it does in most industrial regions. Prompt medical attention to village patients reduced case fatality to 4 percent (Urrutia and Mata, 1974). The demonstrated change in disease behavior was used in strong justification of

Table 12.11
Distribution of 276 Measles Cases, by Age
at Onset and Number and Percentage of
Cases, February 1964–January 1972

Age	Number of cases (percentage)
0–5 months	6 (2.2)
6–11 months	47 (17.0)
12–17 months	23 (8.3)
18–23 months	38 (13.8)
2 years	62 (22.5)
3 years	37 (13.4)
4 years	22 (8.0)
5–9 years	39 (14.1)
10–19 years	2 (0.7)
20+ years	0

mass vaccination of the Guatemalan population under five years of age (Mata et al., 1974c).

Whooping Cough   The disease is associated historically with a high mortality in villages of the region, indeed globally in preindustrial countries. As illustrated in figure 2.8, whooping cough was responsible for a number of the peaks in mortality occurring in Santa María Cauqué at widely spaced intervals; the last outstanding instance was in 1942. An immunization program to protect the population of the village had been under way during the Nutrition-Infection Study (Scrimshaw et al., 1967b) and the Cauqué study, but with little success. An outbreak developed with devastating results in 1968, through a chance importation of the infection into the village. This led to a propagated case within three weeks in a home several blocks removed from the residence of the imported case. Within a month new cases appeared singly or multiply in a number of village families and evolved rapidly into an outbreak of serious proportions illustrated in table 12.12. The occurrence of cases in almost all blocks of the village is evidence of the general and high susceptibility of the population. The epidemic reached a peak in May, three months after the first case, then declined and ended four months later. Attack rates were high for all ages except those more than ten years old, a behavior in agreement with the long absence of the disease from the village. Attack rates were usually higher for females than for males. Case fatality ratio was of the order of 15 percent; it was much greater among infants and preschool children than school children, and was particularly high in the second year.

Table 12.12
Whooping Cough Epidemic: Cases, Deaths, Attack Rates, and Fatalities, by Age and Sex, 1968

Age, years	Population		Cases		Deaths		Percentage of attack rate			Percentage of case fatality ratio		
	Male	Female	Male	Female	Male	Female	Male	Female	Total	Male	Female	Total
<1	24	30	7	12	2	3	29	40	35	29	25	26
1	19	26	8	10	2	6	42	38	40	25	60	44
2	26	30	7	18	0	3	27	60	45	0	17	12
3	18	12	8	6	0	1	44	50	47	0	17	7
4	27	29	4	7	0	0	15	24	20	0	0	0
5–9	109	92	9	13	0	0	8	14	11	0	0	0
10–14	78	87	1	3	0	0	1	3	2	0	0	0
Total	301	306	44	69	4	13	15	23	19	9	19	15

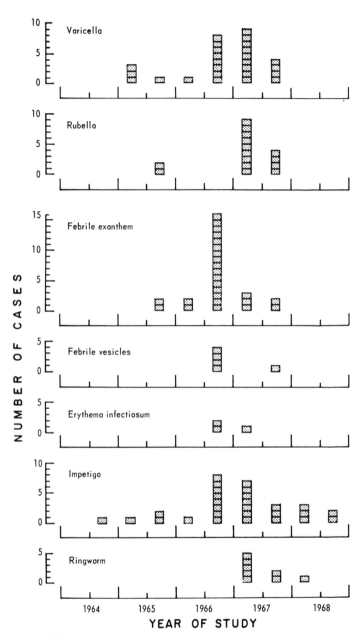

Figure 12.2
Infectious diseases, 45 cohort children, first three years of life, 1964–1968. Most cohort children were 18 months old or more during 1966 and 1967, a time when incidence of all communicable diseases was high.

Other Infectious Diseases   The impact of other communicable diseases on the cohort children is presented in figure 12.2. The information is assessed necessarily with the realization that it represents only the experience of the cohort children from birth to three years of age. The main point is that communicable diseases which ordinarily strike only once in a lifetime show, in this environment, a major occurrence in the second and third years (1966 and 1967), a time when the incidence of all communicable diseases was high. This was true for varicella (21 children among the 45 were infected in those years), rubella (13), and febrile exanthem (23). Even infectious diseases of bacterial and mycotic nature such as impetigo and ringworm occurred with excess frequency in the second and third years of life.

Nutrition-Infection Interaction

The substance of this chapter and of the preceding one has been to demonstrate how the force of infection is able to act deleteriously on the body so intensively that no possibility remains of escaping its notice. Infectious disease therefore becomes a highly significant feature in the matrix of causality governing the genesis of malnutrition and deficits in growth and development.

In the Cauqué study individual variability in rates of infectious diseases was apparently related to differences in resistance and nutrition that were established in infancy and in early childhood and to which infectious diseases themselves contributed. Infection and infectious diseases affect the nutritional status of the child, but it is difficult to measure exactly how much a deficient nutritional status results from infectious diseases or predisposes to them. The practical implication is that many illnesses could be prevented by diminishing opportunities for exposure to infectious agents, thereby contributing to an improved nutritional state and better growth through measures such as increased availability and quality of water, sewer installation, and public education programs on preparation and handling of food, and waste disposal.

An intensive discussion on nutrition-infection interactions pointed out their importance for public health (Scrimshaw et al., 1968a). The most important effects are those consequent to anorexia and fever, to damage to the intestinal mucosa and its function, to rapid transit of food through the intestine, and to altered cell metabolism (Beisel, 1972). Diarrheal and respiratory diseases are the main contributors to nutritional depletion. More recent evidence has shown that even asymptomatic infections—and these are decidedly common—have an effect on cellular metabolism. Virtually every cell function is known to be altered as a consequence of infection. In addition to accepted classical effects, an occurrence of iron and zinc sequestration has been demonstrated, as well as alterations in synthesis of cholesterol and other lipids. Furthermore, synthesis of acute-phase reactant proteins is known to

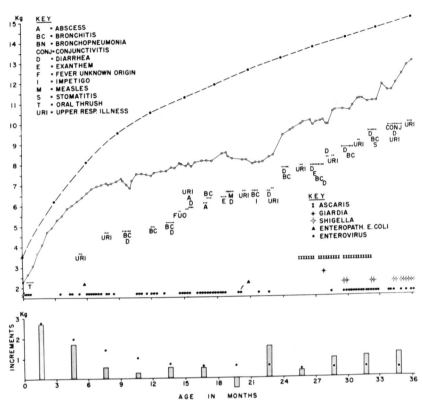

Figure 12.3a
Weight, infections, and infectious diseases of male Child 44. *Above:* solid line represents
weight of child; broken line shows median of the INCAP standard (1956). Length of horizontal lines indicates duration of infectious disease. Each dot marks 1 week positive for
a particular infectious agent. *Below:* observed weight increments (vertical bars) and
expected median increments (dots) of the standard (Mata et al., 1971c).

increase; their role in metabolism has yet to be firmly set, but they represent
some kind of nutrient diversion that contributes, with other deleterious
phenomena, to nutrient wastage (Beisel, 1972).

To investigate the relation of infection and infectious disease to nutritional status, data on weight, diet, and morbidity were displayed graphically
and in summary tables for each of the cohort children and for 50 other
children. This detailed characterization of associated weight changes and
occurrence of infectious disease was made possible by the closely approximated and serially repeated examinations of each child. Children 12 and 44
of the cohort are selected as examples for clinical description of infection and
growth. Child 44 was one of the cohort with a better growth rate (figure
12.3a). Despite an initial low birth weight this boy grew relatively well for

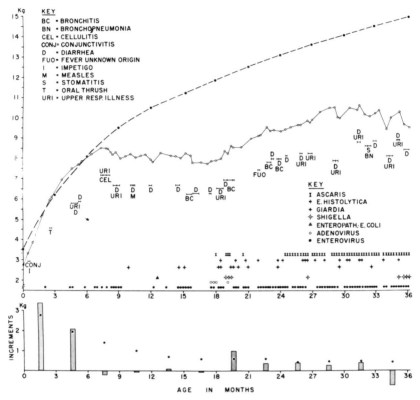

Figure 12.3b
Weight, infections, and infectious diseases of male Child 12. *Above:* solid line represents
weight of child; broken line shows median of the INCAP standard (1956). Length of horizontal lines indicates duration of infectious disease. Each dot marks 1 week positive for
a particular infectious agent. *Below:* observed weight increments (vertical bars) and
expected median increments (dots) of the standard (Mata et al., 1971c).

the first six months, although during the neonatal period he had several virus
infections and after three months became a continued shedder of enteroviruses.

While the load of intestinal infection was not as impressive as for most
village children, an excess frequency of respiratory tract illnesses occurred.
Weaning began at 6 months and was completed at 27 months; dietary supplements were typically deficient in calories and high-quality protein. The
weight curve departed from the reference standard around the sixth postnatal
month. Weight increments were calculated at three-month intervals and compared with the expected increments of the standard weight curve. Height also
departed from reference standards at about the same time. The first episode
of marked weight loss coincided with a combined attack of bronchitis and

diarrheal disease when approximately nine months old. Thereafter, periods of weight stagnation followed bouts of bronchitis, diarrhea, nonspecific exanthem, and measles.

Infections with *Ascaris, Giardia*, and *Shigella* appeared at the end of the second and during the third years. Total weight gain during the second year was remarkably small. The child grew well in the third year, exceeding expectations, although variations in weight gain were noted in association with a variety of infectious disease. However, no catch-up effect was observed. It is to be emphasized that prospective study of Cauqué children into the tenth year of life has demonstrated a persistent stunting of weight and height.

Child 12, presented in figure 12.3b, is an instance of deflection far more pronounced than the preceding example. Again, despite a low birth weight, this boy grew well for the first six months. Intestinal infections during the first six months were as frequent as with Child 44; growth, however, was as good or better than the mean standard. A succession of virus infections began at six months, and infections with *Entamoeba histolytica* and *Shigella* were recorded at 18 months. This date marked the initiation of a period of intense infection by a variety of agents often associated with clinical manifestations. The first weight faltering in this child promptly followed an attack of cellulitis and upper respiratory illness. Another episode of diarrhea and upper respiratory illness then occurred, and later one of measles with diarrhea.

A concentration of infection with ordinary pathogenic agents occurred at the onset of weaning and an associated poor supplementary feeding. During the next 12 months, weight faltering became so intense as to result in virtual arrest of growth. At 18 months slight improvement in growth was noted but stunting persisted throughout the remainder of the second year and during the third year. A renewed series of infections at the end of the third year resulted in more periods of weight loss and still further deterioration of nutritional status. This child had more infections, more infectious diseases, longer periods of weight faltering, and smaller weight increments than did Child 44. At the end of three years levels of weight and height were significantly less.

Great variability was also observed among host responses to the activity of particular agents. For instance, figure 12.4 illustrates the growth of a non-cohort child, a girl of low birth weight who grew satisfactorily for the first 10 weeks as is the expectancy for breast-fed infants. She then contracted an acute respiratory disease, became anorexic, and gained no appreciable weight for four weeks. Meningitis developed at 15 weeks with *Streptococcus pneumoniae* isolated from the cerebrospinal fluid. During this attack the child gained no weight but did respond to treatment. With continued breast-feeding she attained at 44 weeks a weight that matched the mean value for village children. Subsequent inadequate food supplements and a succession of

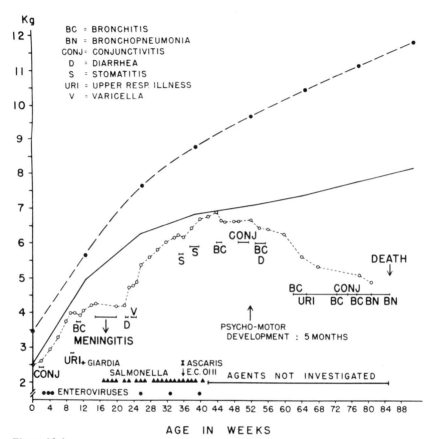

Figure 12.4
Weight, infections, and infectious diseases of female Child 19. *Broken top* line represents the INCAP standard; *solid* line shows the mean weight curve for Cauqué children; *bottom broken* line is observed weights of the child.

respiratory and intestinal infections led to marked debility with an eventually terminal infectious disease. Severe and persisting psychomotor retardation, recognized shortly after recovery from meningitis, persisted until death (Mata et al., 1972c). Autopsies were not feasible under village conditions; localized brain abscess, encephalitis, and terminal septicemia were conjectured but not established.

A variety of infectious diseases produces an effect on growth curves incapable of precise measurement. A common difficulty also exists in determining whether the growth deficit is due primarily to the infectious disease or to malnutrition. However, the assessment itself is of importance in demonstrating the impact of infection on the growth curve. Measles and whooping cough, both common communicable diseases caused by agents of high

Table 12.13
Weight Loss of Patients Surviving an Attack of Measles or Whooping Cough, by Age, 1965–1971

Age, years	Measles							Whooping Cough				
	Number of children	Absolute weight loss, g	Percentage weight loss at onset					Number of children	Absolute weight loss, g	Percentage weight loss at onset		
			< 2	2–4	5–9	10+				< 2	2–4	5+
< 1	42	201 ± 152[a]	18 (43)[b]	14 (33)	10 (24)	0		7	510 ± 666[a]	2 (29)[b]	0	5 (71)
1	32	316 ± 227	12 (38)	11 (34)	8 (25)	1 (3)		8	446 ± 373	1 (13)	4 (50)	3 (38)
2	26	327 ± 178	7 (27)	12 (46)	6 (23)	1 (4)		19	589 ± 693	5 (26)	11 (58)	3 (16)
3	8	469 ± 302	2 (25)	2 (25)	4 (50)	0		10	421 ± 617	5 (50)	4 (40)	1 (10)
4	9	210 ± 139	7 (78)	2 (22)	0	0						
5+	5	171 ± 88	4 (80)	1 (20)	0	0						
Total	122		50 (41)	42 (34)	28 (23)	2 (2)		44		13 (30)	19 (43)	12 (27)

[a]Mean ± S.D.
[b]Number of cases (percentage).

pathological potential, serve to illustrate this impact. Invasion of a susceptible child by the measles virus and its subsequent propagation results invariably in clinical disease. Weight loss during disease thus relates to the infectious process, presumably the result of host-parasite interaction.

Table 12.13 shows loss of weight among 122 children who survived an attack of measles and for whom complete weight data were available. Arbitrarily, a weight loss of less than 2 percent during the acute attack was considered inconsequential. Weight loss of 2 to 4 percent was classed as moderate and of 5 to 9 percent as severe; a loss of 10 percent or more was considered extreme. Loss of weight increases with age up to the fourth year of life. Severe and extreme losses of weight expectedly were most frequent among three year olds and thereafter in one and two year olds in that order. The more severe effects involved children who contracted measles during the weaning process when disturbed nutrition is specially common. The important consideration, however, is the excessive frequency with which children lost as much as 5 percent or more of body weight after measles, about one-fourth of those attacked.

Figure 12.5 illustrates the behavior of whooping cough in a village girl: A represents weight loss and B the expected weight gain the child would have had during the period of recuperation if not attacked by this disease; B is proportional to duration of recuperation of weight loss. Onset at 39 weeks set off a loss of weight that extended through a prolonged convalescence and a recuperation that required approximately 38 weeks. Whooping cough among children with a preceding growth retardation characteristically has a long period of weight recuperation before full recovery from respiratory symptoms. In this regard, assessment of weight loss in the manner described for measles or other diseases of rapid resolution is not wholly adequate for whooping cough because of the prolonged disability.

Forty-four children who survived a bout of whooping cough had complete weight data until full recovery and often weekly during the acute stage. Frequency and extent of weight loss are shown in table 12.13. Overall, age did not have a marked influence on the magnitude of absolute weight loss. Only two year olds showed a tendency to larger weight loss. The proportionate loss of weight, however, was larger in infants and one-year old children. The magnitude of weight loss at equivalent ages at attack are notably greater for whooping cough than for measles. Since the nutritional status at onset was better for infants than for one year olds, this experience with whooping cough contributes to evaluation of the relative place of infectious disease among factors involved in malnutrition and growth retardation.

Although no clear association was evident between reduced food intake and magnitude of weight loss, there is no doubt that these contribute importantly to a deteriorated nutritional status. Anorexia is a common symptom of infectious disease, sometimes in the absence of fever, but more often with

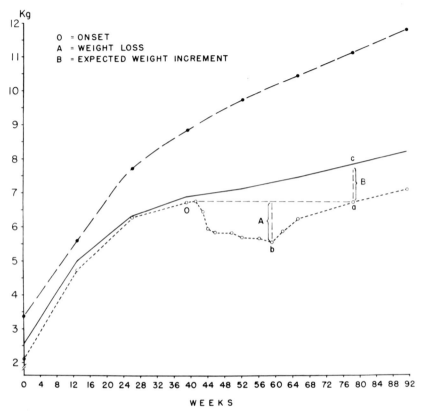

Figure 12.5
Deterioration of the nutritional status of female Child 177 after an attack of whooping cough. *Broken top* line corresponds to the INCAP standard; *solid* line shows the mean weight curve for Cauqué children; *bottom broken* line is observed weights of the child. *O* = onset of disease; *A* = weight loss; *B* = weight gain expected in period equivalent to the length of recuperation if not attacked by the disease. To estimate this amount, the mean weight curve for Cauqué children was used; the curve of the child was assimilated to such a curve at the time of onset.

Table 12.14
Consumption of Tortilla During Whooping Cough, 21 Children, 1968

Child number	Age, years–months	Percentage of consumption[a] by month of disease			Percentage of weight loss[b]
		1st	2nd	3rd	
22	3–5	43[c]	84	108	0
54	3–0	93	79	82	0
37	3–2	41[c]	94	90	0
52	2–11	108	109	149	0
59	2–11	130[d]	200	200	0
76	2–7	94	90	92	1
11	3–8	133	111	102	1
16	3–8	110	122	142	2
35	3–3	98	45[c]	105	2
24	3–5	52[c]	109	105	2
23	3–5	95	54[c]	90	2
31	3–5	96	122	117	2
69	2–7	99	91	97	2
83	2–5	55[c]	39[c]	103	4
91	2–2	100	100	60[c]	4
49	3–0	78	80	69[c]	4
34	3–2	139	57[c]	80	5
88	2–3	98	89	98	5
80	2–5	100	91	100	6
94	2–3	113	154	224	12
18	3–6	33[c]	36[c]	74[c]	22

Note: Adapted from Mata et al., 1972b.
[a]Percentage consumption in relation to intake before onset, considered as 100 percent.
[b]As in table 12.13.
[c]Reduction by at least 25 percent of usual intake.
[d]Increase by more than 25 percent of usual intake.

fever and vomiting also present. Anorexia was present in marked degree in measles and other febrile exanthems, diarrheal disease, respiratory disease, and fever of undetermined origin. Often the duration was for days and sometimes weeks and it was not uncommonly associated with asymptomatic infections (for example, those of *Ascaris*), when first established in one and two year olds.

Table 12.14 summarizes the consumption of tortilla by 21 surviving children, two to four years old, during an attack of whooping cough. Tortilla contributes about a half of calories and total protein to the diet of the child. A significant reduction during illness by at least 25 percent of the usual level consumed was evidenced by five of the children in the first month of disease. Three additional children reduced their intake during the second month and two more in the third month. Overall, a half of affected children had reduced their intake of maize, a behavior paralleled for beans and other foods. The child with the most marked loss also had a very low food intake during the three months of the disease. However, several children lost significant amounts of weight despite adequate food intake, and similar behavior was noted with other infectious diseases, particularly dysentery.

Malnutrition and the Outcome of Infectious Disease
The observed differences in growth curves of individual children can be explained in part by variations in the degree of exposure to infectious agents and the resulting diversity in frequency and severity of clinical manifestations. Conversely, differences in nutrition and growth among children could result in a variety of responses to the developing infectious process.

While the frequent occurrence of infectious disease stems mainly from a large community dosage of infectious agents, many of the clinical manifestations depend on an underlying malnutrition. Evidence in support of this statement was derived in the Cauqué study from the behavior of identical twins. The smaller of a pair showed the greater rate of morbidity and the most days of illness. By episodes, by number of illnesses, and by days of disease the smaller twin had more of each, a behavior seemingly not too dependent on birth weight because in both instances those values were rather close (table 12.15). During the first year of observation both twins experienced a comparable number of episodes but Twin 124 had the more complex morbidity, and the larger twin (Twin 125) more days of illness. The twins behaved differently, however, in the second and third years with the lighter twin manifesting more episodes and days of illness. This is demonstrated in figure 12.6, which uses only those disease episodes from table 12.15 involving an outstanding loss of weight.

Twin 125 had the larger birth weight of the monozygotic pair and grew better, especially after the first year. He also fared better in the response to infection; or conversely, because of lesser morbidity, his growth was better.

Table 12.15
Infectious Diseases, Pair No. 1 of Twins, Birth to Age Three Years, 1966–1969

Age, weeks	Twin 124			Twin 125		
	Episodes	Illnesses	Days	Episodes	Illnesses	Days
< 1 year						
0–12	5	6	43	5	5	48
13–25	3	4	29	3	4	60
26–38	4	9	44	2	5	30
39–51	3	5	24	3	5	37
Total	15	24	140	13	19	175
1–2 years						
52–64	3	3	24	1	2	21
65–77	3	4	44	1	1	28
78–90	1	5	105	1	5	87
91–103	0	0	0	0	1	5
Total	7	12	173	3	9	141
2–3 years						
104–116	3	3	12	2	3	10
117–129	1	3	13	2	3	8
130–142	2	5	34	2	2	8
143–155	4	4	34	4	2	12
Total	10	15	93	10	10	38
Grand Total	32	51	406	26	38	354

Numeral 1 in figure 12.6 indicates the first marked weight loss of the twins at 49 weeks of age, related to diarrhea with mucus in Twin 124 and to diarrhea with moderate dehydration in Twin 125. Numeral 2 marks the appearance of whooping cough in Twin 125 at 77 weeks and in Twin 124 after an appropriate incubation. Both events were followed by weight loss, most pronounced in Twin 124.

At 154 weeks Twin 124 developed laryngotracheobronchitis of seven days duration; three weeks later Twin 125 had an acute diarrheal disease of 11 days. These events are identified in figure 12.6 by Numeral 3; the infectious agents were not determined. Weight loss was proportionately greater for Twin 125, who was the heavier, but weight recuperation was prompter in this twin. Numeral 4 identifies a bronchitis and a diarrhea of 10 days duration in Twin 124 at age 206 weeks, associated with distinct weight loss and a protracted convalescence. The other twin had three days of diarrhea in the same week and his weight suffered less. In the course of time differences in weight of the two twins became progressively divergent. Although both twins shared the same environment with striking similarity in rates of infection and infectious disease, the variations in clinical response could well be due to differences in

288   Results

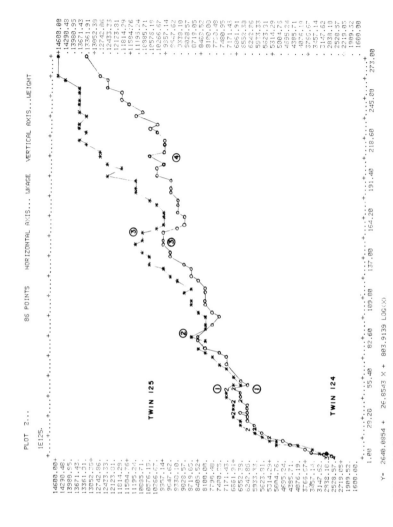

Figure 12.6
Growth curves of monozygotic twins, cases 124 and 125, first five years of life. The horizontal axis
shows age in weeks; the vertical axis represents weight in grams. Numerals indicate events involving
weight loss (see text).

Table 12.16
Frequency and Duration of Diarrhea and Bronchopneumonia as Complications of Measles, 1964–1972

Onset of associated illness, days	Number of cases	Diarrhea		Bronchopneumonia	
		Frequency	Duration, days	Frequency	Duration, days
4+ days before measles onset[a]	9	7[b]	16.1 (7.5)[c]	2[b]	4.0[c]
3 days before to 3 days after measles onset	87	67	6.6 (4.9)	20	3.9 (1.3)
4–6 days after measles onset	26	20	4.6 (3.7)	59	3.6 (0.9)
7–14 days after measles onset	7	5	3.1 (1.1)	18	3.5 (1.8)

Note: 129 cases of diarrhea and 98 cases of bronchopneumonia were studied.
[a]But still present at onset of measles.
[b]Percentage
[c]Mean ± S.D.

host susceptibility or dosage, rather than to differences in growth pattern. Conceivably, better weight and growth pattern express a greater ability to cope with infections, in turn a reflection of individuality in the development of the immune system and other defense mechanisms.

Further evidence of the deleterious effects of malnutrition on the outcome of illness came from the frequent chronicity of disease, particularly diarrhea, respiratory tract infections, and whooping cough; from the undue frequency of complications in measles, whooping cough, and dysentery, giving multiple associated illnesses and symptoms; from the higher case fatality of several diseases, including measles; and from the often prolonged clinical course and convalescence.

The explanation for greater frequency of complications of common communicable diseases could rest in opportunistic invasion by other infectious agents that prey on a debilitated host. Field data from the region suggest, however, that such complications as the diarrhea of measles, varicella, and other communicable diseases are indeed more a particular response of the malnourished host to the specific infection (Scrimshaw et al., 1966; Salomon et al., 1966) than a function of common pathogens or indigenous or opportunist invaders.

Table 12.16 shows the occurrence and duration of the two most common clinical complications of measles in this region, namely, diarrhea and bronchopneumonia, by date of appearance in relation to onset of the measles

Table 12.17
Elapsed Time from Onset of Whooping Cough to Return to Original Weight, 44 Children, 1968

Time, weeks	Number of cases	Percentage
0–4	6	14
5–8	8	18
9–12	8	18
13–16	4	9
17–24	7	16
25+	11	25

Table 12.18
Weight Loss During Measles as a Function of the Degree of Malnutrition at Onset, 114 Cases, 1965–1972

			Percentage of Patients with Weight Loss of:[a]			
Degree of malnutrition	Number of children	Absolute weight loss, g	< 2%	2–4%	5+%	Total with 2+%
Well-nourished	8	96 ± 136[b]	63	38	0	38
I	35	297 ± 338	43	34	23	57
II	60	743 ± 741	35	43	22	65
III	19	258 ± 65	21	32	47	79

[a]Percentage of weight at onset of illness.
[b]Mean ± S.D.

exanthem. Diarrhea occurred more frequently during prodromes and the early exanthematic phase than later. Its duration then was relatively short (averaging five to seven days) compared with diarrheas during incubation or before exposure. These data suggest that diarrhea during the prodromes and exanthem of measles is related to the virus infection itself and is thus distinct from the prevailing or endemic diarrheas of other origin. Bronchopneumonia was frequent during measles prodromes and more so during the exanthem,* yet with no differences in mean duration under the two conditions.

A clinical course prolonged beyond usual limits is another feature of certain infectious diseases in malnourished children. Table 12.17 displays the duration of whooping cough among 44 children from onset to complete

---

* The etiology of bronchopneumonia could be independent of measles virus, as studies in industrial regions indicate, with the greater frequency in this region accounted for by the enhanced host susceptibility of a malnourished population. Some cases could well be of giant cells, the result of a depressed T-immunocyte function (Mata and Faulk, 1973) particularly in view of the tendency of measles virus to persist in cells of malnourished subjects (Scheifele and Forbes, 1972).

Table 12.19
Correlation between Weight Loss during Whooping Cough, Outcome of the Disease, and Child Characteristics, 44 Surviving Children less than Four Years Old, 1968

Variable	Correlation coefficient	P
Age of child, at onset	−0.336	< 0.05
Time to recover weight loss	0.785	< 0.001
Duration of whooping cough	0.135	> 0.05
Duration of associated diarrhea	0.346	< 0.05
Duration of bronchopneumonia	0.657	< 0.01

Note: Weight loss considered as in table 12.14.

return to basal weight before onset. In one half of the cases disability lasted for more than 12 weeks; in one-fourth it exceeded 25 weeks. This prolonged convalescence, while primarily the result of the initial whooping cough and its associated weight loss, was extended in many instances by the sequence of other infectious diseases which characteristically appear in debilitated or depleted individuals living under poor environmental conditions.

The relationship of malnutrition, as defined at the beginning of this chapter, to the outcome of measles is presented in table 12.18. Despite a great variability, absolute weight losses in general were lowest in well-nourished children and greater in individuals classed as second-degree malnourished (II). The most malnourished, however, did not lose as much. A proportional weight loss of less than 2 percent was judged inconsequential; weight loss was more pronounced in malnutrition; in fact, 47 percent of children with third-degree malnutrition showed an acute weight loss of 5 percent or more; well-nourished children had no such loss.

The degree of malnutrition at onset and duration of the disease, however, apparently had no relation to total weight depletion during whooping cough (table 12.19); this was probably due to the death of the most severely malnourished children who had the disease (many could not be weighed at the time of death or even shortly before). Factors related to the degree of weight loss in whooping cough were age of child, duration of associated diarrhea and bronchopneumonia, and time to recover weight loss. The highest correlation was with time to recover weight loss.

The exaggerated levels of measles fatality among malnourished village children appear unrelated to any genetically determined susceptibility (Gordon et al., 1965a: Scrimshaw et al., 1968a) but related to a lesser capacity of the malnourished host to resist infection (Chandra, 1972; Awdeh, 1972; Faulk et al., 1974). Evidence exists that the cellular immune response of malnourished children to measles virus is impaired (Mata and Faulk, 1973).

Rates for acquired disease increase with age past the neonatal period to attain high values in the second year of life and in the first half of the third. Without discounting the importance of sanitation and living conditions, the high rates of disease in the second year suggest strongly that acute infection is then intertwined with malnutrition. The second year is the time the child becomes overtly malnourished. Thus a logical solution would be to improve nutrition at that time of life. The present world food situation poses doubts, however, as to the feasibility and cost of an answer based on food programs. The discussions in chapters 5 and 10 show that diets in the village are not wholly bad; much could be accomplished by better use of available foods. Furthermore, recent evidence has indicated that improved diets of children with high morbidity and mortality rates, with no action toward infection control and prevention, do not result in a beneficial effect on the nutritional status (Parrilla-Ríos, 1973); programs aimed at education, hygiene, and control of infection, however, have produced dramatic results in better health and nutritional status of the child population (Hollister et al., 1955; Aguirre and Pradilla, 1973). In the final analysis infection stands out as the target that can be attacked through community effort without resorting to outside resources.

A comprehensive survey of the Central American population revealed that the main nutritional problems of Guatemala are protein-calorie malnutrition (PCM), deficiencies of vitamin A and riboflavin, and anemias (INCAP-OIR, 1969a). In the village of Santa María Cauqué PCM was recognized mainly on the basis of retarded physical growth. The other deficiencies were evident from biochemical determinations of blood and urine. Although studies of blood and urine in populations such as Santa María Cauqué confirm suboptimal levels of a variety of nutrients, such studies do not reflect the real problem owing to the host's capacity to adapt metabolically to chronic malnutrition and to infection (PAHO, 1971). This is particularly true of children surviving the early environmental stresses past five years of age. Thus, data on physical growth, childhood mortality, occurrence of infectious diseases and of severe forms of malnutrition will provide more adequate indexes of population nutritional state. This chapter will focus on malnutrition as evidenced by anemia, growth retardation, and severe PCM. As will be seen, malnutrition and nutritional abnormalities in Santa María Cauqué were clearly related to the total configuration of biological, social, psychological, and economic characteristics of parents and children.

Anemias and Other Nutritional Deficiencies
Iron deficiency anemia occurs in the highlands of Guatemala in the absence of hookworm infection (Viteri et al., 1973a), due to the low availability of iron in the predominantly vegetarian diet and to the exceedingly high rates of infection which provide a mechanism for iron sequestration even with subclinical infections (Beisel, 1972).

Table 13.1
Hemoglobin Levels, Packed Red Cell Volume, and Mean Corpuscular Hemoglobin
Concentration Levels, 30 Children, Birth to Age Four Years, 1964–1970

Age, years	Number of cases	Hemoglobin, g/100ml	Packed red cell volume, %	Mean corpuscular hemoglobin concentration
1	21	11.60 (1.59)[a] 7.0–13.9	36.03 (3.26) 31.0–42.0	32.60 (2.06) 30.0–38.0
2	25	11.41 (1.01) 9.7–13.0	34.50 (2.95) 29.0–40.0	32.70 (2.19) 29.0–39.0
3	25	11.83 (0.75) 10.9–13.1	35.39 (1.82) 32.0–39.0	33.34 (1.81) 30.0–37.0
4	9	12.04 (0.63) 11.2–13.2	37.13 (1.46) 35.0–40.0	32.43 (1.32) 32.0–35.0

Age, years	Number of cases	Hemoglobin, g/100ml				
		< 10	10	11	12	13
1	21	1 (5)[b]	6 (29)	4 (19)	5 (24)	5 (24)
2	25	1 (4)	9 (36)	8 (32)	5 (20)	2 (8)
3	25	0	3 (12)	12 (12)	9 (36)	1 (4)
4	9	0	0	3 (33)	5 (56)	1 (11)

Age, years	Number of cases	Mean corpuscular hemoglobin concentration				
		29	30	31	32	33+
1	20	0	4 (20)[b]	3 (15)	4 (20)	9 (45)
2	22	2 (9)	4 (18)	2 (9)	3 (14)	11 (50)
3	25	1 (4)	0	5 (20)	4 (16)	15 (60)
4	7	0	1 (14)	1 (14)	2 (29)	3 (43)

[a]Mean (S.D.); below, minimum-maximum values.
[b]Number of children (percentage).

Cultural beliefs of the villagers of Santa María Cauqué made collection of
blood difficult; studies were limited to determination of hemoglobin and
hematocrit in selected children of the cohort. Table 13.1 summarizes mean
hematologic values for cohort children observed prospectively from age one
to age four. Anemia was frequent in the first three years, particularly among
one year olds, many of whom had hemoglobin values as low as seven or eight
grams per 100 milliliter. Interestingly enough, none of the four year olds had
anemia. According to WHO (1972a) and the International Committee for
Standardization in Hematology (1971), hemoglobin values below 11 grams
per 100 milliliter and mean corpuscular hemoglobin concentration (MCHC)
below 31 are indicative of anemia in children six months to three years of
age. MCHC values below 31 were detected in one to three year olds but not
in children four years of age.

The distribution of hemoglobin and MCHC are also shown, respectively, in table 13.1. Thirty-four percent of all one year olds and 40 percent of two year olds had anemia by the above criteria. The situation improved in the third year and particularly in the fourth year of life. Twenty percent of one year olds and 27 percent of two year olds also exhibited low values of MCHC.

The nutrition survey revealed other abnormalities in hematologic and biochemical parameters (INCAP-OIR, 1969a); Cauqué children did not show hypoproteinemia, except under severe infectious stress (Viteri et al., 1973b).

These results give evidence that malnutrition is more common in the first two years of life, but that deficiencies reflected in biological parameters such as hemoglobin concentration improve in the third year and are rare in the fourth. It appears that once a child has fully adapted to an adult type of diet and has been exposed and immunized to the common communicable diseases he or she recovers from the anemia of the first two years.

As for severe vitamin A deficiency, only one case of night blindness was recognized and no cases of xerophthalmia, keratomalacia, or blindness attributable to that deficiency were documented during the eight-year period. The village had only two blind persons, one a newborn who developed *Shigella* conjunctivitis in the course of severe dysentery of the infant and his mother. The other was an elderly person with cataracts.

The nutrition survey in Guatemala did not show overall deficiencies of calcium, iodine, ascorbic acid, niacin, or thiamin. Dietary calcium is improved by the customary treatment of corn with lime, in making tortillas, which also improves the nutritional value of corn in other ways (Bressani et al., 1958b; Katz et al., 1974). Iodine deficiency is not a problem because of fortification of all salt for human consumption with potassium iodate (Ascoli and Arroyave, 1970). Ascorbic acid is provided by the frequent consumption of a variety of fruits and vegetables. Limited amounts of dietary vitamin D are supplemented by full exposure of the population to sunlight which promotes the conversion of the provitamin in the skin. The Cauqué study did, however, find prevalent calorie deficiency and protein deficiency which appear to be high priority problems. The underlying factors are the low socioeconomic development, with poverty and poor education the main components.

Physical Growth Retardation
Among the abnormalities in physical growth of Cauqué children the most obvious were the periods of weight loss and growth arrest incident to infectious disease, anorexia, and food scarcity. The result is early retardation of physical growth or stunting. The deterioration in nutritional status becomes evident by examining the proportion of children lagging behind the percentiles of an accepted standard. Table 13.2 shows the distribution of all village children observed prospectively during the study period with reference to the Denver standard for weight and height (Hansman, 1970). In the

Table 13.2
Cohort Children, by Age and Percentiles of the Denver Weight and Height Standards, 1964-1972

Age, months	Number of cases	Denver weight percentiles					
		< 3rd	3rd–	16th–	50th–	84th–	100th–
Birth	408	25	44	27	4	0	0
3	375	19	27	36	13	5	0
6	374	33	37	23	6	1	0
12	332	78	17	4	1	0	0
18	276	85	13	2	0	0	0
24	249	88	10	2	0	0	0
30	207	87	11	2	0	0	0
36	204	83	15	2	0	0	0
Age, months	Number of cases	Denver height percentiles					
		< 3rd	3rd–	16th–	50th–	84th–	100th–
Birth	407	44	32	22	2	0	0
3	186	65	21	11	3	0	0
6	184	77	18	4	1	0	0
12	166	94	5	1	0	0	0
18	130	97	2	1	0	0	0
24	141	97	3	0	0	0	0
30	109	99	1	0	0	0	0
36	129	98	2	0	0	0	0

Note: Figures show percentage under the 3rd Denver weight and height percentiles.

discussion that follows, only percentiles shown in tables 13.2 and 13.3 were considered. It will be noted that most children fall below the Denver percentiles for weight, between 6 and 18 months of age, to such an extent that at 18 months the majority of children were below the 16th percentile (table 13.2). The situation was worse for height; stunting of most children had occurred by one year of age.

As children grew older they varied in the position they occupied in relation to the standard. Table 13.3 shows that 6 percent of 12 month olds moved up one percentile in weight, while 24 percent stepped down. Among 18 month olds no child showed improvement; 41 percent remained in the same percentile as at 12 months, while the remainder moved to a lower percentile. Decline to a lower percentile was more frequent for height than weight. Data shown in chapter 9 indicate that the stunting continues throughout childhood, but that it does not get much worse; in fact, growth curves of children become relatively parallel to the standard.

Table 13.3
Shifting of Weight and Height of Cohort Children, Denver Weight and Height Percentiles,
Birth to Age Three Years, 1964–1972

	Percentage		
Age, months	Remained in Denver Percentile	Moved up	Moved down
Weight			
6	59	24	17
12	49	6	24
18	41	0	59
24	86	0	14
30	76	0	24
36	85	0	15
Height			
6	50	19	31
12	32	1	67
18	27	1	72
24	25	0	75
30	25	0	75
36	27	1	71

Table 13.4
FAO/WHO Classification of Protein-Calorie Malnutrition, 1971

	Body weight as percentage of standard[a]	Edema	Deficit weight for height[b]
Underweight child	80–60	No	< 10%
Nutritional dwarfing	< 60	No	< 10%
Marasmus	< 60	No	⩾ 10%
Kwashiorkor	80–60	Yes	⩾ 10%
Marasmic-Kwashiorkor	< 60	Yes	⩾ 10%

[a]50th percentile of standard (see text).

[b]Weight for height $= \dfrac{\text{Weight of child}}{\text{Weight of normal child of same height}} \times 100.$

Table 13.5
Incidence of Severe PCM, 45 Cohort Children, Birth to Age Three Years, 1964–1969

Year of life	Number of children	Marasmus[a]	Kwashiorkor	Marasmic-Kwashiorkor	Total PCM
First	45	6 (13)[b]	0	0	6 (13)
Second	44	6 (14)	3 (7)	3 (7)	12 (27)
Third	43	0	3 (7)	1 (2)	4 (9)

[a]Classification of PCM is described in the text and in table 13.4.
[b]Number of new cases (rounded percentage). A case found in one year and continuing into the next was counted only in the year it first appeared.

Severe Protein-Calorie Malnutrition

The classification of severe protein-calorie malnutrition (PCM) was according to FAO/WHO recommendations (1971) with some modifications (table 13.4). The INCAP weight standards (INCAP, 1956) were used instead of the Harvard standards. To class a case as marasmus a deficit in weight for height of at least 10 percent was required in addition to a deficit in body weight for age of at least 40 percent. For epidemiological purposes these arbitrary criteria gave as good an estimate of marasmus as other classifications (Waterlow, 1973). In the following presentation the "underweight" and "nutritional dwarf" classes will not be discussed; reference is made only to the severe forms of PCM.

Table 13.5 shows incidence of forms of severe PCM among the cohort children in the first three years of life. The incidence and prevalence of marasmus and other forms of PCM described below are high. Parental attitudes toward malnutrition differ from those observed toward infectious diseases such as measles and whooping cough. Parents do not appear particularly concerned about marasmus because thin children are the most common occurrence during the weaning period. Thus chronic underweight has been incorporated into the village imagery as a natural occurrence. If a child develops edema, the mother does become preoccupied with the poor appetite of the child and the swelling. Advice on dietary management, however, is ordinarily accepted by the mother only when edematous PCM is relatively far advanced.

Marasmus is the most common form of severe PCM, appearing as early as the first year of life even in breast-fed children. It is a deficiency of long duration, lasting months or years; in Cauqué children it was always associated with exceedingly high rates of infectious disease. Incidence figures reveal that all new cases occurred in the first two years. Also the incidence of marasmus was similar in both sexes. Kwashiorkor and marasmic kwashiorkor, with high rates, were less frequent but more severe and required more intensive medical attention.

Table 13.6
Incidence of Edematous PCM, All Cohorts Born after 11 February, 1964, by Year of
Study and Class of Malnutrition, 1964–1972

Year	Kwashiorkor	Marasmic-Kwashiorkor	Total PCM
1964	0[a]	0	0[b]
1965	0	0	0
1966	1	2	3 (9)
1967	6	2	8 (25)
1968	1	3	4 (13)
1969	5	2	7 (22)
1970	2	2	4 (13)
1971	4	2	6 (19)
Total cases	19	13	32

[a]Number of cases.
[b]Number of cases (percentage frequency).

The presence of edema permits a ready characterization of kwashiorkor
(K) and marasmic kwashiorkor (M-K) in large population groups. The M-K
patients originally had marasmus and developed edema after occurrence of
an infectious process. This type of PCM was more easily recognized than
other types of severe PCM because of its characteristic clinical feature,
severity and high case fatality (Autret and Béhar, 1955).

Table 13.6 shows the incidence of K and M-K by year. The absence of
cases in 1964 and 1965 is due to the fact that severe edematous PCM tends to
appear after the first year of life and the first cohorts of children were recruited in those years. Marasmus is observed in Cauqué infants (table 13.5),
but cases of this disease were not included in the tabulation by year.

Table 13.7 shows the incidence by age, to indicate that weanlings (18 to
35 month olds) are the most severely affected. Two marasmic infants past the
first six months of life developed edema and were classed as marasmic
kwashiorkor patients.

For certain purposes kwashiorkor was arbitrarily subdivided into two
varieties: prekwashiorkor to characterize underweight children brought to the
clinic with the skin changes apparent; and kwashiorkor, where skin changes
and edema had become established. There was an equal susceptibility of the
sexes (table 13.8) although the prekwashiorkor and kwashiorkor male-to-
female ratios indicate a greater severity of the condition among females.

Mortality of K and M-K did not differ strikingly from that observed in
recuperation centers and hospitals (Cook, 1971). Table 13.9 shows 5 deaths
among 32 cases of PCM, a case fatality of 15.6 percent. The case fatality
excluding the prekwashiorkor patients was 22 percent. Deaths were always
associated with infectious diseases of known seriousness, for instance, acute

Table 13.7
Incidence of Edematous PCM, All Cohort Children Born after 11 February, 1964, by
Age and Class of Malnutrition, 1964–1970

Age			Marasmic-	
Years	Months	Kwashiorkor	Kwashiorkor	Total PCM
< 1	6–11	1[a]	1	2 (6)[b]
1	12–17	2	1	3 (9)
	18–23	4	8	12 (38)
2	24–29	4	0	4 (13)
	30–35	6	0	6 (19)
3	36–41	1	2	3 (9)
	42–47	0	0	0
4	48–53	0	0	0
	54–59	0	0	0
5	60–65	0	1	1 (3)
	66–71	0	0	0
6	72–77	1	0	1 (3)
Total cases		19	13	32

[a]Number of cases.
[b]Number of cases (percentage frequency).

diarrheal disease, again emphasizing the important role of infection. Treatment was generally done in the home though there were some hospitalized cases. Emphasis was on maintaining breast-feeding as long as the child was not anorexic, and on giving fluids to compensate for water losses due to diarrhea. Formula preparations were given under supervision by the nurse if the child had anorexia; dietetic advice was provided in all cases. Pneumonia, septicemia, and dysentery required the use of antibiotics.

The distribution of K and M-K by months is shown in figure 13.1. Pre-kwashiorkor was evenly distributed throughout the year. The lack of correlation between appearance of marasmus and season of the year could arise from a generalized poverty independent of seasonal influence of food crops and income.

Kwashiorkor was concentrated in June through September. The combination of all cases depicts a distribution of most cases in the rainy season. A period of food scarcity or serious economic depression likewise often heralds the appearance of kwashiorkor. It also occurs most frequently after the harvest of maize, string beans, and cabbage (see table 2.5) and when plants or vegetables that complement the village diet are most abundant. Due to an insect pest, black beans have not been planted regularly in Santa María in the last 10 years by most families. Black beans are purchased from March through August when sale of crops provides cash.

Table 13.8
Severe PCM, All Cohorts Born after 11 February 1964, by Sex and Class of Malnutrition,
1964–1972

Sex	Pre-Kwashiorkor[a]	Kwashkorkor[b]	Marasmic-Kwashiorkor	Total PCM
Male	7	2	7	16
Female	2	8	6	16
M/F ratio	3.5	0.3	1.2	1.0

[a]Weight deficit and edema.
[b]With skin changes.

Table 13.9
Childhood Deaths from Severe PCM, 1964–1972

Number of child	Age, months	Sex	Year of death	Class of PCM	Concurrent illness
67	23	F	1967	Kwashiorkor	Bronchopneumonia, diarrhea
77	18	F	1968	Marasmic-Kwashiorkor	Whooping cough, atelectasia
255	23	M	1970	Marasmic-Kwashiorkor	Bronchopneumonia
214	39	F	1971	Kwashiorkor	Diarrhea, dehydration
325	18	M	1971	Marasmic-Kwashiorkor	Diarrhea, dehydration

Note: Fatality: Five among 23 cases of edematous PCM with skin changes = 22.0
percent. Five among 32 total edematous PCM = 15.6 percent.

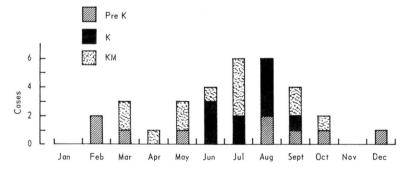

Figure 13.1
Edematous protein-calorie malnutrition, by month, all cohorts, birth to age three years,
1964–1973. Number and percentage of total PCM from January to December: 0(0),
2(6), 3(9), 1(3), 3(9), 4(13), 6(19), 6(19), 4(13), 2(6), 0(0), 1(3).

The peak incidence of edematous PCM in months in which food is more available suggests that there were other causes of this deficiency in the village. One such factor is infectious disease, particularly measles, diarrhea, and respiratory infections which occur more frequently at the end of the dry season and the beginning of the rainy season, that is, a few months before edematous PCM occurs with greatest frequency. In the presence of a relative abundance of food, however, kwashiorkor coincides with the peak incidence of measles, diarrheal disease, respiratory infection, and other kinds of infection. The relationship of food availability, marketing, and cash to malnutrition deserves serious investigation. Although there must be other social factors contributing to the occurrence of severe PCM, they were not unearthed by the Cauqué study.

In August 1974 an epidemic of severe PCM began, with 10 cases of edematous PCM and two deaths in August and September, one-third of the number seen during the entire eight years of the Cauqué study. Similar outbreaks occurred in neighboring villages. The Cauqué epidemic is being investigated. No differences among matched families with and without severe cases of PCM have been noted in socioeconomic status, food availability, and dietary intake. The only difference has been the appearance of acute diarrhea, with dehydration, a few weeks or months before appearance of severe PCM. Strains of toxigenic *Escherichia coli* have been isolated from patients with gastroenteritis and identified by recognized techniques (Evans et al., 1973).

The recent increase in cost of living, adjustments in maternal behavior incident to temporary migration of working males away from the village, and the resultant economic and social disruption of family life may be playing a role in the present outbreak of severe PCM, although the occurrence of the epidemic toxigenic organism appears to be the most likely precipitating factor.

It is important to note that malnutrition occurs primarily in children from 6 to 36 months of age, coinciding with the period when communicable diseases of childhood and calorie-deficient diets are at their highest levels.

Hematological values reveal anemia as a nutritional disease of the first year of life that becomes more acute and prevalent in the second. Displacement of weight and height of individual children to lower percentiles again indicates the first two years of life as critical. Marasmus begins to appear toward the end of infancy and becomes more frequent in the second year. Since breast-feeding is universal in this culture, the appearance of marasmus at such early ages is further evidence of the lack of adequate food supplementation, particularly calories, and of the burden of infectious diseases. The same observation holds for the edematous varieties of PCM.

Data presented in chapters 11 and 12 showed the highest rates of infection and infectious diseases occurring from 6 to 24 months of age. The combined effect of deficient diets and infection is primarily responsible for the high mortality in the first two years of life. This interaction finds clear epidemiological expression in the syndrome of weanling diarrhea (Gordon et al., 1963) and in the second year death rate (Béhar et al., 1958; Gordon et al., 1967) so characteristic of cultures similar to Santa María Cauqué.

Once children are immunized (by attack or artificially) and learn to eat the foods available in the village, malnutrition becomes a lesser problem. Thus the high prevalence of malnutrition reported for the general population of Central America, based on deficits of weight and height is an overestimation (INCAP-OIR, 1969a, 1969b; INCAP-CDC, 1972). A more realistic appraisal of malnutrition based on weight for height relationships or on prospective epidemiologic studies of health and malnutrition shows the problem to be one of preschoool ages and less extensive among school children, adolescents, and working adults. These considerations, along with greater appreciation of the role of infection and the role of total amount of food or calories (versus that of the protein component alone), provide a basis for a redefinition of type of infection, target populations, and priorities for action (Gopalan et al., 1973; Levinson, 1974; Sukhatme, 1974; Valverde et al., 1975; Waterlow et al., 1960).

Chapter 14
Multivariate Analysis of Physical Growth

This chapter summarizes multivariate analyses performed on sets and subsets of the data from the Cauqué study, using variables describing characteristics of mother, child, and environment against those of the child's physical growth. The clinical, epidemiological, and statistical evidence provided in preceding chapters pointed out an association of many of these variables with the growth retardation of Cauqué children. The intent now is to measure mathematically the likely contribution of individual elements and to determine the combinations of variables capable of predicting significant segments of variances of growth.

The village environment presents conditions that interfere with optimal expression of childhood growth potential. Among them, cultural and economic conditions determine a high risk of infection and an inadequate diet, resulting in high childhood mortality, deficient anthropometry, and poor health of pregnant women. Thus, a large proportion of infants show growth retardation at birth, a finding strongly correlated with maternal characteristics.

In general, village children begin to manifest physical growth retardation in the second half of the first year, or even earlier. This behavior relates in part to birth weight and gestational age. The main factors contributing to physical growth retardation, however, are inadequate feeding of infants and children and excessive rates of infection. Other environmental factors such as family stability, parental education, and maternal-infant interaction influence growth patterns but because of the difficulty in quantitating them by the

* This chapter was written jointly with Richard A. Kronmal.

usual methods of medical measurement, they have regularly received less emphasis.

Preceding chapters have shown that physical growth of children correlates with maternal age and maternal weight and height and with gestational age and birth weight. Food intake excluding breast milk showed a poor correlation with physical growth, but breast-feeding as expressed in the variable "weaning age" was strongly correlated with growth. Infectious disease had a definite effect on physical growth as evidenced by its impact on the weight curve, by the resulting reduced food intake, by weight loss during illness, and by the slow convalescence after attack.

Variables Employed in Multivariate Analysis
Step-wise regression analyses (SWRAs) for physical growth were performed using parameters b and c of the curve fitted by the model $y = a + bx + c \log x$, using the weight data for the first three years of life of each individual. Parameter c primarily reflects the period of early growth or growth deceleration while parameter b summarizes growth throughout most of the remainder of the period. Growth in the first months, however, influences to a certain extent the magnitude of b.

For the analyses, variables were grouped arbitrarily in various classes—maternal, newborn, and child—notwithstanding that their complex interrelations often made clear distinction of these factors impossible.

Maternal variables were age, weight, height, birth interval, number of previous deliveries, duration of pregnancy (equivalent to gestational age), and socioeconomic index as defined in chapters 5 and 7. The abbreviations of these variables are given in table 14.1. Newborn variables were sex, birth weight, birth length, birth head circumference, and gestational age as defined in chapter 6. Child variables were weaning age and various measures of diet, infection, and morbidity. Weaning age is the age in months of the child at completed weaning as described in chapter 10. Diet variables—derived from the calorie curve—were the intercept a reflecting onset of supplemental feeding, and the slope b which summarizes mean rate of caloric intake of individual children.

Intestinal infection variables were rates of occurrence of viruses, bacteria, or parasites for individual children, computed for the first, second, and third years of life and for the three years combined. Rates were calculated by dividing the number of weeks positive for a particular agent or groups of agents by the number of weekly specimens examined in a particular period of life. Rates were calculated for agents of recognized pathogenic potential as listed in table 14.1 with their abbreviations. *Dientamoeba fragilis* was not considered because numbers were few. Rates for enteroviruses, adenoviruses, and *Shigella sonnei* in the second and third years of life were similar for all children and were consequently excluded.

Table 14.1
Variables and Abbreviations for Step-Wise Regression Analysis

Variable	Abbreviations
Maternal, newborn, and child variables	
Maternal:	
Age, years	MAGE
Weight, kg	MWT
Height, cm	MHT
Birth interval	BINTER
Number of previous deliveries	DELIV
Duration of pregnancy (gestational age), weeks	DPREG (GAGE)
Socioeconomic index	SECI
Newborn:	
Sex: 1, male; 2, female	ISEX
Weight, g	BWT
Length, cm	BHT
Head circumference, cm	BHEAD
Child:	
Weaning age, months	WAGE
Calorie intercept, *a*	DINT
Calorie slope, *b*	DSLOPE
Intestinal infection variables	
Entamoeba histolytica	EHISTO1, EHISTO2, EHISTO3, EHISTOT[d]
Giardia lamblia	GIARD1, GIARD2, GIARD3, GIARDT
Ascaris lumbricoides	ASCAR1, ASCAR2, ASCAR3, ASCART
Trichuris trichiura	TRICH1, TRICH2, TRICH3, TRICHT
Shigella dysenteriae[a]	SDYS1, SDYS2, SDYS3, SDYST
Shigella flexneri[a]	SFLEX1, SFLEX2, SFLEX3, SFLEXT
Shigella boydii[a]	SBOYD1, SBOYD2, SBOYD3, SBOYDT
Shigella sonnei	SSONN1
Enteroviruses[b]	ENTER1
Adenoviruses[b]	ADENO1

Variable (days of disease)	Codes[c]	Abbreviations
Infectious disease variables		
All infectious diseases and illnesses	All	DILL1, DILL2, DILL3, DILLT[d]
Diarrheal disease	211, 212, 213	DIARR1, DIARR2, DIARR3, DIARRT
Severe diarrhea	213, 1502, 1506	SVD1, SVD2, SVD3, SVDT
Respiratory disease	102, 109, 116	RESP1, RESP2, RESP3, RESPT
Diseases of ear, mouth, and skin	403, 503–505, 902–905, 1002, 1003	EMS1, EMS2, EMS3, EMST

Variable (days of disease)	Codes[c]	Abbreviations
Systemic disease	121, 921–926, 928, 930, 931, 1103, 1105, 1309	SYST1, SYST2, SYST3, SYSTT
Bacterial and yeast disease	102, 103, 109, 116, 121, 212, 213, 403, 505, 601, 602, 801, 902–905, 914, 919, 926, 1002, 1003, 1105, 1107	BACT1, BACT2, BACT3, BACTT
Viral disease	101, 113–115, 211, 301, 501– 504, 921–925, 928, 930, 931, 1103, 1309	VIR1, VIR2, VIR3, VIRT

[a]All serotypes.
[b]All isolates grouped by presumptive criteria (table 4.10).
[c]Codes of infectious diseases as outlined in appendix C.
[d]1, 2, 3, and T at end of abbreviation denote first, second, third, and first three years of life respectively.

For morbidity, days of illness were computed for each child for the first, second, and third years of life, and for the three years combined, and expressed as a percentage of the total days of observation. Rates were calculated for groups of illnesses or for all infectious diseases combined. Rates of total days of illness for the second and third years also were similar for all children and were excluded.

Step-wise regression analyses were made for the cohort children because maternal, newborn, child and growth variables were measured for most of them. The regressions were done on 39 cases only because data on one or more of these variables were missing for six children, this being within usual experience in field work. One child migrated before three years of age; therefore, no information on weaning age was available. Two children died before age three years, and their growth curves could not be obtained and fitted in the same fashion as those of children completing three years. Two other children who developed severe protein-calorie malnutrition were hospitalized and removed from the study in the course of the third year of life. One child lacked information on gestational age.

Correlations for Parameter c

Tables 14.2, 14.3, and 14.4 show correlations among variables used in the regression of the c parameter of the growth curve. Table 14.2 has correlation coefficients for child variables indicating that growth in the first months is better with larger maternal weight (MWT) but is inversely related to maternal

Table 14.2
Correlations among the Estimated Parameter c of the Weight Curve and Maternal and Child Variables, 39 Cases

	MAGE[a]	MHT	MWT	BINTER	DELIV	ISEX	BWT	BHT	BHEAD	GAGE	WAGE	DSLOPE	DINT
c	-0.424[b]	-0.082	0.346[c]	-0.090	-0.316[c]	-0.246	0.033	-0.001	0.164	-0.010	-0.400[b]	0.086	-0.076
MAGE		-0.103	0.028	0.502[b]	0.890[b]	0.201	-0.067	-0.161	-0.141	-0.065	0.615[b]	-0.131	-0.023
MHT			0.363[c]	0.080	-0.013	-0.011	0.195	0.166	0.100	0.209	-0.064	0.137	-0.024
MWT				0.074	0.016	-0.228	0.260	0.224	0.210	0.296	0.046	0.210	-0.181
BINTER					0.524[b]	-0.183	-0.204	-0.194	0.238	-0.286	0.459[b]	0.037	-0.121
DELIV						0.029	0.009	-0.053	-0.025	-0.037	0.464[c]	0.057	-0.119
ISEX							-0.195	-0.318	-0.384[c]	-0.100	0.201	-0.503[b]	0.342[c]
BWT								0.836[b]	0.879[b]	0.725[b]	-0.298	0.289	-0.254
BHT									0.786[b]	0.706[b]	-0.322[c]	0.421[b]	-0.336[c]
BHEAD										0.634[b]	-0.273	0.394[c]	-0.282
GAGE											-0.208	0.129	-0.130
WAGE												-0.049	-0.126
DSLOPE													-0.774[b]

[a]See abbreviations in table 14.1.
[b]P < 0.01.
[c]P < 0.05.

Table 14.3
Correlations among the Parameter c of the Weight Curve and Child's Infection Variables, 39 Cases

	EHISTO1[a]	GIARD1	ASCAR1	TRICH1	SDYS1	SFLEX1	SBOYD1	SSONN1	ENTER1	ADENO1
c	-0.077	-0.310	-0.010	-0.144	0.206	-0.193	0.280	-0.091	-0.208	0.144
EHISTO1		0.046	0.917[b]	-0.023	-0.034	-0.038	-0.027	-0.027	-0.141	0.124
GIARD1			0.071	0.163	-0.108	0.500[b]	-0.037	-0.085	0.260	-0.392[c]
ASCAR1				0.009	0.100	-0.074	-0.052	-0.052	-0.152	0.206
TRICH1					-0.059	-0.066	-0.046	-0.046	-0.194	-0.139
SDYS1						0.048	-0.033	-0.033	-0.118	0.274
SFLEX1							-0.037	-0.037	0.182	-0.030
SBOYD1								-0.026	-0.047	-0.201
SSONN1									0.386[c]	-0.076
ENTER1										-0.201

[a] See abbreviations in Table 14.1.
[b] $P < 0.01$.
[c] $P < 0.05$.

Table 14.4
Correlations among the Parameter c of the Weight Curve and Morbidity Variables, 39 Cases

	DILL1[a]	RESP1	BACT1	SYST1	EMS1	SVD1
c	−0.043	−0.438[b]	0.203	0.094	0.332[c]	0.176
DILL1		−0.120	0.102	0.085	−0.135	0.583[b]
RESP1			0.239	0.255	−0.040	0.090
BACT1				0.167	0.698[b]	0.319[c]
SYST1					0.020	0.322[c]
EMS1						0.035

[a] See abbreviations in table 14.1.
[b] $p < 0.01$.
[c] $p < 0.05$.

age (MAGE), number of deliveries (DELIV), and weaning age (WAGE). These associations may have biological meaning. It is expected that young mothers have less depletion of their nutritional state and therefore secrete more milk resulting in more rapid child growth. On the other hand, the number of deliveries which in poorly nourished women deplete the nutritional state, is a negatively correlated factor. It should be stressed that weaning age is well correlated with maternal age, birth interval, and number of deliveries, seemingly indicating that prolonged breast-feeding is associated with a deteriorated nutritional state.

Table 14.3 shows the correlation among the estimated parameter c and the child's infection variables. Rates for the first year were used because parameter c reflects growth in the first year. Considered independently, none of the rates was significantly correlated with growth deceleration.

Among causes of morbidity, days of respiratory disease in the first year (RESP1) correlated negatively with parameter c (table 14.4). Again, rates were those of the first year of life.

Table 14.5 has a summary of the variables eventually entering in multivariate analyses, with the significance attached to them. Days of respiratory disease in the first year (RESP1) were negatively correlated with birth length (BHT) and positively correlated with weaning age (WAGE); the coefficients of respiratory disease and weaning age were of similar size and identical sign with the dependent variable c. The negative correlation with respiratory disease indicates a direct effect of infection on growth; that with weaning age is the result of a depleted maternal nutrition retarding early growth and prolonging breast-feeding. On the other hand, infants suffering from frequent respiratory disease could grow more slowly and therefore stay at the breast longer. Maternal height does not correlate with c probably because some taller women, having better nutrition, secrete more milk and their children therefore wean earlier.

Table 14.5
Correlations among the Parameter c of the Weight Curve and Selected Variables,
39 Cases

	RESP1[a]	MAGE	BHT	MWT	GIARD1	MHT	WAGE
c	-0.438[b]	-0.424[b]	0.001	0.346[c]	-0.310	-0.082	-0.400[b]
RESP1		0.104	-0.433[b]	-0.301	0.372[c]	0.065	0.326[c]
MAGE			-0.161	0.028	0.082	-0.054	0.615[b]
BHT				0.244	-0.270	0.166	-0.327[c]
MWT					-0.095	0.363[c]	0.046
GIARD1						-0.010	0.418[b]
MHT							-0.064

[a]See abbreviations in table 14.1.
[b]$P < 0.01$.
[c]$P < 0.05$.

Multivariate Analyses for Parameter c

For the analyses, the SWRA using SPSS and BMD package programs and the
technique of "all possible combinations" for choosing the best subsets by
Mallow's Cp package programs were employed for both c and b. These different methods gave remarkably similar answers and resulted in the same
group of variables accounting for a large portion of the variance of growth.
On the other hand, the SWRAs were made using 39 cases with complete data
and 27 independent variables. Under such conditions it is quite possible that
some variables, particularly those entering late in the equation, do so by
chance relationships between their values and that of the dependent variable.
Thus, the use of a large number of variables in small samples could capitalize
on chance; however, in this particular case dozens of tests were made in small
subsets of the variables, and the results resembled those of analysis made with
all variables. Table 14.6 presents a step-wise regression analysis for the estimated parameter c of the weight curve; since parameter c primarily reflects
growth deceleration, rates of infection and disease for the second and third
years of life were excluded. The intercept and slope of the calorie curve also
were excluded because they were calculated from the food supplements to
breast milk given to Cauqué children at two to six months of age and in small
amounts.

Days of respiratory infection in the first year of life (RESP1) showed a
negative regression coefficient and a significant F value accounting for 19 percent of the total variance of c. This implies that infants who grew better had
fewer days of respiratory disease or vice versa. Maternal age added 14.5 percent to the explanation of the variance. The coefficient of this variable was
negative, suggesting that the younger the mother the faster was the infant's
rate of growth in the early months. Young mothers have a greater tendency
to deliver preterm infants who often grow faster in the first months. Also,

Table 14.6
Step-Wise Regression Analysis for the Estimated Parameter c of the Weight Curve,
39 Cases

Variable in order of entry[a]	Regression coefficient (B)	Standard error of B	F value	Level of significance, P	Percentage RSQ	Percentage RSQ
RESP1	−256.72	80.66	10.13	.003	19.2	19.2
MAGE	−164.35	46.64	12.41	.001	33.7	14.5
BHT	−39.87	16.56	5.79	.022	40.7	7.0
MWT	140.42	61.02	5.29	.028	48.7	8.0

Note: Constant = 25682.28.
[a]Variables entered: MHT, BINTER, DELIV, ISEX, BWT, BHEAD, GAGE, WAGE, EHISTO1, GIARD1, ASCAR1, TRICH1, SDYS1, SFLEX1, SBOYD1, SSONN1, ENTER1, ADENO1, DILL1, BACT1, SYST1, EMS1, SVD1.

milk output by primiparae appears adequate since the young mother has not yet been nutritionally depleted through a succession of pregnancies and lactation periods as have older women. Birth length and maternal weight added 7 and 8 percent, respectively, to the total variance of c; the F values were significant. The coefficient of birth length was negative, suggesting that some small babies also tended to grow faster as indicated above. On the other hand, the coefficient for maternal weight was positive, indicating that the heavier the mother the better the initial infant growth, again with nutritional implications.

A total of 48.7 percent of the variance of parameter c was accounted for by the four variables. It is evident that other factors among the list at the end of table 14.6 are likely contributors, but because they are confounded with variables entering into the equation their F's were nonsignificant. The important consideration is that maternal variables and respiratory disease could predict, alone, almost a half of the total variance of growth as expressed in parameter c.

Correlations for Parameter b
Correlations among variables and the estimated parameter b are presented in tables 14.7, 14.8, and 14.9. Only maternal age and weaning age showed significant correlations with b (table 14.7). Infection and morbidity variables in general did not correlate higher with b, although some showed moderate r factors with negative sign, for instance, rates of $E.$ $histolytica$ in the first three years (EHISTOT), disease of the ear, mouth, and skin in the first year (EMS1) and systemic diseases in the first three years (SYSTT) (tables 14.8 and 14.9).

A summary of the variables entering into the equation by multivariate analysis is given in table 14.10. Again, weaning age was the outstanding

Table 14.7
Correlations among the Estimated Parameter b of the Weight Curve and Maternal and Child Variables, 39 Cases

b	MAGE	MHT	MWT	BINTER	DELIV	ISEX	BWT	BHT	BHEAD	WAGE	GAGE	DSLOPE	DINT
	0.346c	0.175	-0.112	-0.036	0.283	0.178	0.026	0.004	0.025	0.403c	0.020	0.065	0.038
MAGE		-0.054	0.028	0.502c	0.890b	0.201	-0.067	-0.161	-0.141	0.583b	-0.065	-0.131	-0.023
MHT			0.363c	0.080	-0.013	-0.011	0.195	0.166	0.100	-0.121	0.209	0.137	-0.024
MWT				0.074	0.016	-0.228	0.266	0.224	0.210	0.010	0.296	0.210	-0.181
BINTER					0.524b	-0.183	-0.204	-0.194	-0.238	0.435b	-0.286	0.037	-0.121
DELIV						0.029	0.009	-0.053	-0.025	0.394c	-0.037	0.057	-0.119
ISEX							-0.195	-0.318c	-0.384c	0.227	-0.100	-0.503b	0.342c
BWT								0.836b	0.879b	-0.311c	-0.130	0.289	-0.254
BHT									0.786b	-0.339c	0.706b	0.421b	-0.336c
BHEAD										-0.292	0.394c	-0.282	-0.240
WAGE											-0.240	-0.049	-0.126
GAGE												0.129	-0.130
DSLOPE													-0.774b

[a]See abbreviations in table 14.1.
[b]$P < 0.05$.
[c]$P < 0.01$.

Table 14.8
Correlations among the Estimated Parameter b of the Weight Curve and Child's Infection Variables, 39 Cases

	EHISTOT[a]	GIARDT	ASCART	TRICHT	SDYST	SFLEXT	SBOYDT	SSONN1	ENTER1	ADENO1
b	-0.218	-0.069	-0.026	0.082	-0.027	-0.279	0.131	0.024	0.104	-0.061
EHISTOT		-0.004	0.091	0.464[b]	-0.264	-0.080	0.021	-0.134	-0.354[c]	-0.238
GIARDT			0.239	0.118	-0.009	0.118	0.270	-0.130	-0.128	0.203
ASCART				0.122	-0.077	-0.128	0.227	-0.125	0.107	0.192
TRICHT					0.067	-0.099	0.026	-0.072	0.036	-0.224
SDYST						0.083	0.044	0.140	0.210	0.101
SFLEXT							-0.033	0.198	0.258	-0.256
SBOYDT								-0.096	-0.270	0.352[c]
SSONN1									0.386[c]	-0.076
ENTER1										-0.201

[a] See abbreviations in table 14.1.
[b] $P < 1.01$.
[c] $P < 0.05$.

Table 14.9
Correlations among the Estimated Parameter b of the Weight Curve and Child's
Morbidity Variables, 39 Cases

	DIARRT[a]	SVDT	RESPT	EMS1	SYSTT	BACTT	VIRT	DILL1
b	0.046	−0.041	0.161	−0.254	−0.208	−0.196	0.096	0.074
DIARRT		0.836[b]	0.152	−0.006	0.217	0.678[b]	0.794[b]	0.631[b]
SVDT			0.139	0.116	0.285	0.716[b]	0.625[b]	0.593[b]
RESPT				−0.102	−0.075	0.277	1.014	0.093
EMS1					0.217	0.371[c]	0.014	−0.135
SYSTT						0.601[b]	0.414[b]	0.218
BACTT							0.572[b]	0.421[b]
VIRT								0.530[b]

[a]See abbreviations in table 14.1.
[b]$P < 0.01$.
[c]$P < 0.05$.

variable, and this in turn was related to birth interval (BINTER) and number
of previous deliveries (DELIV).

Multivariate Analyses for Parameter b

Step-wise regression analyses were made again for 39 cases and 29 independent variables (table 14.11). All analyses with subsets of variables showed
similar results to those presented in the table. Rates of infection and infectious disease for each of the three years or for the first year in some instances,
were used in the regressions, keeping the number of predictive variables under
30. Yearly rates did not add more to the explanation of the variance of b
than did the rates for the three years combined. An exception was the use of
the rate for the first year of enteroviruses (ENTER1), adenoviruses
(ADENO1), S. sonnei (SSONN1), and days of illness (DILL1) for reasons already given.

Weaning age had the highest predictive capacity of growth rate, accounting
for 16.3 percent of the total variance of parameter b. The regression coefficient was positive, indicating better growth in this part of the curve with
prolonged breast-feeding. Birth interval entered second, contributing an
added 5.5 percent more to the variance. The coefficient, however, was negative, probably because it reflected the effect of birth interval once weaning
age—to which it is highly correlated—is taken into account. Maternal height
(MHT) explained an additional 7 percent of the variance and the coefficient
was positive, that is, child growth in this segment of life was better if the
mother was taller.

Infections with *E. histolytica*, *S. flexneri*, and adenoviruses were negatively correlated with b and added more than 20 percent to the total sum of
the R^2 values. Number of previous deliveries was positively correlated
and explained 6.6 percent of the total variance. Again this variable could be a

Table 14.10
Correlations among the Estimated Parameter *b* of the Weight Curve and Maternal and Infection Variables, 39 Cases

	WAGE[a]	BINTER	MHT	DELIV	EHISTOT	SFLEXT	ADENO1
b	0.403[b]	-0.036	0.175	0.283	-0.218	-0.279	-0.061
WAGE		0.435[c]	-0.121	0.394[b]	-0.048	-0.230	0.029
BINTER			0.080	0.524[c]	-0.223	-0.085	0.254
MHT				-0.013	0.115	0.145	-0.031
DELIV					-0.139	-0.053	0.202
EHISTOT						-0.080	-0.238
SFLEXT							-0.256

[a]See abbreviations in table 14.1.
[b]$P < 0.05$.
[c]$P < 0.01$.

Table 14.11
Step-Wise Regression Analysis for the Estimated Parameter *b* of the Weight Curve, 39 Cases

Variable in order of entry[a]	Regression coefficient (B)	Standard error of B	F value	Level of significance, P	Percentage RSQ	Percentage RSQ
WAGE	65.37	15.89	16.91	.000	16.3	16.3
BINTER	-30.62	10.28	9.86	.006	21.8	5.5
MHT	69.75	24.58	8.05	.008	28.7	6.9
EHISTOT	-190.33	52.07	13.35	.001	37.9	9.1
DELIV	102.37	47.27	4.68	.039	44.5	6.6
SFLEXT	-90.01	28.73	9.81	.004	51.6	7.1
BHEAD	25.30	12.46	4.11	.052	54.9	3.2
DINT	2.85	1.15	6.13	.020	59.6	4.7
ADENO1	-25.11	12.77	4.18	.050	63.8	4.2

Note: Constant = -16665.29.
[a]Other variables entered: MAGE, MWT, ISEX, BHT, BWT, GAGE, DSLOPE, GIARDT, ASCART, TRICHT, SDYST, SBOYDT, ENTER1, DIARRT, SVDT, RESPT, EMST, SYSTT, BACTT, VIRT.

reflection of increased maternal experience in child care with age. It had been shown before that number of deliveries also correlated with parity and with an increase in socioeconomic level. Head circumference at birth showed a positive regression coefficient but had an F value of borderline significance. The slope of supplemental foods (DSLOPE) did not enter into the regression.

Overall, 63.8 percent of the total variance of b was accounted for by nine of the variables regressed. When maternal socioeconomic index was included, it entered into the equation in second place after weaning age, with a positive regression coefficient of no significant F value. In the regression with socioeconomic index most of the variables entering in the analysis summarized in table 14.11 also entered in similar order. The total percent sum of R^2 values was 75.8.

Considerable broad evidence has accumulated showing that environmental factors influence growth and development. It can be assumed that differences in phenotypic manifestations of growth among populations of similar growth potential are due to differences in environmental stimuli; history shows that improved socioeconomic conditions correlate with positive secular changes in physical growth. Within a population differences in height and weight attained at specified ages usually correlate well with social class, taller and heavier individuals tending to appear more frequently under better living conditions.

Most observers agree that the growth retardation observed in less developed societies is the result of negative environmental factors, primarily infection and deficient diet. (Sociocultural variables were not investigated intensively in the Cauqué study. Most of them are confounded with biological variables that were measured. Social factors not measured by the study conceivably could have improved the prediction of childhood physical growth.*)

The association of diet (consumption of nutrients) with growth cannot be discounted; weaning age had the highest predictive capacity of physical growth performance. However, little correlation was obtained when the parameters of the calorie "curve" were tested against those of the physical growth curve. A possible explanation could be lack of data on the nutrient value of breast milk; another is the similarity of the dietaries among children

---

* Recognition of the role of infection and environmental sanitation has broadened the concept that malnutrition is not purely a dietary problem but has an infectious component (Scrimshaw et al., 1968a). Infection and hygiene, however, rarely have been considered along with the food problem in the assessment of the health of a society or in the establishment of recommendations for action toward improvement (Mata et al., 1972b; Beghin, 1969). The socioeconomic approach to the malnutrition problem is progressively being recognized, although it still meets with neglect or apprehension because of the formidable barriers inherent in the social structures and political systems that prevail in most preindustrial nations.

and to a lesser extent the variability in amounts of supplemental foods within the diets of individual children.

Weaning age is a complex variable that intrinsically relates not only to nutrient intake by mother and child but also to host resistance to infection— particularly with intestinal pathogens—and to such factors as fertility and child spacing. The last two, in turn, may be associated intimately with maternal nutritional state and health.

Factors of great significance for growth are infection and infectious disease. Their role in the pathogenesis of malnutrition and growth retardation is readily apparent from the wealth of clinical and epidemiological evidence presented in past chapters and from the statistical evidence here introduced. Step-wise regression analyses with many variables summarizing infectious experiences showed that they account for a large and significant part of the variance of physical growth. In the first months of life, when the child is breast-fed and protected from infection by maternal passive immunity and anti-infectious factors in breast milk, the impact of infection may pass unnoticed. Nevertheless, respiratory disease in the first year was negatively correlated with parameter c, showing that infants who grew more slowly had more respiratory disease.

Infection variables had a good capacity of predicting growth; they explained a good part of the variance of a and b. Entering into the equation with significant negative coefficients were rates of *E. histolytica, S. flexneri*, and adenoviruses. Interestingly enough, total days of disease, or days of specific groups of illnesses failed to enter into the equation. A likely explanation is the exceedingly high morbidity characteristic of all village children. Another reason is a methodological failure to discriminate effectively the severe from the mild episodes in the summarization of data.

What emerges from mathematical analyses is not only a prediction of a significantly large portion of the variance of growth, but a keen appreciation of the complexity of the problem. The small size of the sample and the lack of quantitation of some of the variables preclude a definite conclusion on the contribution of many factors. Nevertheless, the existence of interlaced activities of a whole range of variables relating to the mother, the newborn, feeding practices, and infectious processes is clearly evident.

Quantitation of the exact contribution of individual factors is possible by instituting controlled intervention studies. In the meantime, available information provides a basis for practical action directed toward a comprehensive improvement of the childhood environment, particularly including maternal education, child care and feeding, and the control and prevention of infectious disease.

PART IV
SYNOPSIS, INTERVENTIONS, PRIORITIES, AND FUTURE ALTERNATIVES

Chapter 15
Synopsis, Interventions, Priorities, and Future Alternatives

This book describes the health and growth of children in a typical highland village of Guatemala in the 1960s. My duty, however, is to go beyond a historical account of village and population to interpret some of the findings of the study. A wealth of information collected over nine years of prospective field investigation revealed that fundamental problems of underdevelopment affect most aspects of the health of the population and limit possibilities for improvement. Although Indian traditions permeate village life, they have not ruled out a degree of influence by western culture. The present health problems have their roots more in the prevailing poverty, low state of community development, and population growth than in the innate culture of the Mayan Indian.

Summary of Findings
The Cauqué study revealed that more than 40 percent of infants are of low birth weight and that four-fifths of them experience fetal growth retardation. This reflects an inadequate maternal environment and has implications for both childhood survival and growth and development. Neonatal mortality by birth weight was that of advanced countries. However, fetal maturity continues to influence postneonatal, infant, and preschool mortality, although nutritional and infectious factors play the most distinct part.

Also, the marked deficit in observed physical growth correlated with birth weight and gestational age of the newborn, and even more strongly with the exceedingly high rates of infection and dietary deficiencies.

Mild and chronic malnutrition is a common finding at all stages of growth, including those of pregnancy and lactation. No increase in maternal food intake was observed during pregnancy and lactation; infection and infectious disease were frequent during gestation. Cultural and ecological factors determined that all children are breast-fed for two or three years. Supplementation of the diet of breast-fed children begins at two to six months with provision of fluids and gruels of poor biological value and questionable hygiene; solid foods, mainly tortillas, beans, and vegetables, are introduced later. The change from breast milk to an adult type of diet is a protracted process. Mothers do not have food supplements of good quality nor do they possess the knowledge and facilities to prevent infection. The acceptance of bulky and low-nutrient foods and the risks of infection predispose to weanling diarrhea, growth retardation, and related phenomena of infants and toddlers.

The mechanisms determining prolonged lactation are not well known. The Cauqué study showed that children who grow more slowly during the first months of life tend to be weaned later. Conversely, children with more rapid early growth are weaned earlier. Biological factors such as maternal nutrition and rate of child growth seem to influence duration of breast-feeding. Cultural factors also are important; they account for the absolute ability in nursery—even by primiparae—and they influence prolonged breast-feeding. They also account for the limited maternal knowledge of food preparation and food hygiene and of the diversity of foods that can complement the caloric intake of children.

Infection, particularly gastrointestinal, stands out as a main, if not the most important, factor in damaging the intestinal mucosa and in malabsorption, nutrient wastage, and related phenomena. This study did not reveal a remarkably deficient diet except for calories; however, their amount and quality were not markedly inadequate when related to the weight of the child. The incidence of infection is excessively high compared with that of more advanced societies. The small infant is relatively protected from infections—particularly intestinal—through transplacental immunity, factors in breast milk, and indigenous intestinal microflora. After the first months of life, resistance factors fade and the child begins a series of clinically debilitating episodes. The usual effects of the interaction of infection and deficient diet are weanling diarrhea and repetitive acute respiratory disease, with longer duration of disease, frequent weight loss, increased case fatality, and growth retardation. The critical period is from six to thirty months; protein-calorie malnutrition, growth retardation, and mortality are most evident then.

After three years of age the child has become immune to the commoner community infections; he fares better with the village diet. The body replenishes some of its reserves, growth improves, and mortality decreases sharply; however, individuals remain stunted and with evidence of mild chronic malnutrition. The relation of infection to malnutrition is thus evident. Malnutrition mainly appears in infants and preschool children. Older children, adolescents, and adults are less affected. However, severe malnutrition may appear again in old age, primarily due at that time to a limited ability to obtain foods.

The prospective nature of the study permitted assessment of changes in host and environment over a span of nine years. In general, biological characteristics such as fetal growth, postnatal physical growth, dietary intake, and behavior of infectious diseases remained rather stable during the study. Likewise, some environmental factors showed marked stability while others deteriorated. For instance, land area per capita and wages as a function of cost of living remained rather fixed or decreased. The absence of significant improvements in physical, biological, and sociocultural factors is taken as the reason for a lack of observable improvement with time in nutrition, mortality, and growth of children.

In the causation of malnutrition, infection plays a major role. Thus, the ultimate causes are the low socioeconomic development, deficient education and environmental sanitation, and scarcity of economic resources. A small improvement of the environment has resulted in fewer deaths with no corresponding decrease in births, and a resulting growth rate of more than 3 percent per year with an ensuing saturation of the land. The village demographic situation is indeed not too different from that of the country as a whole and other areas of Central America. Population projections for the year 2000 based on current growth rates are 15 million inhabitants for Guatemala, a population density of 145 per square kilometer; for Central America, including Panama, the projection is 47 million people and a density of 94 per square kilometer. El Salvador and Guatemala face the more pressing situation in view of their current relatively large populations and limited usable territory.

Since the Indian participates to a significant degree in the money economy, inflation, the energy crisis, and recession are affecting rural life, making control and prevention a more difficult task.

Considerations of Possible Interventions
Historically, poverty and underdevelopment have been attributed to a tendency of the Indian to remain encased in his own traditions, customs, and beliefs, and to his inability to assimilate progress effectively. However, the lowlands of Guatemala where the population is almost wholly of Spanish descent, or a mixture of Indian and Spanish, reveal a similar or even worse underdevelopment than that in the Indian environment. Hence, it is illogical to consider the historical background of the Mayans as mainly responsible for their slow progress. It is my belief that the tropical ecosystem has been a negative factor, making development more difficult; on the other hand, adequate mechanisms to transfer knowledge and resources on education, hygiene, and nutrition have not been developed.

Tradition in the Indian culture has strong positive values. The Indian has managed to survive adverse environmental conditions—a fact well illustrated by the present demographic growth—and produce individuals of good biological and human quality. Positive cultural values are revealed in childbirth, breast-feeding, and social aspects of village life.

As a biologist and student of public health I cannot avoid recognizing the health problems of the village and other similar localities and asking if feasible solutions can be evolved and implemented. However, the danger exists in the tendency of health professionals to assess the problem from the single biological viewpoint, often the first step in a series of errors. What the biologist overlooks is that the individual he examines is a member of a society in which 50 percent of the people are illiterate, sanitary provisions are inadequate, housing is deficient, and nutrition is poor. Above all, most people in this society have a low economic capacity because of continued dependence on a subsistence agriculture based on small plots of land or on peasant labor in the large landholdings.

The most pressing problem is related equally to the population increase (with the attendant restricted availability of land, food shortage, inflation, and recession) and to the low level of education and the lack of technology, both of which are accentuated by the different acculturation of urban and rural groups and by ethnic prejudice.

To recommend interventions capable of improving the health and growth of village children calls for responsibility and careful analysis. A missionary attitude often results in prescription of independent food supplementation, immunization, and family planning programs. A medical conscience has placed undue emphasis upon hospitalization and the establishment of nutrition recuperation centers in the management of severe malnutrition. Whether influenced by goodwill or emotion, such actions commonly fail to grasp the nature of the problem and are not always exempt from prejudice. All too often they lack information or conviction as well as adequate logistics for implementation and evaluation.

A decision to intervene in a village like Santa María Cauqué is difficult because practically every variable susceptible to individual modification—whether biological, economic, or nutritional—is related to some other, and intervention in one will not necessarily be associated with benefits in another but even may result in long-range deleterious effects.

The complexities of recommending public health action are illustrated by several examples. The first concerns birth weight. It is not clear that improved food intake during pregnancy will lead regularly to significant increase in fetal growth in villages such as Santa María Cauqué where the incidence of low birth weight infants is about 40 percent. A stunted growth of women is probably the main determinant of the low birth weight, with food intake during pregnancy having a more limited effect. Thus, the improvement of fetal growth requres a combined emphasis on the health and growth of infants, children, and adolescents, so that taller and better-nourished generations of women will gestate larger fetuses.

A second example relates to child feeding practices. The custom in Santa María Cauqué is to breast-feed for prolonged periods, adding supplemental foods of low nutritive and poor hygienic quality after two to six months of lactation. Due to the relationship between child growth and weaning age, an increase in food intake by lactating women and in nutritive and wholesome food supplements to the child will probably induce earlier weaning for several reasons. Infants growing better will empty the breasts more rapidly; because better food supplements are accepted more readily, teeth will erupt earlier and the child will adapt to solid foods more readily. Thus, to improve the nutrition of breast-fed infants and children will inevitably result in more rapid growth and earlier weaning. However, if the environment is not improved in terms of sanitation, children will continue to be exposed to infection while the period of protection by breast milk is shortened. Furthermore, earlier weaning will inevitably lead to shorter birth intervals and more frequent pregnancy unless some means of family planning is adopted.

A third example pertains to immunization programs directed against such diseases as whooping cough and measles. As isolated efforts these measures benefit the overall nutritional state and contribute to a lesser childhood mortality. Likewise, vector control programs reduce malaria and other arthropod-transmitted diseases. However, differences of opinion exist as to the benefits of such interventions because they stimulate demographic growth with no necessary assurance of a better quality of life.

Another example pertains to the treatment and control of disease. In many areas of the world great emphasis has been, and still is, given to programs of outpatient and mobile clinics and other types of therapeutic action. While mortality is reduced by these means, morbidity is little affected, because that element is determined by the quality of the environment and the nutritional state of the host. When medical care programs are soundly organized, they accomplish for the childhood population a reduction in deaths from diarrhea, severe protein-calorie malnutrition, and the complications of measles, whooping cough, and other diseases; they also will promote survival of infants with dehydration, and even tetanus and meningitis. Such activities may stimulate response to the need for prevention but the overall effect of such programs in terms of reducing frequency of disease is limited. Unaccompanied by community development, they contribute to survival of children who often are poorly conditioned to function optimally and yet are a factor in demographic growth and perhaps a burden to society.

A final example relates to prevention of infection through control of fecal waste. Latrine programs have had great emphasis because, by fecal disposal, many parasitic diseases are controlled. However, latrine programs implemented without concomitant introduction of household water, sanitary education, and perhaps an enhanced income to promote the use of soap can have negative effects. First, the orthodox position assumed in defecation in latrines distributed in our villages favors soiling of perianal areas. Second, there is a tendency to use paper or leaves when a latrine is available—a non-indigenous custom—thus favoring contamination of the hands with fecal bacteria. If household water and education are not made available, gains in control of parasitic infection can be neutralized or overwhelmed by an increase in diarrheal disease.

Many interventions by international or governmental action or by scientific organizations have shown that family planning, nutrition supplementation, immunization, and even agricultural extension have often failed to improve nutrition and growth significantly in the absence of improved education and living standards.

Recognition of Health Priorities

Santa María Cauqué and hundreds of similar villages in Central America obviously would benefit from an overall improved environment. This comprises better opportunities for education and increases in food availability, in child care and family planning, in environmental sanitation and personal hygiene, and in prevention of infection. Accumulated scientific knowledge provides specific recommendations for each of these activities.

Education is the most pressing need in community development. Difficulties encountered in improving the education of the Indian population stem from an inability to cross the cultural barrier. Even for the ladino or mestizo populations of Guatemala and other Central American nations, no adequate knowledge exists as to how people think and what they need to learn and in what way. Teaching systems and practices are those established in Guatemala City after being transferred from Europe, the United States, or other advanced societies. Why village children should enter school at age seven or why school programs do not emphasize ruralism, village life, and the history of the Mayan are questions that have not been asked enough. Examination of curricula shows orthodox educational programs that fail to grasp rural problems or those of the society and the nation as a whole. They insure continued cultural allegiance to Europe or North America and often promote the barriers between urban and rural populations.

Details of what needs to be taught in village schools are beyond the scope of this discussion. In general, a sense of Indian identity or at least a sensitivity to Indian culture will be needed to analyze present needs and to design, implement, and evaluate new programs for Indians and ladinos. It appears logical that rural children should know of their ancestral civilizations in order to enhance their dignity. Teaching should emphasize agricultural practices, food habits, housing, personal hygiene, sanitation, and the conservation of the environment—all elements necessary to promote health and survival—yet care should be taken not to destroy or degrade important traditions and beliefs. The linguistic identity of the Indian should be preserved and used to teach relevant concepts.

Another equally important aspect pertains to food availability which is intimately related to land distribution. With population growth the amount of land per family in villages has become insufficient to produce the necessary food; it has effectively decreased by 20 percent over the last ten years. The saturation of the land has not been mitigated by diversified crop planning activities for the rural Indians and ladinos nor by improved agricultural production. A significant part of crops is lost to rodents, insects, and fungi due to poor methods of grain storage. At the village level agricultural technology as well as granaries can be improved by studying local conditions and materials. This requires technological information resulting from specific research. If granaries alone were improved, food availability would increase by 20 or 30 percent; a lesser fluctuation in food prices and in speculation and food imports is an added consideration.

A third equally important factor is community development by improved health services, environmental sanitation, and social mechanisms that organize and stimulate the people to higher levels of living and welfare. In this regard little is known due to an inability to recognize the needs of the rural Indian and ladino.

To change rural school programs requires a reorientation of methods for the training of teachers and professionals in vocational schools and universities and the creation of paraprofessional schools to train personnel at intermediate levels, with greater capacity to help the people in greatest need. University programs are stressed because traditionally more freedom, liberalism, and social conscience (at least theoretically) are found there, but they have consistently failed to reach the rural population properly. Curricula for professional training are not clearly oriented toward the development of individuals capable of solving the national problems on a priority basis; rather they emphasize training for an industrialized society.

Physicians often know more about treatment of rare and unusual chronic and degenerative diseases than about prevention and treatment of common infections. Their interest in public health and epidemiology is generally scant, and full awareness of national medical priorities is commonly lacking.

Engineers able to build skyscrapers and modern houses have not developed systems to improve dwellings in the countryside, using local materials of low cost; they have not developed simple technologies for sewers, water supply, and electrification systems for rural areas.

Veterinarians may excel in the care and treatment of pets and large animals, but no significant advance has occurred in zootechnics, particularly as applied to animal husbandry in rural areas. Cattle raising as practiced in

Cental America has not resulted in an increased intake of animal protein by most of the population because the product is diverted to foreign markets. Agronomists are trained to produce cash crops, yet interest in improving the quality and yield of corn, beans, and other staple crops is only beginning to emerge. Most seeds for vegetables and other garden foods are imported from abroad.

Lawyers learn orthodox systems of justice, virtually the codes of the Spanish colonizers. No incentive exists to generate sound legislation to effect an agrarian reform, to stabilize prices and wages, and above all, to protect the Indian and the peasant from exploitation and abuse by the elite classes.

When it comes to governmental action, the situation is no better. The true intent of politicians is a matter of continued debate and controversy. Assuming that national leaders all desire the best for their country, the actions taken often leave much to be desired. Governments frequently are established, maintained, and deposed by the power structures and elite groups whose goals and interests are not necessarily to improve the nation in a harmonious way, but rather to increase their own personal power and capital. Great pressures are exerted on the executive, legislative, and judicial branches of government to promote actions beneficial to the interests of business, industry, and more recently multinational complexes.

Regarding research, there is also a need for a better definition of priorities—nutrition, infection, childhood mortality, population growth—and a reorientation of effort. Undue support has been given to clinical and laboratory studies of severe protein-calorie malnutrition and to laboratory studies of food and of infection as well. Relatively little emphasis has been given to long-term epidemiologic studies on causality. The Cauqué study was an effort in that direction; it was limited, however, to diagnosis of the problem and characterization of areas that theoretically could benefit from intervention.

Here is where knowledge is limited or nonexistent. If we are asked how interventions can be carried out, answers will not be available in most instances. Scientists and bureaucrats responsible for advice on specific actions commonly do not know enough about legislation for agrarian reform or about availability of local foods for practical use in supplementation of the diet of the weanling. More importantly, there has been a neglect of methodology pertaining to transfer of available knowledge to target population groups. Few data exist on educational techniques for teaching the Indian and ladino women and children of Guatemala and other Central American nations. Furthermore, the systems of dissemination of scientific information are not always effective in reaching political spheres and the scientific and intellectual community as well.

If one were to outline specific recommendations applicable to present conditions, the following are most likely to yield significant improvements in health:

- Increase in volume of household water to reduce attack of diarrheal disease
- Increase in number of household beds to reduce attack of respiratory disease
- Education in hygiene, on hand and diaper washing, boiling of water, and waste disposal to prevent many infections
- Immunization against measles, whooping cough, tuberculosis, and tetanus
- Control of arthropod-transmitted infections, by plaguicides, better housing, and environmental sanitation
- Health services for treatment of acute infectious disease
- Agrarian reform
- Agricultural extension: education, distribution of seed, use of fertilizer, preservation of grains
- Education in weaning practices and nutrition
- Family planning
- Food price control
- Improvement of wages

Most of these actions require the training of subprofessional personnel in specific disciplines or areas of action, for instance, agricultural extension and nutrition education, health promotion and family planning. The use of paraprofessional personnel represents the only feasible way to solve the bottleneck of delivery of "health and development packages" to the population groups that need them most.

What is evidently needed is a within-country and international redefinition of priorities and of the avenues of required action. Problem solving at the village level requires changes in some areas along with strengthening of inherent traditions. This is possible only with all societal forces working toward that goal. Much could be done if the wealthy and ruling classes of the society were committed to share their time, resources, and knowledge. History tells us that this has rarely occurred. The emphasis necessarily should be on education, agrarian reform, and agricultural practices; on environmental sanitation and housing; and on health services and family planning. In this regard great care should be exerted to avoid generalizations and oversimplification. While in Guatemala an agrarian reform seems appropriate to promote development of the Indian (an inherent agriculturist), in other nations a different kind of action appears indicated, for instance, improved legislation on wages and loans. Even within a country a choice of alternatives is logical, which emphasizes the need to conduct basic research on causality and intervention in individual countries, regardless of their size and extent of development.

Legislation for agrarian reform has been relatively effective in some nations. Education is a complex problem but surmountable, as socialist countries have demonstrated. The same opinion applies to environmental sanitation. Integrated health services targeting on the mother and child are a reality in many areas and serve as effectors of the "packages of health." The important consideration is that all of these actions must be part of a national plan in which Indian and ladino representatives should take part; they must be implemented in a coordinated fashion, and not as independent efforts. This is the holistic approach.

A Question of Alternatives

The dilemma is how rapidly measures should be taken, or whether it is possible to implement them within a framework of peace. The general impression is that most Central American countries are progressing all too slowly. The capital cities generally are buoyant and charming, with a proliferation of industries, buildings, and restaurants and an enlargement of capital and resources. This contrasts with the poverty of rural areas, although even there some slow progress is evident. For example, over the past decade an increase in literacy of 10 percent, a modest tendency toward fewer births, a nationwide system of health centers and roads, and a mass immunization campaign against measles were accomplished. Biological characteristics indicate, however, that there is all too little improvement in the overall quality of life.

Some authorities anticipate that further progress and development can be expected within several generations, while others declare that such will not be the case. Saturation of the land, maintenance of infection levels, and economic depression could bring more malnutrition and infectious disease in the future or maintain the present levels. Guatemala and El Salvador are countries in Central America which could reach a point of no return, that is, a position in which population growth and the accompanying societal stress so increase the numbers of illiterate people that the result is more deforestation, decreased per capita food production, widespread famine and pestilence, or, finally, the more dreaded territorial expansion through war.

The question should not be whether change is occurring but whether the recorded progress will suffice before population numbers become too great. To continue at the present rhythm appears dangerous. The solution is not only in the hands of scientists or health workers but also with national leaders and the population itself.

A degree of international cooperation is definitely required. There must be commitment on the part of the industrial nations to let other nations develop their own systems of government, particularly when such evolution promises significant gains in health and development. International cooperation could be oriented toward more intensive distribution of firsthand technology and scientific knowledge to the less developed nations through enlarged programs for leadership training, through cooperation in the world balance of prices of trade goods, and through aid in strengthening plans considered important by the recipient countries. Aid for defense has contributed to building a world arsenal; more often than not, it has been a deterrent to progress in developing nations that receive such aid.

The most important actions must emanate from the poor nations themselves. They must develop their own scientific and technical capabilities for investigation and attack on their health and development problems. The role of scientists should go beyond that of providing answers to specific questions. All too often the scientific community has been guilty of indifference and lack of leadership in issues pertaining to the welfare and survival of society. Scientists must take a firm position and be outspoken, so that their opinions sensitize policymakers and elite groups.

I believe there already is an awareness among many social circles of an impending need for more rapid progress in Central America. However, at this writing all but one of the region's governments are ruled by military bodies, often most concerned with maintaining the status quo. The hope remains that many, even the military, may become cognizant of existing difficulties and activate the needed social reforms.

Alternatives are political upheaval or the acceptance of a level of population density and underdevelopment from which society will escape with difficulty. Both alternatives potentially involve bloodshed and much suffering. The first does not necessarily guarantee the desired changes and benefits.

While our investigation identified health and growth problems of children and their causes, it extended beyond that: an attempt to provide answers to some of the questions, and especially a recognition of socioeconomic factors as essential to any sound understanding. The governments and nations themselves must decide on the particular applications of current knowledge essential to an effective national policy of development, without inflicting significant alterations on the positive values of the indigenous culture.

Appendix A
Staff

Principal Investigator
Leonardo J. Mata, 1962-1974*

Field Director
Juan J. Urrutia, 1965-1974

Field Staff

Physicians
Juan J. Urrutia, Carlos E. Beteta, 1963-1965

Nurses
Olga Román, 1963-1972; Palmira Dardón, 1963-1972; Catalina Monzón, 1967-1972

Dietitian
Bertha García, 1964-1972

Laboratory Technicians
Raúl Fernández, 1962-1972; Elba Villatoro, 1965-1972

Field Workers
Gustavo Linares, 1963-1972; Emma Blanco, 1963-1972

Midwives
Juana Cutzán, 1963-1972; Candelaria Valle, 1963-1972

Domestic Helpers
Julia Chiroy; Juana Zil; Hercilia Chiroy; Manuela García; Josefa Chiroy; Juliana Díaz; Isabel Alvarez

* Period of employment in the Cauqué study.

Laboratory Staff

Microbiologists
Leonardo J. Mata, 1962–1972; María L. Mejicanos, 1966–1972; Armando Cáceres, 1968–1972; Grace Greenwood, 1971–1972

Laboratory Technicians
Olegario Pellecer, 1963–1972; Luis A. Sánchez, 1963–1969; Roberto Rosales, 1964–1972; Adelaida Comparini, 1965–1968; Gloria Restrepo, 1968–1970; Rafael Godínez, 1969–1972; Horacio Mazariegos, 1971–1972

Laboratory Helpers
Eudelia Ortíz, 1962–1968; Mélida de Tenas, 1962–1971; Josefina Hernández, 1964–1972; Gustavo Arango, 1965–1968; Luisa Juanta, 1965–1972; José Luis González, 1968–1971

Students
Amanda Negreros, 1963–1965; David C. Dale, 1965; Celina Carrillo, 1967; Miriam Cordón, 1967–1971; Robert Morhart, 1968; Laura I. Galich, 1968–1969; Richard G. Wyatt, 1969; Richard Rheinbolt, 1969; David Martin, 1970; Dan Cherkin, 1973; Wendie Branwell, 1973

Other Staff

Biostatistician
Richard Kronmal, 1972–1974

Data Processor
Claire Joplin, 1972–1974

Programmers
Constantino Albertazzi, 1964–1969; Eduardo Arellano, 1967–1974; Jerry Kronmal, 1972; Ruth Corddry, 1972–1974; Estelle Russek, 1973–1974

Secretaries
Ada Luz Colmenares, 1965–1967; Christa Haeussler, 1967–1969; Marion Landsberger, 1969–1971; Ana Leticia Molina, 1971; Patricia Solé, 1971–1973; Patricia Morales, 1973

Data Clerks
Armando Maldonado, 1968–1971; Hugo Gudiel, 1969–1972; Arturo Monasterio, 1971–1972; Benjamín Mejía, 1974

Special Staff, Part-Time

Audiovisual Aids
German Sojo, 1964–1974; Elio Cuéllar, 1964–1972

Editorial Services
Amalia de Ramírez, 1964–1972

Photographers
Barnie Cole, 1964; Guillermo Lucero, 1965–1974; Jill Gibson, 1968

Appendix B
Advisors and Consultants

Chin, Tom D. Y., Director, Ecological Investigations Program, Center for Disease Control, Kansas City, Kansas.

Cravioto, Joaquín, Chief, Department of Scientific Investigations, Hospital del Niño del IMAN, Mexico, D.F.

Dubos, René, Professor and Scientist, The Rockefeller University, New York.

Edsall, Geoffrey, Professor and Chairman, Department of Microbiology, London School of Hygiene and Tropical Medicine, London, England.

Ewing, William H., Chief, Enteric Bacteriology Unit, Center for Disease Control, Atlanta, Georgia.

Fox, John P., Professor of Epidemiology, University of Washington, School of Public Health and Community Medicine, Seattle, Washington.

Frenkel, Jack, Professor of Pathology and Oncology, University of Kansas Medical Center, Kansas City, Kansas.

Gangarosa, Eugene J., Chief, Bacterial Diseases Branch, Center for Disease Control, Atlanta, Georgia.

Golubjatnikov, Rjurik, Chief, Immunology Section, State Laboratory of Hygiene, Madison, Wisconsin.

Gordon, John E., Senior Lecturer, Department of Nutrition and Food Science, Massachusetts Institute of Technology, and Professor of Preventive Medicine and Epidemiology, Emeritus, Harvard University, Cambridge, Massachusetts.

Herrmann, Kenneth L., Chief, Viral Exanthems Unit, Center for Disease Control, Atlanta, Georgia.

Johnson, Karl M., Director, Middle America Research Unit, Gorgas Memorial Institute, Canal Zone, Panama.

Katz, Michael, Professor, Tropical Medicine and Pediatrics, The Faculty of Medicine, Columbia University, New York, New York.

Keusch, Gerald T., Associate Professor of Medicine, Mount Sinai Hospital, Mount Sinai School of Medicine, New York, New York.

Kogon, Alfred, Associate Professor of Epidemiology, University of Washington, School of Public Health and Community Medicine, Seattle, Washington.

Kronmal, Richard A., Associate Professor of Biostatistics, University of Washington, School of Public Health and Community Medicine, Seattle, Washington.

Mayorga, Rubén, Professor of Mycology, Universidad de San Carlos de Guatemala, Guatemala.

McGregor, Ian A., Director, Medical Research Council Laboratories, Gambia.

Melvin, D. Mae, Chief, Parasitology Training Unit, Center for Disease Control, Atlanta, Georgia.

Olarte, Jorge, Chief of Research, Hospital Infantil de Mexico, Mexico, D.F.

Pérez-Miravete, Adolfo, General Director, Public Health Research, Secretary of Public Health and Assistance, Mexico, D.F.

Read, Merrill S., Program Director, Growth and Development Branch, National Institute of Child Health and Human Development, Bethesda, Maryland.

Schaedler, Russell W., Chairman, Department of Microbiology, The Jefferson Medical College of Philadelphia, Pennsylvania.

Scrimshaw, Nevin S., Department Head, Nutrition and Food Science, and Professor of Human Nutrition, Massachusetts Institute of Technology, Cambridge, Massachusetts.

Stark, Charles R., Chief, Epidemiology Branch, Office of Epidemiology and Biometry, National Institute of Child Health and Human Development, Bethesda, Maryland.

Trejos, Alfonso, Chief of Laboratories, Hospital San Juan de Dios, Costa Rica.

Villanueva, Mario, Chief, Clinical Laboratory, Hospital Herrera Llerandi, Guatemala.

Weller, Thomas H., Director, Center for the Prevention of Infectious Diseases, Harvard School of Public Health, Boston, Massachusetts.

Appendix C
Code for Signs, Symptoms, Illnesses,
Diseases, and Injuries, 1964–1972

Table C.1
Illnesses, Diseases, and Injuries

	Item	Key[a]	Code
Respiratory	Upper respiratory tract illness	(ID)	0101
(01)	Tonsillo-pharyngitis, with exudate	(ID)	0102
	Purulent rhinitis (febrile nasopharyngitis)	(ID)	0103
	Pharyngitis	(ID)	0109
	Acute laryngitis	(ID)	0111
	Acute laryngotracheobronchitis	(ID)	0113
	Bronchitis	(ID)	0114
	Bronchiolitis	(ID)	0115
	Pneumonia, bronchopneumonia	(ID)	0116
	Whooping cough	(ID)	0121
	Aspiration pneumonia	(O)	0120
Gastrointestinal	Diarrhea	(ID)	0211
(02)	Diarrhea, with mucus	(ID)	0212
	Diarrhea, with blood and mucus	(ID)	0213
Eye	Conjunctivitis	(ID)	0301
(03)	Hordeolum, lid abscess	(ID)	0302
Ear	Otitis externa, infection of retroauricular canal and/or		
(04)	cellulitis of ear	(ID)	0401
	Otitis media, suppurative	(ID)	0403
Mouth	Primary herpes simplex	(ID)	0501
(05)	Recurrent herpes simplex	(ID)	0502
	Stomatitis, other forms	(ID)	0503
	Herpangina	(ID)	0504
	Thrush	(ID)	0505
	Apical abscess	(ID)	0506
Genitourinary	Urinary infection (pyelonephritis)	(ID)	0801
(08)	Balanoposthitis	(ID)	0802

Table C.1 (continued)

	Item	Key[a]	Code
Skin	Impetigo, newborn	(ID)	0901
(09)	Impetigo, vesicles, pustules, crusts	(ID)	0902, 0903
	Abscess, furuncle	(ID)	0904
	Cellulitis	(ID)	0905
	Necrosis	(ID)	0910
	Secondary infections (of wound, burn, laceration)	(ID)	0914
	Secondary infection (of eczema, dermatitis, urticaria)	(ID)	0919
	Eczema and/or intertrigo	(O)	0916
	Dermatitis (contact)	(O)	0917
	Urticaria, papulous	(O)	0918
	Wound	(T)	0911
	Burn	(T)	0912
	Laceration	(T)	0913
Exanthems	Measles (Rubeola)	(ID)	0921
(09)	Rubella (German measles)	(ID)	0922
	Chickenpox (Varicella)	(ID)	0923
	Exanthem subitum (Roseola infantum)	(ID)	0924
	Erythema infectiosum	(ID)	0925
	Scarlet fever	(ID)	0926
	Herpes simplex (excluding lips)	(ID)	0928
	Undifferentiated febrile exanthem	(ID)	0930
	Undifferentiated febrile vesicles	(ID)	0931
Scalp	Impetigo	(ID)	1002
(10)	Abscess	(ID)	1003
	Mycosis (ringworm)	(ID)	1004
Other	Mumps	(ID)	1103
(11, 12, 13)	Nonspecific fever	(ID)	1105
	Omphalitis	(ID)	1107
	Tenosynovitis	(ID)	1309
	Pre-Kwashiorkor	(ND)	1202
	Kwashiorkor	(ND)	1203
	Fracture	(T)	1301
	Contusion, bruise	(T)	1303

[a]ID = infectious disease; ND = nutritional disease; T = trauma or injury; and O = other.

Table C.2
Signs and Symptoms

Item	Key[a]	Code
Atelectasia, lung	(ID)	0117
Vomiting	(ID)	0203
Colic and/or tenesmus	(ID)	0204
Expulsion of helminths	(ID)	0216
Rectal prolapse	(ID)	0221
Dehydration	(ID)	0251
Glossitis	(ID, ND)	0508
Cheilitis	(ID, ND)	0509
Adenitis, lymphadenitis	(ID)	0601
Adenitis, suppurated lymphadenitis	(ID)	0602
Convulsions	(ID, O)	0703
Temperature, °C		
rectal oral		
37.5–38.4 37.0–37.9	(ID)	1401
38.5–39.4 38.0–38.9	(ID)	1402
39.5–40.4 39.0–39.9	(ID)	1403
40.5+ 40.0+	(ID)	1404
Diarrhea		
Number of stools per day		
4–6	(ID)	1501
7–9	(ID)	1502
10–12	(ID)	1503
13–15	(ID)	1504
16–20	(ID)	1505
21+	(ID)	1506
Anorexia		1601
Despondency and/or irritability		1602

[a]ID = infectious disease; ND = nutritional disease; and O = other.

Table C.3
Additional Symptoms and Diseases Recorded in Pregnant Women

Item	Key[a]	Code
Hepatitis	(ID)	1101
Protein-calorie malnutrition	(ND)	1251
Edema of lower extremities	(O)	1381
Rhinitis, atrophic	(O)	104
Gastritis	(O)	201
Irritable colon	(O)	206

[a]ID = infectious disease; ND = nutritional disease; and O = other.

Table C.4
Treatment

	Item	Code
Supportive	Not treated	1701
	Kaolin-pectin and/or placebo for diarrheal disease	1702
	Aspirin	1703
	Expectorant	1704, 1707
	Oral rehydration	1705
	Venous rehydration	1706
	Nasal drops	1708
	Antispasmodics	1709
	Antinauseants	1711
	Bronchodilators	1712
	Ointment (without antibiotics)	1731
	Ointment (with antibiotics and/or corticosteroids)	1732
	Antiseptics	1733
	Gentian violet	1734
	Colirium without antibiotic	1735
	Ophthalmic ointment with antibiotics	1736
	Surgical drain	1738
	Methyl salicylate	1739
Specific	Penicillin	1751
	Chloramphenicol	1752
	Tetracyclines	1753
	Erythromycin	1754
	Ampicillin	1756
	Sulfonamides	1757
	Nalidixic acid	1759
	Nystatin	1760
	Paromomycin	1761
	Hydroxyquinolein	1763
Other	Piperazine	1781
	Vitamins	1783
	Dietary treatment	1785
	Digitalis	1787
	Phenobarbital	1788

Appendix D
Variables of the Cauqué Study

I. Census
 1. Year
 2. Population
 3. Sex
 4. Age
 5. Family relationship
 6. Ethnic group
 7. Literacy
 8. Schooling
 9. Wearing of shoes
 10. Occupation
 11. Language
 12. Real estate[a]
 13. Kind of floor
 14. Kind of walls
 15. Kind of roof
 16. Number of rooms
 17. Cooking fire
 18. Water supply
 19. Feces disposal
 20. Garbage disposal
 21. Land usage

II. Vital Statistics
 1. Year
 2. Birth
 3. Death
 4. Cause of death
 5. Population estimates
 6. Age
 7. Sex

III. Socioeconomic Index
 1. Identification of family
 2. Score[a]

IV. Pregnant Woman
 1. Identification [a]
 2. Age
 3. Marital status
 4. Date of examination
 5. Reason for enrolling
 6. Date of last menstruation
 7. Obstetrical experience
 8. Number of examinations
 9. Trimester
 10. Illnesses in trimester
 11. Diagnosis[a]
 12. Duration of pregnancy
 13. Method for assessing duration of
  pregnancy
 14. Number of pregnancies
 15. Number of deliveries
 16. Number of abortions
 17. Number of living children
 18. Number of dead children
 19. Number of stillbirths
 20. Birth interval
 21. Weight
 22. Body length
 23. Arm circumference
 24. Leg circumference
 25. Tricipital skinfold thickness

V. Newborn
1. Identification
2. Sex
3. Birth date
4. Hour of birth
5. Birth order
6. Birth weight
7. Birth length
8. Birth head circumference
9. Birth thorax circumference
10. Age at examination
11. Informant
12. Appearance
13. Crying
14. Respiration
15. Defecation
16. Umbilical, strangulations
17. Temperature
18. Skeleton
19. Fracture
20. Skin
21. Mucosa
22. Lungs
23. Heart
24. Nervous system
25. Moro's reflex
26. Muscle tone
27. Congenital malformations[a]
28. Duration of labor
29. Type of delivery
30. Presentation
31. Rupture of membranes
32. Early neonatal death

VI. Child Growth
1. Identification
2. Age
3. Sex
4. Date of examination
5. Weight
6. Height
7. Head circumference
8. Thorax circumference
9. X-ray of hand wrist[a]
10. Health condition

VII. Diet of Mother
1. Identification
2. Age
3. Trimester of pregnancy
4. Date of study
5. Calories
6. Nutrients[a]
7. Frequency of intake of foods
8. Quantity of food

VIII. Diet of Child
1. Identification
2. Sex
3. Age
4. Date of study
5. Calories
6. Nutrients[a]
7. Frequency
8. Quantity
9. Lactation
10. Weaning age

IX. Illnesses and Injuries of Child
1. Identification
2. Sex
3. Age
4. Date of examination
5. Weight near onset
6. Weight near end of episode
7. Symptom or sign[a]
8. Infectious disease[a]
9. Nutritional disease[a]
10. Other disease[a]
11. Trauma or injury[a]
12. Number of episode
13. Duration of symptom
14. Duration of disease
15. Duration of episode[a]
16. Severity
17. Death
18. Cause of death[a]

X. Laboratory Specimens
1. Identification of child
2. Number of specimen
3. Date of collection
4. Hour specimen produced
5. Age of specimen
6. Number of order
7. Type of examination
8. Health status of child
9. Kind of specimen
10. Diversification of specimen

XI. Infection Variables

A. Fecal Specimens
1. Date of collection
2. Age of subject
3. Health condition of subject
4. Type of specimen
5. Physical characteristics
6. Acidity
7. Blood and mucus
8. Occult blood

B. Blood Specimens
1. Date of collection
2. Age of subject
3. Health condition of subject
4. Type of specimen

C. Kind of study
  1. Viruses
  2. Pathogenic bacteria
  3. Indigenous flora
  4. Yeasts
  5. Parasites
  6. Immunoglobulins
  7. Antibodies
  8. Hematology

D. Viruses
  1. Enterovirus-like
  2. Adenovirus-like
  3. Paralytogenic (infant mice) agent
  4. Poliovirus[a]
  5. Echovirus[a]
  6. Coxsackievirus[a]
  7. Adenovirus (group)

E. Bacteria
  1. *Shigella dysenteriae*[a]
  2. *Shigella flexneri*[a]
  3. *Shigella boydii*[a]
  4. *Shigella sonnei*
  5. Enteropathogenic *Escherichia coli*[a]
  6. *Salmonella*[a]
  7. Indigenous flora[a]
  8. *Staphylococcus*[a]
  9. *Streptococcus*[a]
  10. *Mycobacterium tuberculosis*
  11. *Streptococcus pneumoniae*
  12. *Neisseria gonorrhoeae*
  13. Other

F. Parasites
  1. *Ascaris lumbricoides*
  2. *Trichuris trichiura*
  3. *Entamoeba histolytica*
  4. *Dientamoeba fragilis*
  5. Other *amebae*[a]
  6. *Giardia lamblia*
  7. Other flagellates[a]
  8. Other helminths[a]

G. Immunoglobulins
  1. IgG
  2. IgM
  3. IgA
  4. Secretory IgA

H. Antibodies
  1. *Toxoplasma gondii*
  2. *Treponema pallidum*
  3. *Salmonella*[a]
  4. *Shigella*[a]
  5. Enteropathogenic *Escherichia coli*
  6. Polioviruses
  7. Reoviruses
  8. Herpesviruses
  9. Cytomegaloviruses

XII. Other: Hematology
  1. Hemoglobin
  2. Hematocrit

Note: For definition of variables, refer to text.
[a]Each item includes (or is made of) several variables, from two to as many as twenty or more.

Appendix E
Anthropometric Data

Table E.1
Population in Growth Study, 1964–1972

Age	Cohorts							
	1964	1965	1966	1967	1968	1969	1970	1971
Birth	37	45	46	59	57	53	67	60
6 mo	32	44	40	53	53	54	60	38
1 yr	30	40	45	49	52	52	57	7
1 yr 6 mo	25	45	40	37	48	45	36	0
2 yr	24	43	38	41	53	47	5	
2 yr 6 mo	28	43	35	34	43	24	0	
3 yr	27	47	37	39	50	4		
3 yr 6 mo	28	43	37	38	25	0		
4 yr	27	44	38	29	2			
4 yr 6 mo	27	45	37	23	0			
5 yr	27	45	36	3				
5 yr 6 mo	27	43	22	0				
6 yr	27	45	9					
6 yr 6 mo	27	24	0					
7 yr	27	4						
7 yr 6 mo	24	0						

Table E.2
Mean Weights and Heights, All Cohort Children, by Age, 1964–1972

Age	Weight, g		Height, cm	
	Number of cases	Mean ± S.E.	Number of cases	Mean ± S.E.
1 wk	409	2,624 ± 20	346	46.6 ± 0.13
4 wk	347	3,299 ± 30	327	48.9 ± 0.15
3 mo	375	5,050 ± 39	186	55.3 ± 0.21
6 mo	374	6,267 ± 43	184	60.5 ± 0.20
9 mo	352	6,829 ± 48	167	63.9 ± 0.23
1 yr	332	7,069 ± 50	166	66.0 ± 0.27
1 yr 6 mo	276	7,801 ± 56	130	70.2 ± 0.27
2 yr	251	8,617 ± 69	143	73.6 ± 0.31
2 yr 6 mo	207	9,481 ± 83	109	77.1 ± 0.36
3 yr	204	10,371 ± 87	129	80.1 ± 0.32
3 yr 6 mo	171	11,251 ± 99	109	83.7 ± 0.38
4 yr	155	11,711 ± 108	89	86.0 ± 0.39
4 yr 6 mo	132	12,865 ± 120	100	89.3 ± 0.42
5 yr	111	13,471 ± 136	92	91.8 ± 0.43
5 yr 6 mo	92	14,175 ± 170	81	94.1 ± 0.49
6 yr	81	14,899 ± 180	78	96.8 ± 0.56
6 yr 6 mo	51	15,877 ± 242	51	99.9 ± 0.64
7 yr	31	17,233 ± 287	31	103.6 ± 0.86

Table E.3
Mean Weights of Annual Cohorts, by Age, 1964–1971

Age	Cohorts							
	1964	1965	1966	1967	1968	1969	1970	1971
1 wk	2,702[a] (388)	2,694 (363)	2,585 (370)	2,680 (367)	2,574 (407)	2,519 (553)	2,642 (423)	2,642 (329)
6 mo	6,501 (712)	6,180 (908)	6,256 (806)	6,326 (693)	6,271 (878)	6,095 (905)	6,227 (860)	6,404 (805)
1 yr	7,341 (738)	6,881 (826)	7,158 (824)	7,113 (924)	7,125 (933)	6,929 (1,012)	6,931 (936)	7,539 (1,218)
1 yr 6 mo	7,887 (992)	7,597 (862)	7,778 (851)	7,944 (969)	7,867 (1,001)	7,692 (942)	7,923 (909)	
2 yr	8,938 (1,103)	8,262 (989)	8,448 (988)	8,873 (1,179)	8,600 (1,115)	8,645 (1,114)	9,221 (997)	
2 yr 6 mo	9,754 (1,076)	9,351 (1,103)	9,339 (1,085)	9,693 (1,383)	9,298 (1,119)	9,631 (1,484)		
3 yr	10,588 (1,099)	10,118 (1,222)	10,204 (1,234)	10,652 (1,286)	10,401 (1,247)	10,296 (1,921)		
3 yr 6 mo	11,394 (1,197)	11,001 (1,302)	10,971 (1,255)	11,588 (1,367)	11,421 (1,315)			
4 yr	12,070 (1,475)	11,789 (1,137)	11,956 (1,549)	12,307 (1,457)	12,211 (1,743)			
4 yr 6 mo	12,906 (1,549)	12,722 (1,238)	12,640 (1,441)	13,460 (1,197)				
5 yr	13,800 (1,511)	13,317 (1,277)	13,351 (1,591)	14,271 (761)				
5 yr 6 mo	14,697 (1,577)	13,981 (1,503)	13,912 (1,864)					
6 yr	15,243 (1,676)	14,796 (1,557)	14,378 (1,765)					
6 yr 6 mo	16,109 (1,522)	15,616 (1,930)						
7 yr	16,978 (1,524)	18,952 (904)						

[a]Mean, g; below (S.D.).

Table E.4
Mean Heights of Annual Cohorts, by Age, 1964–1971

Age	Cohorts							
	1964	1965	1966	1967	1968	1969	1970	1971
1 wk	47.5[a]	47.1	46.9	46.9	46.3	45.5	46.7	46.9
6 mo	61.6	60.4	59.8	61.7	60.2	56.4	60.3	60.7
1 yr	67.6	65.4	65.6	*	*	64.9	65.9	66.8
1 yr 6 mo	71.1	69.6	66.4	*	*	69.9	70.9	
2 yr	73.9	72.8	73.5	*	73.9	73.1	75.3	
2 yr 6 mo	77.9	77.2	75.0	*	76.9	76.8		
3 yr	80.3	80.3	79.3	79.7	80.1	80.1		
3 yr 6 mo	84.2	83.7	82.2	83.9	83.3			
4 yr	86.3	86.2	86.3	86.3	84.6			
5 yr	92.1	91.9	91.4	93.7				
6 yr	97.6	96.6	95.5					
7 yr	103.4	104.6						

*Incomplete data.
[a]Mean, cm.

Table E.5
Mean Head Circumference, Annual Cohorts of 1964 and 1965, by Age, 1964–1972

	1964		1965		Total	
Age	Number of cases	Mean, cm (S.D.)	Number of cases	Mean, cm (S.D.)	Number of cases	Mean, cm (S.D.)
1 wk	35	33.2 (1.5)	43	32.9 (1.4)	78	33.1 (1.4)
4 wk	34	35.1 (1.6)	38	34.9 (1.4)	72	34.9 (1.5)
3 mo	32	38.9 (1.3)	34	38.5 (1.7)	66	38.7 (1.5)
6 mo	32	41.5 (1.3)	31	40.9 (1.6)	63	41.2 (1.5)
9 mo	30	43.0 (1.3)	27	42.4 (1.6)	57	42.7 (1.5)
1 yr	26	43.9 (1.3)	28	42.9 (1.6)	54	43.4 (1.5)
1 yr 3 mo	20	44.5 (1.3)	27	43.6 (1.7)	47	43.9 (1.6)
1 yr 6 mo	18	44.7 (1.3)	27	44.2 (1.5)	45	44.4 (1.5)
1 yr 9 mo	16	45.1 (1.6)	27	44.6 (1.6)	43	44.8 (1.6)
2 yr	17	45.5 (1.5)	27	44.8 (1.6)	44	45.1 (1.6)
2 yr 3 mo	17	45.9 (1.3)	26	45.2 (1.7)	43	45.5 (1.6)
2 yr 6 mo	17	46.2 (1.2)	25	45.7 (1.7)	42	45.9 (1.5)
2 yr 9 mo	17	46.4 (1.2)	25	45.9 (1.6)	42	46.1 (1.5)
3 yr	23	46.4 (1.5)	25	46.3 (1.6)	48	46.3 (1.5)
3 yr 3 mo	17	46.8 (1.1)	24	46.6 (1.6)	41	46.7 (1.4)
3 yr 6 mo	19	46.8 (1.1)	24	47.1 (1.6)	43	47.0 (1.4)
3 yr 9 mo	17	47.2 (1.0)	23	47.1 (1.5)	40	47.2 (1.3)
4 yr	17	47.3 (1.2)	24	47.5 (1.6)	41	47.4 (1.4)
5 yr	17	48.3 (1.2)	24	48.0 (1.7)	41	48.1 (1.5)
6 yr	17	48.6 (1.1)	24	48.5 (1.6)	41	48.6 (1.4)
7 yr	17	49.4 (1.0)	4	50.7 (2.7)	21	49.6 (1.5)

Table E.6
Mean Thorax Circumference, Annual Cohorts of 1964 and 1965, by Age, 1964–1972

	1964		1965		Total	
Age	Number of cases	Mean, cm (S.D.)	Number of cases	Mean, cm (S.D.)	Number of cases	Mean, cm (S.D.)
1 wk	35	31.5 (1.9)	43	30.0 (1.6)	78	30.7 (1.9)
4 wk	34	34.3 (2.3)	38	32.9 (2.3)	72	33.6 (2.4)
6 mo	32	41.0 (1.7)	31	39.8 (2.1)	63	40.4 (1.9)
1 yr	26	42.6 (2.2)	28	40.7 (2.3)	54	41.6 (2.4)
1 yr 6 mo	18	43.9 (2.4)	27	42.7 (2.2)	45	43.2 (2.3)
2 yr	17	45.5 (2.3)	27	44.3 (2.3)	44	44.7 (2.4)
2 yr 6 mo	17	47.9 (1.4)	25	47.1 (2.7)	42	47.4 (2.3)
3 yr	22	48.8 (1.7)	25	48.6 (2.8)	47	48.7 (2.3)
3 yr 6 mo	19	51.1 (2.6)	24	49.1 (2.4)	43	49.9 (2.7)
4 yr	17	50.9 (2.2)	24	51.0 (2.5)	41	50.9 (2.4)
5 yr	17	53.2 (2.2)	24	52.7 (2.6)	41	52.9 (2.4)
6 yr	17	53.9 (2.3)	24	54.4 (2.4)	41	54.2 (2.3)
7 yr	17	56.3 (2.3)	4	59.2 (2.8)	21	56.9 (2.6)

Table E.7
Population of Singletons Studied Prospectively, Cohorts Defined by Birth Weight, 1964–1972

Age	Birth weight, g				
	< 2,001	2,001–2,500	2,501–3,000	3,001+	Total
1 wk	25/33[a]	140/118	197/162	40/36	402/339
2 wk	23/23	117/115	161/157	38/37	339/332
3 wk	22/22	111/111	154/154	35/35	322/322
4 wk	21/21	117/113	165/150	34/34	337/318
3 mo	19/19	128/64	177/81	40/23	364/117
6 mo	16/6	123/62	180/85	39/22	358/175
9 mo	13/5	114/52	176/80	34/22	337/159
1 yr	14/8	104/47	165/82	35/21	318/158
1 yr 3 mo	13/7	94/41	156/74	33/18	296/140
1 yr 6 mo	12/7	89/38	139/69	28/16	268/130
1 yr 9 mo	10/6	81/37	130/62	28/16	249/121
2 yr	10/7	78/43	123/67	28/17	239/134
2 yr 3 mo	11/7	74/39	113/60	26/14	224/120
2 yr 6 mo	10/6	65/33	101/56	24/12	200/107
2 yr 9 mo	8/4	66/36	101/58	26/14	201/112
3 yr	7/6	65/45	96/58	23/15	191/124

[a]Cases with weight/cases with height.

Table E.8
Weight of Singletons, Birth to Age Three Years, Prospective Study of Cohorts Defined by Birth Weight, 1964–1972

Age	Birth weight, g < 2,001	2,001–2,500	2,501–3,000	3,001+	Total
1 wk	1,702 (302)[a]	2,385 (164)	2,812 (191)	3,209 (179)	2,634 (400)
2 wk	1,816 (395)	2,605 (209)	3,067 (232)	3,444 (253)	2,865 (462)
3 wk	1,976 (465)	2,806 (258)	3,299 (274)	3,686 (277)	3,081 (504)
4 wk	2,182 (481)	3,019 (326)	3,554 (348)	3,903 (378)	3,318 (545)
3 mo	3,777 (671)	4,740 (557)	5,302 (603)	5,672 (580)	5,066 (732)
6 mo	5,044 (779)	5,966 (709)	6,439 (716)	7,057 (611)	6,282 (822)
9 mo	5,938 (588)	6,493 (817)	6,944 (810)	7,731 (812)	6,832 (805)
1 yr	6,165 (546)	6,776 (852)	7,160 (818)	7,938 (870)	7,076 (910)
1 yr 3 mo	6,323 (754)	7,124 (911)	7,511 (874)	8,371 (777)	7,432 (969)
1 yr 6 mo	6,784 (517)	7,470 (848)	7,939 (873)	8,539 (918)	7,794 (937)
1 yr 9 mo	6,979 (587)	7,839 (861)	8,375 (968)	8,958 (1,081)	8,210 (1,025)
2 yr	7,396 (631)	8,159 (879)	8,769 (1,062)	9,649 (1,005)	8,616 (1,107)
2 yr 3 mo	7,556 (777)	8,565 (972)	9,285 (985)	9,975 (1,431)	9,042 (1,170)
2 yr 6 mo	7,851 (821)	9,031 (1,005)	9,702 (1,057)	10,529 (1,245)	9,491 (1,205)
2 yr 9 mo	8,504 (895)	9,564 (947)	10,149 (1,096)	11,003 (1,319)	10,001 (1,196)
3 yr	9,022 (1,108)	9,940 (1,012)	10,544 (1,157)	11,626 (1,217)	10,413 (1,249)

[a]Mean (S.D.), g.

Table E.9
Height of Singletons, Birth to Age Three Years, Prospective Study of Cohorts Defined by Birth Weight, 1964-1972

Age	Birth weight, g				
	< 2,001	2,001-2,500	2,501-3,000	3,001+	Total
1 wk	41.6 (2.0)[a]	45.4 (1.3)	47.7 (1.2)	49.3 (1.0)	46.7 (2.3)
2 wk	42.2 (2.3)	46.2 (1.4)	48.5 (1.3)	50.4 (1.8)	47.5 (2.5)
3 wk	43.1 (2.2)	47.2 (1.4)	49.4 (1.3)	50.9 (1.1)	48.3 (2.3)
4 wk	43.7 (2.1)	47.8 (1.9)	50.1 (1.3)	51.8 (1.2)	49.0 (2.5)
3 mo	50.3 (3.4)	54.2 (2.1)	56.3 (1.9)	57.7 (2.1)	55.4 (2.7)
6 mo	55.8 (3.7)	59.4 (2.1)	61.5 (2.1)	62.5 (2.1)	60.7 (2.6)
9 mo	59.5 (3.7)	62.5 (2.6)	64.7 (2.4)	66.4 (1.9)	64.0 (2.9)
1 yr	62.8 (2.3)	64.6 (2.7)	66.7 (2.4)	68.6 (2.3)	66.1 (2.9)
1 yr 3 mo	64.1 (2.6)	66.7 (3.0)	68.5 (2.6)	71.2 (2.5)	68.1 (3.2)
1 yr 6 mo	65.4 (1.0)	68.7 (2.2)	71.0 (2.9)	72.5 (2.8)	70.2 (3.1)
1 yr 9 mo	67.1 (2.0)	70.7 (2.5)	72.9 (3.3)	74.6 (2.8)	72.2 (3.4)
2 yr	69.5 (2.9)	72.2 (2.8)	74.1 (3.8)	76.4 (3.3)	73.5 (3.7)
2 yr 3 mo	70.6 (3.4)	74.0 (2.9)	75.2 (5.7)	77.2 (3.5)	74.8 (4.8)
2 yr 6 mo	72.4 (3.3)	76.4 (3.1)	77.8 (4.1)	77.9 (2.6)	77.1 (3.8)
2 yr 9 mo	75.2 (2.9)	77.8 (2.8)	79.5 (3.9)	80.1 (3.6)	78.9 (3.7)
3 yr	77.3 (3.4)	78.9 (3.4)	80.7 (3.8)	82.4 (2.9)	80.1 (3.7)

[a]Mean (S.D.), cm.

Table E.10
Head Circumference of Singletons, Birth to Age Three Years, Prospective Study of
Cohorts Defined by Birth Weight, 1964–1972

Age	Birth weight, g				
	< 2,001	2,001–2,500	2,501–3,000	3,001+	Total
1 wk	29.2 (1.9)[a]	32.3 (0.8)	33.5 (0.8)	34.5 (0.9)	32.9 (1.6)
	23	118	162	36	339
3 wk	30.5 (2.2)	33.6 (0.8)	34.9 (0.9)	35.7 (1.2)	34.2 (1.6)
	22	111	154	35	322
3 mo	34.9 (2.7)	38.1 (0.9)	39.2 (0.9)	39.6 (1.4)	38.6 (1.7)
	7	28	40	12	87
6 mo	38.2 (2.7)	40.7 (1.2)	41.6 (1.0)	42.2 (1.4)	41.2 (1.4)
	3	27	37	11	78
1 yr	41.3 (1.7)	42.8 (1.2)	43.8 (1.1)	45.6 (1.9)	43.5 (1.5)
	3	21	34	10	68
1 yr 6 mo	43.2 (2.1)	43.7 (1.2)	44.6 (1.1)	45.6 (2.1)	44.4 (1.4)
	2	17	24	6	49
2 yr	43.7 (2.1)	44.5 (1.4)	45.6 (1.3)	46.2 (1.6)	45.3 (1.6)
	2	19	28	9	58
2 yr 6 mo	44.2 (2.0)	45.2 (1.3)	46.3 (1.0)	47.0 (2.2)	45.9 (1.5)
	2	14	21	6	43
3 yr	45.0 (1.4)	45.5 (1.4)	46.8 (0.8)	47.4 (1.9)	46.4 (1.5)
	3	20	27	10	60

[a]Mean (S.D.), cm; below, number of cases.

Table E.11
Thorax Circumference of Singletons, Birth to Age Three Years, Prospective Study of Cohorts Defined by Birth Weight, 1964–1972

Age	Birth weight, g				
	< 2,001	2,001–2,500	2,501–3,000	3,001+	Total
1 wk	26.2 (1.6)[a]	29.6 (1.3)	31.3 (1.1)	32.7 (1.0)	30.5 (1.9)
	23	118	162	36	339
3 wk	27.9 (2.9)	31.4 (1.3)	33.3 (1.3)	34.5 (1.1)	32.4 (2.1)
	22	111	153	35	321
3 mo	34.3 (2.5)	37.5 (1.8)	39.3 (1.7)	39.7 (1.4)	38.3 (2.3)
	7	28	39	12	86
6 mo	37.1 (2.3)	39.7 (1.9)	40.8 (1.6)	41.6 (1.1)	40.4 (1.9)
	3	27	37	11	78
1 yr	39.9 (0.4)	41.1 (2.2)	42.1 (2.4)	43.3 (2.1)	41.9 (2.4)
	3	21	34	10	68
1 yr 6 mo	42.6 (1.9)	42.4 (2.3)	43.4 (2.2)	44.7 (1.9)	43.2 (2.3)
	2	17	24	6	49
2 yr	42.4 (0.2)	44.4 (2.1)	44.9 (2.4)	46.9 (2.2)	44.9 (2.4)
	2	19	28	9	58
2 yr 6 mo	44.1 (3.3)	46.8 (2.4)	47.6 (1.8)	48.8 (2.2)	47.4 (2.3)
	2	14	21	6	43
3 yr	47.2 (2.1)	48.1 (2.5)	48.7 (1.9)	50.0 (2.3)	48.6 (2.3)
	3	20	26	10	59

[a]Mean (S.D.), cm; below, number of cases.

Table E.12
Weight of Singletons, Birth to Age Three Years, Prospective Study of Cohorts Defined
by Gestational Age, 1964–1972

Age	Gestational age, weeks				Total
	< 35	35–36	37–38	39+	
1 wk	1,511(180)[a]	1,923(475)	2,513(374)	2,712(320)	2,615(401)
2 wk	1,558(264)	2,102(540)	2,742(442)	2,956(363)	2,937(372)
3 wk	1,606(380)	2,310(544)	2,944(492)	3,175(401)	3,252(315)
4 wk	1,829(450)	2,486(556)	3,173(564)	3,408(456)	3,397(462)
3 mo	3,726(248)	4,079(999)	4,970(755)	5,140(671)	5,203(545)
6 mo	4,983(183)	5,443(1,025)	6,293(828)	6,328(789)	6,434(659)
9 mo	5,846(131)	6,229(931)	6,808(887)	6,861(895)	7,253(647)
1 yr	6,136(246)	6,339(883)	7,241(994)	7,103(889)	7,231(805)
1 yr 3 mo	6,222(390)	6,459(1,072)	7,595(876)	7,471(958)	7,469(758)
1 yr 6 mo	6,756(400)	7,028(992)	7,916(927)	7,828(931)	7,885(644)
1 yr 9 mo	7,072(524)	7,202(1,195)	8,275(1,216)	8,267(979)	8,112(717)
2 yr	7,588(720)	7,703(1,183)	8,328(1,139)	8,715(1,094)	8,434(566)
2 yr 3 mo	7,568(138)	7,940(1,427)	8,636(1,377)	9,155(1,112)	8,886(818)
2 yr 6 mo	8,443(338)	8,280(1,459)	9,239(1,573)	9,610(1,134)	9,215(904)
2 yr 9 mo	9,018(184)	9,108(1,783)	9,735(1,302)	10,086(1,159)	9,647(939)
3 yr	10,121[b]	9,734(2,040)	10,135(1,272)	10,478(1,214)	10,016(1,140)

[a]Mean (S.D.), g.
[b]One child.

Table E.13
Height of Singletons, Birth to Age Three Years, Prospective Study of Cohorts Defined by Gestational Age, 1964–1972

Age	Gestational age, weeks		Total
	< 37	37+	
1 wk	42.1 (2.6)[a]	46.9 (1.9)	46.7 (2.3)
	22	308	330
2 wk	42.6 (2.8)	47.8 (2.0)	47.5 (2.5)
	22	302	324
3 wk	43.4 (2.8)	48.7 (1.9)	48.3 (2.4)
	20	296	316
4 wk	44.3 (3.0)	49.4 (2.0)	49.1 (2.4)
	19	292	311
3 mo	51.1 (4.4)	55.6 (2.4)	55.4 (2.7)
	9	164	173
6 mo	57.3 (3.9)	60.8 (2.4)	60.6 (2.6)
	9	162	171
9 mo	60.5 (3.5)	64.2 (2.8)	64.0 (2.9)
	8	148	156
1 yr	63.0 (2.6)	66.3 (2.8)	66.1 (2.9)
	9	147	156
1 yr 3 mo	63.8 (2.1)	68.3 (3.0)	68.0 (3.1)
	7	131	138
1 yr 6 mo	66.1 (1.8)	70.5 (2.9)	70.2 (3.1)
	8	121	129
1 yr 9 mo	67.4 (2.6)	72.4 (3.3)	72.1 (3.4)
	6	114	120
2 yr	69.9 (2.9)	73.8 (3.7)	73.5 (3.7)
	8	125	133
2 yr 3 mo	71.4 (3.4)	75.0 (4.8)	74.8 (4.8)
	8	111	119
2 yr 6 mo	74.3 (4.5)	77.3 (3.7)	77.0 (3.8)
	9	96	105
2 yr 9 mo	77.1 (4.0)	79.0 (3.7)	78.9 (3.7)
	7	103	110
3 yr	79.2 (4.3)	80.3 (3.7)	80.2 (3.7)
	7	112	119

[a]Mean (S.D.), cm; below, number of cases.

Table E.14
Head Circumference of Singletons, Birth to Age Three Years, Prospective Study of
Cohorts Defined by Gestational Age, 1964–1972

| | Gestational age, weeks | | |
Age	< 37	37+	Total
1 wk	29.5 (2.3)[a]	33.1 (1.2)	32.9 (1.6)
	22	308	330
2 wk	30.1 (2.4)	33.8 (1.2)	33.6 (1.6)
	22	302	324
3 wk	30.6 (2.6)	34.5 (1.2)	34.2 (1.6)
	20	296	316
4 wk	31.6 (2.3)	35.1 (1.2)	34.8 (1.5)
	19	291	310
3 mo	35.4 (3.3)	38.8 (1.2)	38.5 (1.7)
	7	78	85
6 mo	39.3 (2.7)	41.3 (1.2)	41.2 (1.4)
	5	71	76
9 mo	41.0 (2.2)	42.9 (1.3)	42.7 (1.4)
	5	64	69
1 yr	42.0 (2.1)	43.6 (1.4)	43.5 (1.4)
	4	62	66
1 yr 3 mo	43.3 (2.3)	44.1 (1.6)	44.0 (1.6)
	3	57	60
1 yr 6 mo	44.0 (2.1)	44.3 (1.4)	44.3 (1.4)
	3	45	48
1 yr 9 mo	44.2 (2.4)	45.0 (1.6)	44.9 (1.6)
	3	53	56
2 yr	44.7 (2.2)	45.3 (1.5)	45.3 (1.6)
	3	54	57
2 yr 3 mo	44.8 (2.4)	45.7 (1.5)	45.6 (1.6)
	3	53	56
2 yr 6 mo	45.1 (2.2)	45.9 (1.4)	45.9 (1.5)
	3	39	42
2 yr 9 mo	45.4 (2.1)	46.2 (1.4)	46.2 (1.5)
	3	49	52
3 yr	45.9 (1.9)	46.4 (1.5)	46.4 (1.5)
	4	55	59

[a]Mean (S.D.), cm; below, number of cases.

Table E.15
Weight of Singletons, Birth to Age Six Years, Prospective Study of Cohorts Defined by
Birth Weight and Gestational Age, 1964–1972

Age	Preterm		Term, small-for-gestational age	Term	
	< 2,001 g	2,001–2,500 g		2,501–3,000 g	> 3,000 g
1 wk	1,551 ± 65[a]	2,327 ± 68	2,366 ± 15	2,812 ± 14	3,207 ± 29
	(16)	(6)	(137)	(190)	(39)
3 mo	3,653 ± 193	4,941 ± 425	4,677 ± 51	5,316 ± 45	5,667 ± 94
	(12)	(5)	(125)	(173)	(39)
6 mo	4,936 ± 221	6,406 ± 237	5,909 ± 67	6,444 ± 54	7,057 ± 100
	(11)	(5)	(118)	(175)	(38)
1 yr	5,957 ± 131	7,299 ± 379	6,739 ± 84	7,174 ± 64	7,959 ± 150
	(10)	(4)	(99)	(162)	(34)
2 yr	7,361 ± 249	8,539 ± 936	8,122 ± 100	8,777 ± 97	9,695 ± 191
	(8)	(3)	(73)	(120)	(27)
3 yr	9,080 ± 532	10,951 ± 1,465	9,827 ± 112	10,545 ± 121	11,680 ± 260
	(5)	(3)	(60)	(93)	(22)
4 yr	10,240 ± 694	12,792	11,413 ± 194	12,246 ± 154	13,174 ± 405
	(4)	(1)	(37)	(64)	(17)
5 yr	11,600 ± 738	15,180	12,800 ± 218	13,868 ± 191	14,469 ± 486
	(4)	(1)	(30)	(50)	(11)
6 yr	12,901 ± 838	18,468	13,927 ± 267	15,467 ± 247	15,585 ± 554
	(4)	(1)	(21)	(33)	(10)

[a]Mean ± S.E., g; below (number of children).

Table E.16
Height of Singletons, Birth to Age Six Years, Prospective Study of Cohorts Defined by
Birth Weight and Gestational Age, 1964–1972

	Preterm		Term, small-for-gestational age	Term	
	< 2,001 g	2,001–2,500 g		2,501–3,000 g	> 3,000 g
1 wk	40.6 ± 0.4[a]	45.2 ± 0.5	45.3 ± 0.1	47.7 ± 0.1	49.3 ± 0.2
	(15)	(6)	(117)	(156)	(35)
3 mo	48.7 ± 0.1	56.0 ± 0.8	53.9 ± 0.2	56.3 ± 0.2	57.7 ± 0.5
	(6)	(3)	(63)	(79)	(22)
6 mo	55.1 ± 0.2	60.9 ± 1.1	59.2 ± 0.3	61.6 ± 0.2	62.5 ± 0.5
	(5)	(3)	(59)	(82)	(21)
1 yr	61.9 ± 0.8	66.7 ± 0.7	64.4 ± 0.4	66.7 ± 0.3	68.7 ± 0.5
	(6)	(2)	(46)	(81)	(20)
2 yr	69.5 ± 0.1	71.3 ± 1.2	72.2 ± 0.4	74.1 ± 0.5	76.5 ± 0.8
	(6)	(2)	(42)	(67)	(16)
3 yr	77.6 ± 0.1	81.4 ± 3.2	78.9 ± 0.5	80.8 ± 0.5	82.4 ± 0.3
	(4)	(3)	(42)	(57)	(14)
4 yr	81.8 ± 0.5	87.1	84.6 ± 0.7	86.9 ± 0.5	88.2 ± 1.0
	(2)	(1)	(26)	(43)	(11)
5 yr	85.2 ± 1.1	93.7	90.4 ± 0.8	92.9 ± 0.6	93.5 ± 1.4
	(3)	(1)	(27)	(45)	(8)
6 yr	92.2 ± 2.1	100.5	96.7 ± 0.9	98.9 ± 0.9	96.9 ± 1.5
	(4)	(1)	(21)	(32)	(10)

[a]Mean ± S.E., cm; below (number of children).

Table E.17
Head Circumference of Singletons, Birth to Age Six Years, Prospective Study of Cohorts
Defined by Birth Weight and Gestational Age, 1964–1972

Age	Preterm		Term, small-for-gestational age	Term	
	< 2,001 g	2,001–2,500 g		2,501–3,000 g	> 3,000 g
1 wk	28.3 ± 0.4[a]	32.0 ± 0.5	32.2 ± 0.1	33.5 ± 0.1	34.5 ± 0.2
	(15)	(6)	(117)	(156)	(35)
3 mo	34.1 ± 1.2	38.6 ± 1.4	37.9 ± 0.2	39.2 ± 0.2	39.6 ± 0.4
	(5)	(2)	(27)	(40)	(11)
6 mo	38.2 ± 1.6	40.8 ± 1.7	40.6 ± 0.2	41.6 ± 0.2	42.1 ± 0.5
	(3)	(2)	(24)	(37)	(10)
1 yr	41.3 ± 0.9	44.4	42.7 ± 0.3	43.8 ± 0.2	44.7 ± 0.7
	(3)	(1)	(19)	(34)	(9)
2 yr	43.7 ± 1.5	46.6	44.4 ± 0.3	45.6 ± 0.3	46.2 ± 0.6
	(2)	(1)	(18)	(28)	(8)
3 yr	45.0 ± 0.8	48.3	45.4 ± 0.3	46.8 ± 0.2	47.3 ± 0.7
	(3)	(1)	(20)	(27)	(9)
4 yr	45.7 ± 1.0	48.6	46.8 ± 0.3	47.5 ± 0.2	48.3 ± 1.2
	(2)	(1)	(12)	(21)	(5)
5 yr	46.4 ± 1.1	50.0	47.4 ± 0.3	48.4 ± 0.2	48.9 ± 1.3
	(2)	(1)	(12)	(21)	(5)
6 yr	47.1 ± 1.1	50.6	47.9 ± 0.3	48.8 ± 0.2	49.4 ± 1.2
	(2)	(1)	(12)	(21)	(5)

[a]Mean ± S.E., cm; below (number of children).

References

Adams, M. S., and J. D. Niswander
Birth weight of North American Indians: A correction and amplification.
Human Biol. 45:351-357, 1973.

Aguirre, A., and A. Pradilla
Newer community approaches in Columbia. In *Nutrition programmes for pre-school children.* Reports of a conference held in Zagreb, Yugoslavia, 23-26 Aug. 1971. D. B. Jelliffe and E. F. P. Jelliffe, eds., pp. 270-279, 1973.

Alden, E. R., T. Mandelkorn, D. E. Woodrum, R. P. Wennberg, C. R. Parks, and A. Hodson
Morbidity and mortality of infants weighing less than 1000 grams in an intensive care nursery. *Pediatrics* 50:40-49, 1972.

Alford, C. A., J. W. Foft, W. J. Blankenship, G. Cassady, and J. M. Benton
Subclinical central nervous system disease of neonates: A prospective study of infants born with increased levels of IgM. *J. Pediat.* 75:1167-1178, 1969.

Althabe, O., G. Aramburú, R. L. Schwarcz, and R. Caldeyro-Barcia
Influence of the rupture of membranes on compression of the fetal head during labor. In *Perinatal factors affecting human development.* PAHO Sci. Pub. 185:143-149, 1969.

American Academy of Pediatrics
Nomenclature for duration of gestation, birth weight and intra-uterine growth. *Pediatrics* 39:935-939, 1967.

American Public Health Association
Control of communicable diseases in man. 11th ed. A. S. Benenson, ed. Washington, D.C., 1970.

Bressani, R., and N. S. Scrimshaw
Effect of lime treatment on *in vitro* availability of essential amino acids and solubility of protein fractions in corn. *J. Agric. Food Chem.* 6:774-778, 1958b.

Cáceres, A., and L. J. Mata
Hemaglutinación indirecta para la investigación de anticuerpos a enterobacteriáceas. *Rev. Lat. Microbiol.* 12:137-144, 1970.

Cáceres, A., and L. J. Mata
Niveles de immunoglobulinas en una población del altiplano guatemalteco. *Bol. Of. San. Pan.* 76:115-124, 1974.

Casey, H. L.
Standardized diagnostic complement fixation method and adaptation to microtest. Part I and II. Public Health Monograph No. 74. PHS Pub. No. 1228, 1965.

Center for Disease Control
Shigella dysenteriae type 1. California 1964-1970. *MMWR* 19:207, 1970.

Chandra, R. K.
Fetal malnutrition and postnatal immunocompetence. *Am. J. Dis. Child.* 4:450-454, 1975.

Chandra, R. K.
Immunocompetence in undernutrition. *J. Pediat.* 81:1194-1200, 1972.

Charles, D., and M. Finland, eds.
Obstetric and perinatal infections. Philadelphia: Lea and Febiger, 1973.

Chase, H. C.
Relationship of certain biologic and socio-economic factors to fetal, infant, and early childhood mortality. II. Father's occupation, infant's birth weight and mother's age. Albany, N.Y.: New York State Dept. of Health, 1962.

Chávez, A., and C. Martínez
Nutrition and development of infants from poor rural areas. III. Maternal nutrition and its consequences on fertility. *Nutr. Rep. Internat.* 7:1-8, 1973.

Cherkin, D. C.
Fertility dynamics in an Indian village of highland Guatemala. Thesis. University of Washington, 1974.

Ciba Foundation
Intrauterine infections. Ciba Fnd. Symposium 10 (new series). Amsterdam: Excerpta Medica, 1973.

Contreras, C., G. Arroyave, and M. A. Guzmán
Estudio comparativo del contenido de proteínas, riboflavina, carotenos y vitamina A de la leche materna entre dos grupos de mujeres de bajo y alto nivel socio-económico. *Arch. Venezol. Nutr.* 12:69-91, 1962.

Cook, R.
Is hospital the place for the treatment of malnourished children? *J. Trop. Ped. Environ. Child. Health* 17:15-25, 1971.

Coronel, J. G., G. Bustamante, and G. Uribe
Prematuridad en nuestro medio. *Pediatría (Rev. Soc. Col. Ped. Puericult.)* 10:275-302, 1968.

Corsa, L., T. F. Pugh, T. H. Ingals, and J. E. Gordon
Premature birth as a problem of human populations. *Am. J. Med. Sci.* 224: 343-360, 1952.

Dale, D. C., and L. J. Mata
Studies of diarrheal disease in Central America. XI. Intestinal bacterial flora in malnourished children with shigellosis. *Am. J. Trop. Med. Hyg.* 17:397-403, 1968.

Davie, R., N. Butler, and H. Goldstein
From birth to seven. The second report of the national child development study (1958 Cohort). The National Children's Bureau, Longman. London: William Cloves & Sons, 1972.

Davies, P. A.
Bacterial infection in the fetus and newborn. *Arch. Dis. Child.* 46:1-27, 1971.

Deacon, W. E., J. B. Lucas, and E. V. Price
Fluorescent treponemal antibody-absorption (FTA-ABS) test for syphilis. *J. Amer. Med. Assoc.* 198:626-628, 1966.

Dingle, J. H., C. F. Badger, and W. S. Jordan
Illness in the home. A study of 25,000 illnesses in a group of Cleveland families. Cleveland: Press of Western Reserve University, 1964.

Dubos, R., R. W. Schaedler, and R. Costello
Composition, alteration and effects of the intestinal flora. *Fed. Proc.* 22:1322-1329, 1963.

Dubos, R., R. W. Schaedler, R. Costello, and P. Hoet
Indigenous, normal, and autochthonous flora of the gastrointestinal tract. *J. Exp. Med.* 122:67-76, 1965.

Duncan, B., L. O. Lubchenco, and C. Hansman
Growth charts for children 0-18 years of age. *Pediatrics* 54:497-501, 1974.

Dunnebacke, T. H., and E. M. Zitcer
Preparation and cultivation of primary human amnion cells. *Cancer Res.* 17:1043-1046, 1957.

Edwards, P. R., and W. H. Ewing
Identification of enterobacteriaceae. Minneapolis, Minn.: Burgess Pub. Co., 1962.

Eichenwald, H. F., ed.
The prevention of mental retardation through the control of infectious diseases. Bethesda, Md.: USDHEW, 1966.

Emanuel, I.
Some preventive aspects of abnormal intrauterine development. *Postgr. Med.* 51:144-149, 1972.

Erhardt, C. L., G. B. Joshi, F. G. Nelson, B. H. Kroll, and L. Weiner
Influence of weight and gestational age on perinatal and neonatal mortality by ethnic group. *Am. J. Pub. Health* 54:1841-1855, 1964.

Evans, D. J., D. G. Evans, and S. L. Gorbach
Production of vascular permeability factor by enterotoxigenic *Escherichia coli* isolated from man. *Infection and Immunity* 8:725-730, 1973.

Fábrega, H.
Disease and social behavior: An interdisciplinary perspective. Cambridge, Mass.: MIT Press, 1974.

Falkner, F.
General considerations in human development. In *Human development*, F. Falkner, ed. London: W. B. Saunders Co., 1966, pp. 10-39.

Faulk, W. P., E. M. DeMaeyer, and A. J. S. Davies
Some aspects of malnutrition on the immune response in man. *Am. J. Clin. Nutr.* 27:638-646, 1974.

Fitzhardinge, P. M., and E. M. Steven
The small-for-date infant. I. Later growth patterns. *Pediatrics* 49:671-681, 1972.

Flores, M., Z. Flores, B. García, and Y. Gularte
Tabla de composición de alimentos de Centro América y Panamá. INCAP, Guatemala, 1960.

Flores, M., B. García, Z. Flores, and M. Y. Lara
Annual patterns of family and children's diet in three Guatemalan Indian communities. *Brit. J. Nutr.* 18:281-293, 1964.

Flores, M., M. T. Menchú, and M. A. Guzmán
Evaluación dietética de familias y preescolares mediante la aplicación de diferentes métodos y técnicas—Area rural de Nicaragua. *Arch. Latinoamer. Nutr.* 23:325-344, 1973.

Flores, M., M. T. Menchú, M. Y. Lara, and M. Béhar
Dieta adecuada de costo mínimo para Guatemala. INCAP, Guatemala, 1969.

Flores, M., and E. Reh
Estudios de hábitos dietéticos en poblaciones de Guatemala. IV. Santa María Cauqué. Supl. No. 2, *Bol. Of. San. Pan. Publ. Cient. INCAP*, pp. 163-173, 1955.

Food and Agriculture Organization, World Health Organization
Expert group on requirements of Vitamin A, Thiamine, Riboflavine and Niacin. WHO Tech. Rep. Ser. 362, 1967.

Food and Agriculture Organization, World Health Organization
Food fortification. Protein-calorie malnutrition. WHO Tech. Rep. Ser. 477, 1971.

Fox, J. P., L. R. Elveback, I. Spigland, T. E. Frothingham, D. A. Stevens, and M. Huger
The virus watch program: A continuing surveillance of viral infections in metropolitan New York families. I. Overall plan, methods of collecting and handling information and a summary of specimens collected and illnesses observed. *Am. J. Epidemiol.* 83:389-412, 1966.

Fox, J. P., C. E. Hall, M. K. Cooney, R. E. Luce, and R. A. Kronmal
The Seattle Virus Watch. II. Objectives, study population and its observation, data processing and summary of illnesses. *Am. J. Epidemiol.* 96:270-285, 1972.

Gangarosa, E. J., D. R. Perera, L. J. Mata, C. Mendizábal-Morris, G. Guzmán, and L. Reller
Epidemic Shiga bacillus dysentery in Central America. II. Epidemiologic studies in 1969. *J. Infect. Dis.* 122:181-190, 1970.

Garn, S. M., and C. G. Rohmann
Communalities of the ossification centers of the hand and wrist. *Am. J. Phys. Anthrop.* 17:319-323, 1959.

Gelfand, H. M., W. W. Heningst, J. P. Fox, and D. R. LeBlanc
Longitudinal studies of enteric viral infections. In *Proc. 6th internat. congr. trop. med. & malaria* 5:265-283, 1958.

Gelfand, H.M., A. H. Holguin, G. E. Marcheti, and P. M. Feorino
A continuing surveillance of enteroviral infections in healthy children in six United States cities. I. Viruses isolated during 1960 and 1961. *Am. J. Hyg.* 78:358-375, 1963.

Gelfand, H. M., L. Potash, D. R. LeBlanc, and J. P. Fox
Revised preliminary report on the Louisiana observations of the natural spread within families of living vaccine strains of poliovirus. In *Live poliovirus vaccines.* PAHO Sci. Pub. 44:203-217, 1959.

Giroud, A.
The nutrition of the embryo. Springfield, Ill.: Charles C. Thomas, 1970.

Gitlin, D., J. Kumate, J. Urrusti, and C. Morales
The selectivity of the human placenta in the transfer of plasma proteins from mother to fetus. *J. Clin. Invest.* 43:1938-1951, 1964.

Goldman, A. S., and C. W. Smith
Host resistance factors in human milk. *J. Pediat.* 82:1082-1090, 1973.

Goldstein, H.
Factors influencing the height of seven year old children—results from the National Child Development Study. *Human Biol.* 43:92-111, 1971.

Gómez, F., R. Ramos-Galván, S. Frenk, J. Cravioto, R. Chávez, and J. Vázquez
Mortality in second and third degree malnutrition. *J. Trop. Pediat.* 2:77-83, 1956.

Gopalan, C.
Protein intake of breast-fed poor Indian infants. *J. Trop. Pediat.* 2:89-92, 1956.

Gopalan, G., M. C. Swaminathan, V. K. Krishan-Kumari, D. Hanumantha-Rao, and K. Vijayaraghavan
Effect of calorie supplementation on growth of undernourished children. *Am. J. Clin. Nutr.* 26:563-566, 1973.

Gorbach, S. L.
Intestinal microflora. *Gastroenterology* 60:1110-1129, 1971.

Gorbach, S. L.
The toxigenic diarrheas. *Hosp. Pract.* 8:103-110, 1973.

Gordon, J. E.
Field epidemiology. *Am. J. Med. Sci.* 246:354-376, 1963.

Gordon, J. E., W. Ascoli, V. Pierce, M. A. Guzmán, and L. J. Mata
Studies of diarrheal disease in Central America. VI. An epidemic of diarrhea in a Guatemalan highland village, with a component due to *Shigella dysenteriae* type 1. *Am. J. Trop. Med. Hyg.* 14:404-411, 1965b.

Gordon, J. E., I. D. Chitkara, and J. B. Wyon
Weanling diarrhea. *Am. J. Med. Sci.* 245:345-377, 1963.

Gordon, J. E., M. A. Guzmán, W. Ascoli, and N. S. Scrimshaw
Acute diarrheal disease in less developed countries. 2. Patterns of epidemiological behavior in rural Guatemalan villages. *Bull. Wld Hlth Org.* 31:9-20, 1964.

Gordon, J. E., A. A. J. Jansen, and W. Ascoli
Measles in rural Guatemala. *J. Pediat.* 66:779-786, 1965a.

Gordon, J. E., V. Pierce, W. Ascoli, and N. S. Scrimshaw
Studies of diarrheal disease in Central America. II. Community prevalence of *Shigella* and *Salmonella* infections in childhood populations of Guatemala. *Am. J. Trop. Med. Hyg.* 11:389-394, 1962.

Gordon, J. E., J. B. Wyon, and W. Ascoli
The second year death rate in less developed countries. *Am. J. Med. Sci.* 254:357-380, 1967.

Greenhill, J. D., and E. A. Friedman
Biological principles and modern practice of obstetrics. Philadelphia: W. B. Saunders Co., 1974, p. 730.

Greenwald, P., H. Funakawa, S. Mitani, T. Mishimura, and S. Takeuchi
Influence of environmental factors on foetal growth in man. *Lancet* 1:1026-1029, 1967.

Greulich, W. W., and S. I. Pyle
Radiographic atlas of the skeletal development of the hand and wrist. 2nd ed. Stanford, Ca.: Stanford University Press, 1959.

Guzmán, M. A., N. S. Scrimshaw, H. Bruch, and J. E. Gordon
Nutrition and infection field study in Guatemalan villages, 1959-1964. VII. Physical growth and development of preschool children. *Arch. Environ. Hlth.* 17:107-118, 1968.

Habicht, J. P., R. Martorell, C. Yarbrough, R. M. Malina, and R. E. Klein
Height and weight standards for preschool children. How relevant are differences in growth potential? *Lancet* 1:611-615, 1974.

Hall, C. E., M. K. Cooney, and J. P. Fox
The Seattle Virus Watch program. I. Infection and illness experience of virus watch families during a community-wide epidemic of echovirus type 30 aseptic meningitis. *Am. J. Pub. Health* 60:1456-1465, 1970.

Hanshaw, J. B., H. J. Steinfeld, and C. J. White
Fluorescent antibody test for cytomegalovirus macroglobulin. *New Engl. J. Med.* 279:566-570, 1968.

Hansman, C.
Anthropometry and related data. In *Human growth and development.* R. W. McCammon, ed. Springfield, Ill.: Charles C. Thomas, 1970, pp. 103-154.

Hardy, J. B.
Birth weight and subsequent physical and intellectual development. *New Engl. J. Med.* 289:973-974, 1973.

Harris, A., A. A. Rosemberg, and L. M. Riedel
A microflocculation test for syphilis using cardiolipin antigen. Preliminary report. *J. Vener. Dis. Inform.* 27:169-174, 1946.

Hollister, A. C., M. D. Beck, A. M. Gittelsohn, and E. C. Hemphill
Influence of water availability on *Shigella* prevalence in children of farm labor families. *Am. J. Pub. Health* 45:354-362, 1955.

Howie, R. N.
Congenital malformations in the newborn: a survey at the National Women's Hospital, 1964-67. *N. Zeal. Med. J.* 71:65-71, 1962.

Hurtado, J. J.
Estudio del crecimiento en lactantes guatemaltecos bien nutridos. *Guatemala Pediátrica* 2:78-94, 1962.

INCAP
Evaluación del estado nutricional. INCAP, Series *Enseñando Nutrición* No. 9, Guatemala, 1956.

INCAP-CDC-HEW
Nutritional evaluation of the population of Central America and Panama, 1965-1967. DHEW Pub. No. (HSM) 72-8120, 1972.

INCAP-LSU
International atherosclerosis project. Standard operating protocol. Text, appendices and forms, 1962.

INCAP-OIR
Evaluación nutricional de la población de Centro América y Panamá. Guatemala. INCAP, Guatemala, 1969a.

INCAP-OIR
Evaluación nutricional de la población de Centro América y Panamá. El Salvador. INCAP, Guatemala, 1969b.

International Committee for Standardization in Hematology
Proposed recommendations for measurements of serum iron in human blood. *Brit. J. Haemat.* 20:451-453, 1971.

Jackson, R. L.
Somatic growth of children in the United States. *Missouri Medicine* October: 807-816, 1969.

Jackson, R. L., and G. Kelly
Growth charts for use in pediatric practice. *J. Pediat.* 27:215-229, 1945.

Jansen, A. A. J.
Birth weight, birth length, prematurity and neonatal mortality in New Guineans. *Trop. Geogr. Med.* 14:341-349, 1962.

Johnston, F. E., M. Borden, and R. B. MacVean
Height, weight, and their growth velocities in Guatemalan private school children of high socio-economic class. *Human Biol.* 45:627-641, 1973.

Jurado-García, E., A. Abarca, C. Osorio, R. Campos, A. Saavedra, J. Alvarez, and J. Parra
El crecimiento intrauterino. I. Evaluación del peso y la longitud corporal fetal en la ciudad de México. Análisis estadístico de 16,807 nacimientos consecutivos de producto único vivo. *Bol. Méd. Hosp. Infant.* (Mexico) 27:163-249, 1970.

Katz, S. H., M. L. Hediger, and L. A. Valleroy
Traditional maize processing technique in the New World. Traditional alkali

processing enhances the nutritional quality of maize. *Science* 184:765-773, 1974.

Kennedy, W. P.
Epidemiologic aspects of the problem of congenital malformations. Birth Defect Original Article, NF Series 8:1-18, 1967.

Kennell, J. H., R. Jerauld, H. Walfe, D. Chesler, N. C. Kreger, W. McAlpine, M. Steffa, and M. H. Klaus
Maternal behavior one year after early and extended post-partum contact. *Develop. Med. Child. Neurol.* 16:172-179, 1974.

Kennell, J. H., and M. H. Klaus
Care of the mother of the High-Risk Infant. *Clin. Obst. Gyn.* 14:926-954, 1971.

Klaus, M. H., and A. A. Fanaroff
Care of the high risk neonate. Philadelphia: W. B. Saunders, 1974.

Klaus, M., R. Jerauld, N. Kreger, W. McAlpine, M. Steffa, and J. H. Kennell
Maternal attachment; importance of the first post-parture-days. *New Engl. J. Med.* 286:460-469, 1972.

Kloene, W., F. B. Bang, S. M. Chakraborty, M. R. Cooper, H. Kulemann, M. Ota, and K. V. Shah
A two-year respiratory virus survey in farm villages in West Bengal, India. *Am. J. Epidemiol.* 92:307-320, 1970.

Kronmal, R. A.
A conversational computer statistical system. Part A. Data processing programs. Part B. Data file creation and utility programs. Seattle, Wa.: Dept. Biostatistics, School of Public Health and Community Medicine, University of Washington, 1974.

Kronmal, R. A., L. Bender, and J. Mortensen
A conversational statistical system for medical records. *J. Roy Stat. Soc.* 19:82-92, 1970.

Laga, E. M., S. G. Driscoll, and H. N. Munro
Comparison of placentas from two socioeconomic groups. II. Biochemical characteristics. *Pediatrics* 49:33-39, 1972.

Lechtig, A., G. Arroyave, J. P. Habicht, and M. Béhar
Nutrición materna y crecimiento fetal (Revisión). *Arch. Latinoamer. Nutr.* 21:505-530, 1971.

Lechtig, A., J. P. Habicht, G. Guzmán, and E.M. Girón
Influencia de la características maternas sobre el crecimiento fetal en poblaciones rurales de Guatemala. *Arch. Latinoamer. Nutr.* 22:255-265, 1972c.

Lechtig, A., J. P. Habicht, E. de León, and G. Guzmán
Influencia de la nutrición materna sobre el crecimiento fetal en poblaciones
rurales de Guatemala. II. Suplementación alimentaria. *Arch. Latinoamer.
Nutr.* 22:117-131, 1972a.

Lechtig, A., J. P. Habicht, G. Guzmán, and E. de León
Morbilidad materna y crecimiento fetal en poblaciones rurales de Guatemala.
Arch. Latinoamer. Nutr. 22:243-253, 1972b.

Lechtig, A., and L. J. Mata
Levels of IgG, IgA and IgM in cord blood of Latin American newborns from
different ecosystems. *Rev. Lat. Microbiol.* 13:173-179, 1971.

Lechtig, A., J. J. Ovalle, and L. J. Mata
Niveles de IgG, IgA, IgM y C3 en niños indígenas de Guatemala durante los
primeros 6 meses de edad. *Rev. Lat. Microbiol.* 14:65-71, 1972d.

Legg, S., M. Davies, R. Prywes, V. Sterk, and P. Weiskopt
The Jerusalem Perinatal Study. 2. Infant deaths 1964-1966. A cohort study
of socio-ethnic factors in deaths from congenital malformations and from
environmental and other causes. *Israel J. Med. Sci.* 5:1107-1116, 1969.

Lennette, E. H., and N. J. Schmidt
Diagnostic procedures for viral and rickettsial diseases. 3rd ed. New York:
APHA, Inc., 1964.

Levinson, F. J.
*Morinda: An economic analysis of malnutrition among young children in
rural India.* Cambridge, Mass.: Cornell/MIT Int. Nutr. Policy Ser., 1974.

Lim, K. A., and M. Benyesh-Melnick
Typing of viruses by combination of antiserum pools. Application to typing
of enteroviruses (Coxsackie and Echo). *J. Immunol.* 84:309-317, 1960.

Lin, C. C., and I. Emanuel
A comparison of American and Chinese intrauterine growth standards. Are
American babies really smaller? *Am. J. Epidemiol.* 95:418-430, 1972.

Love, E. J., and R. A. H. Kinch
Factors influencing the birth weight in normal pregnancy. *Am. J. Obst. Gyn.*
91:342-349, 1965.

Lubchenco, L. O.
Assessment of gestational age and development at birth. *Ped. Clin. N.A.*
17:125-145, 1970.

Lubchenco, L. O., M. Delivoria-Papadopoulos, and D. Searls
Long-term follow-up studies of prematurely born infants. II. Influence of
birth weight and gestational age on sequelae. *J. Pediat.* 80:509-512, 1972a.

Lubchenco, L. O., C. Hansman, and E. Boyd
Intrauterine growth in length and head circumference as estimated from live
births at gestational ages from 26 to 42 weeks. *Pediatrics* 37:403-408, 1966.

Lubchenco, L. O., F. A. Horner, L. H. Reed, I. E. Hix, D. Metcalf, R. Cohig, H. C. Elliott, and M. Bourg
Sequelae of premature birth. *Am. J. Dis. Child.* 106:101-115, 1963.

Lubchenco, L. O., D. T. Searls, and J. V. Brazie
Neonatal mortality rate: Relationship to birth weight and gestational age. *J. Pediat.* 81:814-822, 1972b.

Luna-Jaspe, G. H., M. Arango, J. Díaz, and H. Botero
El peso y la talla del nacimiento en un grupo de niños de clase económica baja. Manizales, Colombia. *Arch. Latinoamer. Nutr.* 19:41-51, 1969.

Luna-Jaspe, H., J. Cravioto, and L. Vega-Franco
Operación Nimiquipalg. VIII. Estudio comparativo de la evolución de la mortalidad entre la ciudad de Nueva York y una aldea rural de Guatemala. *Rev. Col. Méd.*, Guatemala, 16:45-55, 1965.

McGregor, I. A., A. K. Rahman, B. Thompson, W. Z. Billewicz, and A. M. Thomson
The growth of young children in a Gambian village. *Trans. Roy. Soc. Trop. Med. Hyg.* 62:341-352, 1968.

McGregor, I. A., A. K. Rahman, A. M. Thomson, W. Z. Billewicz, and B. Thompson
The health of young children in a West African (Gambian) village. *Trans. Roy. Soc. Trop. Med. Hyg.* 64:48-77, 1970b.

McGregor, I. A., D. S. Rowe, M. E. Wilson, and W. Z. Billewicz
Plasma immunoglobulin concentrations in an African (Gambian) community in relation to season, malaria and other infections and pregnancy. *Clin. Exp. Immunol.* 7:51-74, 1970a.

McKeown, T., and J. R. Gibson
Observations on all births (23,970) in Birmingham, 1947. IV. "Premature birth." *Brit. Med. J.* 2:513-517, 1951.

Malcolm, L. A.
Growth and development in New Guinea—A study of the Bundi People of the Madang District. Institute of Human Biology, Papua, New Guinea, Monograph Ser. No. 1. New South Wales: Surrey Beatty & Sons, 1970.

Mancini, G., A. O. Carbonara, and J. F. Heremans
Immunochemical quantitation of antigens by single radial immunodiffusion. *Int. J. Immunochem.* 2:235-254, 1965.

Martínez, C., and A. Chávez
Nutrition and development in infants of poor rural area. 1. Consumption of mother's milk by infants. *Nutr. Rep. Internat.* 4:139-149, 1971.

Mata, L. J.
Estudio sobre la incidencia de shigelas en Guatemala. *Rev. Biol. Trop.*, Costa Rica, 5:211-230, 1957.

Mata, L. J.
Infección intestinal en niños de áreas rurales centroamericanas y sus posibles implicaciones nutricionales. *Arch. Latinoamer. Nutr.* 19:153-172, 1969.

Mata, L. J.
The relationship of maternal infection to fetal growth and development. In *Symposia of the Swedish Nutrition Foundation XII*, Uppsala, pp. 43-48, 1974.

Mata, L. J., F. J. Aguilar, D. L. Eddins, K. L. Herrmann, J. H. Nakano, and J. R. Aguilar
Vacunación masiva contra el sarampión en la República de Guatemala, 1972. Evaluación de la campaña. *Bol. Méd. Hosp. Infantil* (México) 31:505-517, 1974c.

Mata, L. J., A. Cáceres, R. Fernández, M. F. Torres, M. Cordón, and R. Rosales
Avances sobre el conocimiento de la disentería en Guatemala. *Rev. Lat. Microbiol.* 14:1-10, 1972d.

Mata, L. J., A. Cáceres, and M. F. Torres
Epidemic Shiga dysentery in Central America. *Lancet* 1:600-601, 1971a.

Mata, L. J., C. Carrillo, and E. Villatoro
Fecal microflora in healthy persons in a preindustrial region. *Appl. Microbiol.* 17:596-602, 1969a.

Mata, L. J., and F. Castro
Epidemiology, diagnosis, and impact of Shiga dysentery in Central America. In *Industry and tropical health.* VIII. Proceedings of the 8th Conference. Industrial Council for Tropical Health, 1974, pp. 30-37.

Mata, L. J., M. A. Catalán, and J. E. Gordon
Studies of diarrheal disease in Central America. IX. *Shigella* carriers among young children of a heavily seeded Guatemalan convalescent home. *Am. J. Trop. Med. Hyg.* 15:632-638, 1966.

Mata, L. J., M. Cordón, R. Fernández, M. L. Mejicanos, and J. J. Urrutia
Estudio cuantitativo de la flora fecal en pacientes con disentería Shiga. In *Simposio sobre Disentería Shiga*, PAHO Sci. Pub. 283:95-101, 1974b.

Mata, L. J., and W. P. Faulk
The immune response of malnourished subjects with special reference to measles. *Arch. Latinoamer. Nutr.* 23:345-362, 1973.

Mata, L. J., R. Fernández, and J. J. Urrutia
Infección del intestino por bacterias enteropatógenas en niños de una aldea de Guatemala, durante los tres primeros años de vida. *Rev. Lat. Microbiol. Parasitol.* 11:102-109, 1969b.

Mata, L. J., E. J. Gangarosa, A. Cáceres, D. R. Perera, and M. L. Mejicanos
Epidemic Shiga bacillus dysentery in Central America. I. Etiologic investigations in Guatemala, 1969. *J. Infect. Dis.* 122:170-180, 1970.

Mata, L. J., F. Jiménez, and M. L. Mejicanos
Evolution of intestinal flora of children in health and disease. In *Recent advances in microbiology*, A. Perez-Miravete and D. Peláez, eds. Mexico: Mexican Association of Microbiology, 1971b, pp. 363-374.

Mata, L. J., R. Lüttmann, and L. Sánchez
Microorganismos enteropatógenos en niños con diarrea severa. *Rev. Col. Med.*, Guatemala, 15:176-184, 1964.

Mata, L. J., M. L. Mejicanos, and F. Jiménez
Studies on the indigenous gastrointestinal flora of Guatemalan children. *Am. J. Clin. Nutr.* 25:1380-1390, 1972a.

Mata, L. J., and J. J. Urrutia
Intestinal colonization of breast-fed children in a rural area of low socioeconomic level. *Ann. N.Y. Acad. Sci.* 176:93-109, 1971.

Mata, L. J., J. J. Urrutia, C. Albertazzi, O. Pellecer, and E. Arellano
Influence of recurrent infections on nutrition and growth of children in Guatemala. *Am. J. Clin. Nutr.* 25:1267-1275, 1972c.

Mata, L. J., J. J. Urrutia, and M. Béhar
Infección en la mujer embarazada y en los productos de la concepción. *Arch. Latinoamer. Nutr.* 24:15-45, 1974a.

Mata, L. J., J. J. Urrutia, A. Cáceres, and M. A. Guzmán
The biological environment in a Guatemalan rural community. In *Proc. Western Hemisphere Nutr. Cong. III.* Mt. Kisco, N.Y.: Futura Pub. Co., Inc., 1972b, pp. 257-264.

Mata, L. J., J. J. Urrutia, and B. García
Effect of infection and diet on child growth: Experience in a Guatemalan village. In *Nutrition and infection*, Ciba Fnd. Study group No. 31, Wolstenholme, G. E. W., and M. O'Connor, eds. Boston: Little Brown & Co., 1967a, pp. 112-126.

Mata, L. J., J. J. Urrutia, B. García, R. Bressani, P. Lachance, and M. A. Guzmán
A model for maize fortification with soy bean flour, lysine and other nutrients in a low socioeconomic rural community. In *Nutritional improvement of maize*, Bressani, R., J. E. Braham, and M. Béhar, eds. INCAP, 1972e, pp. 273-287.

Mata, L. J., J. J. Urrutia, B. García, R. Fernández, and M. Béhar
Shigella infection in breast-fed Guatemalan Indian neonates. *Am. J. Dis. Child.* 117:142-146, 1969c.

Mata, L. J., J. J. Urrutia, and J. E. Gordon
Diarrhoeal disease in a cohort of Guatemalan village children observed from birth to age two years. *Trop. Geogr. Med.* 19:247-257, 1967b.

Mata, L. J., J. J. Urrutia, and A. Lechtig
Infection and nutrition of children of a low socioeconomic rural community. *Am. J. Clin. Nutr.* 24:249-259, 1971c.

Mata, L. J., and R. G. Wyatt
Host resistance to infection. *Am. J. Clin. Nutr.* 24:976-986, 1971.

Melnick, J. L.
Tissue culture methods for the cultivation of poliomyelitis and other viruses. In *Diagnostic procedures for virus and rickettsial diseases.* New York: APHA, Inc., 1956, pp. 97-152.

Melvin, D. M., and L. J. Mata
Intestinal parasites in a Mayan-Indian village of Guatemala. *Rev. Lat. Microbiol.* 13:15-19, 1971.

Menchú, M. T., G. Arroyave, and M. Flores
Recomendaciones dietéticas diarias para Centro América y Panamá. INCAP Pub. No. E-709, 1973.

Méndez, J., and C. Behrhorst
The anthropometric characteristics of Indian and urban Guatemalans. *Human Biol.* 35:457-469, 1963.

Mendizábal, C. A., L. J. Mata, E. Gangarosa, and G. Guzmán
Epidemic Shiga dysentery in Central America. II. Magnitude of the outbreak and mortality in Guatemala in 1969. *Am. J. Trop. Med. Hyg.* 20:927-933, 1971.

Miller, F. J. W., W. Z. Billewicz, and A. M. Thomson
Growth from birth to adult life of 442 Newcastle Upon Tyne children. *Brit. J. Prev. Soc. Med.* 26:224-230, 1972.

Monif, G. R. G.
Viral infections of the human fetus. London: Collier-MacMillan Ltd., 1969.

Monto, A. S., and K. M. Johnson
A community study of respiratory infections in the tropics. I. Description of the community and observations on the activity of certain respiratory agents. *Am. J. Epidemiol.* 86:78-92, 1967.

Monto, A. S., and B. M. Ullman
Acute respiratory illness in an American Community. The Tecumseh Study. *J. Amer. Med. Assoc.* 227:164-169, 1974.

Moore, A. E., L. Sabachewsky, and H. W. Toolan
Culture characteristics of four permanent lines of human cancer cells. *Cancer Res.* 15:598-602, 1955.

Morley, D., J. Bicknell, and M. Woodland
Factors influencing the growth and nutritional status of infants and young children in a Nigerian village. *Trans. Roy. Soc. Trop. Med. Hyg.* 62:164-195, 1968.

Narasinga-Rao, B. S., K. Visweswara-Rao, and A. N. Naidu
Calorie-protein adequacy of the dietaries of preschool children in India. *J. Nutr. Dietet.* 6:238-244, 1969.

National Academy of Sciences
Recommended dietary allowances. NAS Pub. 1964, Washington, D.C., 1968.

National Center for Health Statistics
International comparison of perinatal and infant mortality: The United States and six West European countries. USDHEW, PHS-NCHS, Ser. 3, 1967.

Nelson, D. P., and L. J. Mata
Bacterial flora associated with the human gastrointestinal mucosa. *Gastroenterology* 58:56-61, 1970.

Niswander, K. R., and M. Gordon
The women and their pregnancies. USDHEW, Pub. No. (NIH) 73-379, 1972.

Oberndorfer, L., and W. Mejía
Statistical analysis of the duration of breast-feeding. A study of 200 mothers of Antioquia province, Colombia. *J. Trop. Med.* 14:27-42, 1968.

Olson, L. C., V. Lexomboon, P. Sithisarn, and H. E. Nayes
The etiology of respiratory tract infections in a tropical country. *Am. J. Epidemiol.* 97:34-43, 1973.

Ota, W., and F. B. Bang
A continuous study of viruses in the respiratory tract in families of a Calcutta Bustee. I. Description of the study area and patterns of virus recovery. *Am. J. Epidemiol.* 95:371-391, 1972.

Otzoy, S.
Santa María Cauqué. Publicaciones especiales del Instituto Indigenista Nacional de Guatemala. Manuscript, 1949.

Ounsted, M., and M. E. Taylor
The postnatal growth of children who were small-for-dates or large-for-dates at birth. *Develop. Med. Child Neurol.* 13:421-434, 1971.

Palmer, D. F., K. L. Herrmann, and R. E. Lincoln
A procedural guide to the performance of the standardized rubella hemagglutination-inhibition test. Atlanta, Ga.: USDHEW, PHS, CDC, 1970.

Pan American Health Organization
Metabolic adaptation and nutrition. Sci. Pub. No. 222, 1971.

Parks, W. P., L. T. Queiroga, and J. L. Melnick
Studies of infantile diarrhea in Karachi, Pakistan. II. Multiple virus isolations from rectal swabs. *Am. J. Epidemiol.* 85:469-478, 1967.

Parrilla-Ríos, C. M.
Valor nutritivo global de dietas cuyas proteínas provienen predominantemente del maíz y del frijol negro en niños de 2 to 7 años. Interrelación entre morbilidad y nutrición. INCAP, Thesis, 1973.

Plank, S. J., and M. C. Milanesi
Infant feeding and infant mortality in rural Chile. *Bull. Wld Hlth Org.* 48: 203-210, 1973.

Puffer, R. R., and C. V. Serrano
Patterns of mortality in childhood. PAHO Sci. Pub. No. 262, 1973.

Rao, K. S. J., M. C. Swaminathan, S. Swarup, and V. N. Patwardhan
Protein malnutrition in South India. *Bull. Wld Hlth Org.* 20:603-639, 1959.

Remington, J. S.
The present status of the IgM fluorescent antibody technique in the diagnosis of congenital toxoplasmosis. *J. Pediat.* 75:1116-1124, 1969.

Ritchie, L. S.
An ether sedimentation technique for routine stool examinations. *Bull. U.S. Army Med. Dept.* 8:326, 1948.

Rosa, F. W., and M. Turshen
Fetal nutrition. *Bull. Wld Hlth Org.* 43:785-795, 1970.

Rosales, L., C. L. Quintanilla, and J. Cravioto
"Operación Nimiquipalg." III. Epidemiología popular de enfermedades prevalentes en el medio rural de Guatemala. *Guatemala Pediátrica* 4:60-64, 1964.

Rosebury, T.
Microorganisms indigenous to man. New York: McGraw-Hill Book Co., 1962.

Rosen, L.
Reoviruses. In *Diagnostic procedures for viral and rickettsial diseases.* Lennette, E. H., and N. J. Schmidt, eds. New York: APHA, Inc., 1964, pp. 259-267.

Rowe, D. S., S. G. Anderson, and B. Grab
A research standard for human serum immunoglobulins IgG, IgA and IgM. *Bull. Wld Hlth Org.* 42:535-552, 1970.

Rowe, D. S., I. A. McGregor, S. J. Smith, P. Hall, and K. Williams
Plasma immunoglobulin concentrations in a West African (Gambian) community and in a group of healthy British children. *Clin. Exp. Immunol.* 3:63-79, 1968.

Sabin, A. B., M. Ramos-Alvarez, J. Alvarez-Amézquita, W. Pelon, R. H. Michaels, I. Spigland, M. A. Koch, J. M. Barnes, and J. S. Rhim
Live, orally given poliovirus vaccine. Effects of rapid immunization on populations under conditions of massive enteric infection with other viruses. *J. Amer. Med. Assoc.* 173:1521-1526, 1960.

Salber, E. J.
The significance of birth weight, as illustrated by a comparative study of South African racial groups. *J. Trop. Ped.* 1:54-60, 1955.

Salomon, J. B., J. E. Gordon, and N. S. Scrimshaw
Studies of diarrheal disease in Central America. X. Associated chickenpox, diarrheal and kwashiorkor in a highland Guatemalan village. *Am. J. Trop. Med. Hyg.* 15:997-1002, 1966.

Sanjur, D. M., J. Cravioto, L. Rosales, and A. van Veen
Infant feeding and weaning practices in a rural preindustrial setting. A socio-cultural approach. *Acta Paediat. Scand.* Suppl. 200, 1970.

Sarram, M., and M. Saadatnejadi
Birth weight in Shiraz (Iran) in relation to maternal socioeconomic status. *Obstet. Gynec.* 30:367-370, 1967.

Schaedler, R. E., R. Dubos, and R. Costello
The development of the bacterial flora in the gastrointestinal tract of mice. *J. Exp. Med.* 122:59-66, 1965.

Scheifele, D. W., and C. E. Forbes
Prolonged giant cell excretion in severe African measles. *Pediatrics* 50:867-873, 1972.

Scrimshaw, N. S., W. Ascoli, J. J. Kevany, M. Flores, S. J. Icaza, and J. E. Gordon
Nutrition and infection field study in Guatemalan villages, 1959-1964. III. Field procedure, collection of data and methods of measurement. *Arch. Environ. Hlth.* 15:6-15, 1967b.

Scrimshaw, N. S., M. A. Guzmán, M. Flores, and J. E. Gordon
Nutrition and infection field study in Guatemalan villages, 1959-1964. V. Disease incidence among preschool children under natural village conditions, with improved diet and with medical and public health services. *Arch. Environ. Hlth.* 16:223-234, 1968b.

Scrimshaw, N. S., M. A. Guzmán, and J. E. Gordon
Nutrition and infection field study in Guatemalan villages, 1959-1964. I. Study plan and experimental design. *Arch. Environ. Hlth.* 14:657-662, 1967a.

Scrimshaw, N. S., J. B. Salomon, H. A. Bruch, and J. E. Gordon
Studies of diarrheal disease in Central America. VIII. Measles, diarrhea and nutritional deficiency in rural Guatemala. *Am. J. Trop. Med. Hyg.* 15:625-631, 1966.

Scrimshaw, N. S., C. E. Taylor, and J. E. Gordon
Interactions of nutrition and infection. *Am. J. Med. Sci.* 237:367-403, 1959.

Scrimshaw, N. S., C. E. Taylor, and J. E. Gordon
Interactions of nutrition and infection. WHO Monograph Ser. No. 57, 1968a.

Sever, J. L.
Perinatal infections affecting the developing fetus and newborn. In *The pre-*

vention of mental retardation through the control of infectious diseases. Bethesda, Md.: USDHEW, NIH, 1966, pp. 37-68.

Shattuck, G. C., J. C. Bequaert, J. H. Sandground, M. M. Hillferty, and S. D. Clark
A medical survey of the Republic of Guatemala. Washington, D.C.: Carnegie Institute of Washington, 1938.

Smith, G. H.
Income and nutrition in the Guatemalan highlands. Thesis. Dept. Economics and Graduate School, University of Oregon, 1972. Univ. microfilms. Ann Arbor, Mich., 1973.

Solien-González, N. L.
Culture change in a Guatemalan community. *Papers of the Michigan Academy of Science, Arts, and Letters* 62:239-247, 1957.

Stewart, R. J. C.
Small-for-dates offspring: an animal model. In *Nutrition, the nervous system, and behavior.* PAHO Sci. Pub. 251:33-37, 1972.

Stiehm, E. R.
Fetal defense mechanisms. *Am. J. Dis. Child.* 4:438-443, 1975.

Stiehm, E. R. and H. H. Fundenberg
Serum levels of immune globulins in health and disease: A survey. *Pediatrics* 37:715-727, 1966.

Stuart, H. C. and H. V. Meredith
Use of body measurement in the school health program. *Am. J. Pub. Health* 36:1365-1373, 1946.

Sukhatme, P. V.
The protein problem, its size and nature. *J.R. Statist. Soc.* 137:166-199, 1974.

Susser, M., F. A. Marolla, and J. Fleiss
Birth weight, fetal age and perinatal mortality. *Am. J. Epidemiol.* 96:197-204, 1972.

Tanner, J. M., and A. M. Thomson
Standards for birth weight at gestation periods from 32 to 42 weeks, allowin for maternal height and weight. *Arch. Dis. Childhood* 45:566-569, 1970.

Thomson, A. M., W. Z. Billewicz, and F. E. Hytten
The assessment of fetal growth. *J. Obstet. Gynaec. Brit. Cwlth.* 75:903-916, 1968.

Towbin, A.
Central nervous system damage in the human fetus and newborn infant. Mechanical and hypoxic injury incurred in the fetal-neonatal period. *Am. J. Dis. Child.* 119:529-542, 1970.

Tyrrell, D. A. J.
Common colds and related diseases. Baltimore: Williams & Wilkins Co., 1965.

University of Washington
CDC 6400 users guide. 1973.

Urrutia, J. J. and L. J. Mata
Complicaciones del sarampión: experiencia en una zona rural de Guatemala.
Bol. Of. San. Pan. 77:223–230, 1974.

US Department of Health, Education and Welfare
A study of infant mortality from linked records by birth weight, period of gestation and other variables. United States. DHEW Pub. No. (HSM) 72-1055, 1972c.

Usher, R.
Neonatal mortality at the Royal Victoria Hospital and the Province of Quebec. Paper presented at the Conference on Neonatal Intensive Care, 10–12 June 1974, NIH, Washington, D.C.

Valverde, V., W. Vargas, I. Rawson, G. Calderón, R. Rosabal, W. Aguilar, L. F. Gutiérrez, and R. Gutiérrez
La deficiencia calórica en pre-escolares del área rural de Costa Rica. *Arch. Latinoamer. Nutr.* 25:351–361, 1975.

Van Zijl, W. J.
Studies on diarrhoeal diseases in seven countries by the WHO Diarrhoeal Diseases Advisory Team. *Bull. Wld Hlth Org.* 35:249–261, 1966.

Viteri, F. E., M. A. Guzmán, and L. J. Mata
Anemias nutricionales en Centro América. Influencia de infección por uncinaria. *Arch. Latinoamer. Nutr.* 23:33–53, 1973a.

Viteri, F. E., L. J. Mata, and M. Béhar
Métodos de evaluación del estado nutricional proteinico-calórico en pre-escolares de condiciones socio-económicas diferentes. Repercusión nutricional del sarampión en niños crónicamente subalimentados. *Arch. Latinoamer. Nutr.* 23:13–31, 1973b.

Waterlow, J. C.
Note on the assessment and classification of protein-energy malnutrition in children. *Lancet* 2:87–89, 1973.

Waterlow, J. C., J. Cravioto and J. M. L. Stephen
Protein malnutrition in man. In *Advances in protein chemistry*, Vol. 15. New York: Academic Press, 1960.

Weatley, W. B.
A rapid staining procedure for intestinal amoebae and flagellates. *Am. J. Clin. Pathol.* 21:990–991, 1951.

Wegman, M. E.
International trends in postperinatal mortality. *Am. J. Dis. Child.* 121:105–110, 1971.

Weiss, W., and E. C. Jackson
Maternal factors affecting birth weight. In *Perinatal factors affecting human development.* PAHO Sci. Pub. No. 185, 1972.

Weld, J. T.
Candida albicans. Rapid identification in cultures made directly from human materials. *Arch. Dermat. Syph.* 67:473–478, 1953.

Weller, T. H. and F. A. Neva
Propagation in tissue culture of cytopathic agents from patients with rubella-like illness. *Proc. Soc. Exp. Biol. Med.* 111:215–225, 1962.

Wenner, H. A.
Outline of laboratory procedures for the diagnosis of enterovirus infections. In *Diagnostic procedures for viral and rickettsial diseases.* 3rd ed. Lennette, E. H., and N. J. Schmidt, eds. Washington, D.C.: APHA, Inc., 1964, pp. 243–258.

Wiener, G., R. V. Rider, W. C. Oppel, and P. A. Harper
Correlates of low birth weight. Psychological status at eight to ten years of age. *Pediat. Res.* 2:110–118, 1968.

Williams, R. C., and R. J. Gibbons
Inhibition of bacterial adherence by secretory immunoglobulin A: A mechanism of antigen disposal. *Science* 172:697–699, 1972.

World Health Organization
Expert Group on Prematurity–Final Report. WHO Tech. Rep. Ser. No. 27, Geneva, 1950.

World Health Organization
Nutritional anaemias. WHO Tech. Rep. Ser. No. 503, 1972a.

World Health Organization
Public health aspects of low birth weight. In *WHO 3rd Report*, 1961.

Wyatt, R. G., B. García, A. Cáceres, and L. J. Mata
Immunoglobulins and antibodies in colostrum and milk of Guatemalan Mayan women. *Arch. Latinoamer. Nutr.* 22:629–644, 1972.

Yerushalmy, J.
The classification of newborn infants by birth weight and gestational age. *J. Pediat.* 71:164–172, 1967.

Younger, J. S.
Monolayer tissue cultures. I. Preparation and standardization of suspensions of trypsin-dispersed monkey kidney cells. *Proc. Soc. Exp. Biol. Med.* 85:202–205, 1954.

Index

Abortion
   defined, 98
   frequency of, 99, 100, 113, 122, 207–208
Adams, M. S., 135
Adenoviruses, 81, 111, 248, 266, 305, 306, 315, 316
Advisors and consultants, 335–336
Agriculture, village, 17–23, 24, 30–31
Aguirre, A., 292
Alden, E. R., 132
Alford, C. A., 127, 128
Althabe, O., 117
American Public Health Association (APHA), 228, 270
Anemia, 293–295, 302
Animals, domestic. *See* Livestock
Anorexia, 167, 220, 257, 264, 268, 277, 283, 286, 295, 300
Anthropometry, physical
   data on, collection of, 61–67, 89, 346–361
   and growth and development in infancy and early childhood, 167–201, 222, 304–318, 321–322
   of mothers, 98, 101, 137–151
   of newborns, 121–127, 137–151, 305, 317
   of pregnant women, 61–62, 64, 101–104
Antonov, A. N., 135
Arroyave, G., 61, 257, 295
Ascaris, 53–56, 111, 239, 240, 242, 280, 286, 306, 309, 314

Ascoli, W., 257, 295
Ascorbic acid, intake of
   by children, 71, 211–214, 217, 220–222, 295
   by pregnant women, 69, 106–111
Atoles, 205, 322
Autret, M., 257, 299
Awdeh, Z. L., 113, 251, 291

Babson, S. G., 195
Bacteria
   acquisition of, by infants, 132, 229–232
   file, 88
   rates of intestinal infection by, 242–247
Bacteroides, 230, 231, 232, 233
Bailes de la Conquista, 50
Bailey, K. V., 209
Baltimore Biological Laboratory (BBL), 79
Banco de Guatemala, 86
Bang, F. B., 237
Beans, black
   consumption of, 30, 34, 104, 106, 109, 206, 207, 286
   cultivation of, 17, 18, 19, 21, 22, 300
   nutritive value of, 106–111
Beck, D. M., 244, 246, 247
Béhar, M., 56, 163, 170, 257, 299, 303
Behrhorst, C., 169
Beisel, W. R., 113, 277, 278, 293
Bengoa, J. M., 166
Benyesh-Melnick, M., 81
Bergner, L., 143

Beteta, C., 167
Beveridge, W. I. B., 90
Bifidobacteria, 209, 229-233
Biomedical Computer Programs (BMD), 44, 87, 311
Birth interval
  fertility and, 101, 227
  fetal growth and, 138, 142-143, 147, 149, 150-151
  and growth of infants, 227, 305, 310, 312-318
  and weaning, 207, 208
Birth order, fetal growth and, 138, 141, 147, 149, 151
Birth process, 62-63, 98, 115-118, 122-123, 229, 253
Birth rates, 34-39, 46, 55-57
Birth records, 55-57
Birth weight. *See also* Fetal growth
  comparison with industrialized nations, 126, 130, 132, 135, 150, 164-166
  data on, collection of, 121, 346-361
  fetal growth and, 137, 152
  and gestational age, 132-136, 137-151, 152-166, 169-201, 321
  and growth and development in infancy and childhood, 169-201, 220, 304, 305, 321-325
  infant mortality and, 132, 155-159, 164-166
  infection and, 127-132, 264-265
  low (LBW), incidence and implications of, 122, 126, 132-136, 137-151, 152-166, 321
  and maternal factors, 137-151
  and serum immunoglobulins, 129-132
  survival during infancy and early childhood and, 151, 152-166
Bjerkedal, T., 132
Blackwell, R. Q., 143
Blanco, R. A., 192
Blood groups, distribution of, 25
Boeing Computer Facility, 86
Bossak, H. N., 84
Breast-feeding
  and fertility, 99, 101, 208, 226, 227
  and growth and development in infancy and early childhood, 151, 222-227, 253, 302, 305, 310-312, 315, 318
  and maternal health and nutrition, 143, 226, 312
  and newborn survival, 151, 227, 253
  practices, 69-70, 118-120, 165, 202-205, 207-208, 272, 300, 322, 325
  weaning, growth, and, 222-227, 302
  and weaning process, 205-209

Breast milk, nutritional and immune properties of, 69, 110, 209-212, 229, 232-233, 236, 253, 302, 310-312, 317, 318, 322, 325. *See also* Foods, supplemental
Bressani, R., 106, 206, 295
Bronchopneumonia. *See* Respiratory disease
Brucella, 84, 112

Cáceres, A., 84, 112, 128, 265
Cakchiquel, 24, 32, 48, 56
Calcium, intake of
  by children, 71, 217, 219, 295
  by pregnant women, 69, 106-111
Calories
  deficiencies in, 257, 295, 302-303, 322
  intake of, 68
    by children, 34, 70-71, 211-217, 220-223, 322
    and physical growth of infants and children, 214-226, 305, 311, 317, 322
    by pregnant women, 34, 69, 106-111, 144
Candida albicans, 83
Carbonated beverages, purchase of, 21, 34
Casey, H. L., 84
Castro, F., 273
CDC 6400 Users Guide, 87
Center for Disease Control (CDC), 83, 273
Central America, health and population problems of, 3-4, 111, 121, 323, 330, 331
Central American Food Composition Table, 68, 104
Chandra, R. K., 132, 166, 291
Charles, D., 113
Chase, H. C., 165
Chávez, A., 70, 209, 226
Cherkin, D. C., 91
Children, base population (465), annual cohorts of. *See also* Infants; Newborns
  anemia in, 293-295, 302
  anthropometry of, 67, 121-127, 346-361
  birth rates of, 34-39
  birth weights of (*see* Birth weight)
  cohort (45) (*see* Cohort Children)
  control (54) (*see* Control Children)
  death rates of, 34-39, 132, 155-159, 302-303
  diet and feeding practices of, 69-71, 202-227
  disease in (*see* Disease, infectious)

Children, base population (*continued*)
  economic role of, 17, 18
  enrollment and observation of, 4, 59–
    60, 62-64, 67
  growth and development of, 151, 167–
    201, 295-297, 302-303, 304-318
  infection in, 75-76, 127-133
  injury in, 71-75, 258-259, 270
  and intestinal colonization and infection,
    228-253
  maternal interaction with, 98, 118-120,
    165, 203, 207, 227, 314
  survival of, 151, 152-166, 302-303
Chilomastix mesnili, 236, 239, 240
Christmas, celebration of, 50
Ciba Foundation, 132
Climate, 7, 16-17, 24, 110, 209, 257, 300
Clostridia, 229, 230, 231
Clothing, 23, 25, 56, 60
Cofradías, 27, 50, 205
Cohort children
  diseases in, 254-292
  enrollment and observation of, 4, 59–
    60, 63-64
  hemoglobin values in, 294
  intestinal colonization and infection in,
    239-253
  multivariate analyses of, 307-318
  PCM in, 297-302
  physical growth of, 60, 294-297
  supplemental food intake of, 205-208
Collaborative Perinatal Study, 114
Contraception, 99, 208
Contreras, C., 209
Control children, enrollment and obser-
    vation of, 59-60
Conversational Computer Statistical
    System (CCSS), 44, 85, 86-87
Cook, R., 299
Corsa, L., 132
Courtship, 29-30
Coverage, continuous, of village popula-
    tion, 43, 46
Cuerdas, 18, 19
Cultural characteristics, 25-32, 60-61,
    324
Curanderos, 27, 51, 55

Dale, D. C., 78, 83, 250
Data
  collection of, 54-91, 115, 121-123, 127,
    132, 152, 159
  computer analyses of, 54, 86-87
  ethical aspects of use of, 50, 54-55
  facilities for, 44-45
  files, 87-89

  statistical analysis and biological inter-
    pretation of, 89-91
  variables, list of, 342-344
Davies, P. A., 132
Deacon, W. E., 84
Death. *See also* Mortality
  causes of, 159-163, 299, 301
  rates, 34-39, 46, 55-57, 155-159
  records, 55-57
Diarrheal disease. *See also* Intestine, in-
    fection and colonization of
  birth weight and, 155
  case fatality in, 161-164, 208
  data on, collection of, 55-56
  duration and severity of, 270, 289-290
  epidemics of, 34-35, 246, 272-273
  epidemiologic behavior of, 272-273
  and growth, 306, 315
  impact on nutrition of, 110, 227, 277,
    280, 286-291, 301-302
  rates of, 111, 114-115, 259-265
  treatment of, 270-272
Dientamoeba, 242
  fragilis, 111, 242, 243, 305
Diet. *See also* Foods, supplemental; Mal-
    nutrition; Nutrition-infection inter-
    action
  deficiencies in, 34, 109-111, 257, 322
  and fetal growth, 109-111, 143-144,
    150-151
  file, 89
  and growth and development in infancy
    and early childhood, 179, 196, 209–
    227, 304-305, 317-318
  of infants and young children, 69-71,
    202-227, 322
  and newborn survival, 165, 227
  of pregnant women, 67-68, 98, 102,
    104-111, 113, 143-144, 150-151,
    324
Dingle, J. H., 256
Diplococcus, 80
Disease, infectious. *See also* Infection;
    Intestine, infection and colonization
    of
  case fatalities from, 159-164
  code for, 337-341
  data on, collection of, 55-56, 71-75
  defined, 256
  duration and severity of, 270
  epidemiologic behavior of, 272-277
  fetal growth and, 145-147
  and growth and development in infancy
    and early childhood, 179, 196, 220–
    222, 304-318
  malnutrition and outcome of, 3-4, 161–
    166, 277-292, 299-303, 321-322

Disease, infectious (continued)
  nutrition and, 3-4, 98, 161-166, 220,
    227, 257-258, 277-393, 321-322
  rates of, 111-115, 159-164, 259-265
  symptoms of, 256-257, 264, 265-270,
    341
  treatment and prevention of, 51-53, 74,
    270-272, 325, 329, 341
  in twins, history of, 254-256
  village imagery of, 29-29
Disease, noninfectious, 258-259
Dubos, R., 228, 229
Dunnebacke, T. H., 80
Duncan, B., 172
Dysentery. See Diarrheal disease

Earthquake, destruction of Santa María
    Cauqué by, 35
Economy, 17-23, 30-32, 35, 56, 60-61,
    110, 323, 324, 326-330
Education, 6, 32, 33, 56, 60-61, 99, 253,
    291, 295, 304, 318, 323, 324, 326-
    327, 329
Edwards, P. R., 78, 79
EEC. See Escherichia coli
Eichenwald, H. F., 132
Electricity, availability of, 12, 45, 46, 61,
    327
Emanuel, I., 132
Endogamy, high rate of, 25
Endolimax nana, 235, 236, 240
Energy crisis, effect of, 17, 21, 217, 323
Entamoeba coli, 111, 239, 240
Entamoeba histolytica, 111, 235, 238,
    239, 240, 242, 248, 249, 265-266,
    280, 306, 309, 312, 314, 315, 316,
    318
Enteric viruses. See Enteroviruses
Enterobacteriaceae, 229, 231, 236
Enterobius, 242
Enterococci, 232
Enteromonas hominis, 236
Enteroviruses, 80-83, 84, 111, 117, 236,
    248, 252, 265, 305, 306, 309, 314,
    315
Epidemics: 34-38, 59, 257
  of acute respiratory disease, 34-35
  of diarrhea and dysentery, 34-35, 246,
    272-273
  of measles, 34-35
  of protein-calorie malnutrition, 302
  of whooping cough, 34-35, 38, 52, 161,
    274
Erhardt, C. L., 132
Escherichia coli, 229-233, 235, 237, 302
  enteropathogenic (EEC), 78, 79, 83,
    236, 247, 248, 251

Ethnicity, 21-25, 56
Eubacteria, 209, 232-233
Evans, D. J., 302
Ewing, W. H., 78, 79

Fábrega, H., 254
Falkner, F., 195
Family planning measures, 99, 101, 227,
    253, 324-326, 329
Fanaroff, A. A., 165
FAO. See Food and Agriculture Organi-
    zation
Faulk, W.P., 113, 251, 270, 291
Feces. See Hygiene and sanitary practices;
    Intestine, infection and colonization
    of; Laboratory procedures
Feeding practices. See Diet
Fertility
  effect of breast-feeding on, 99, 101, 208,
    226, 318
  of Indians, 24
  of village women, 99, 101
Fetal growth. See also Growth
  assessment of, 121, 137-151
  birth interval and, 138, 142-143
  infection and, 112-113
  maternal variables and, 110, 112-113,
    137-151, 199, 324-325
  retardation (FGR), 113, 121, 135, 158,
    161, 188, 304, 314, 321
  survival and, 152-166, 321
Field operations
  concept and approach, 4, 43-44
  and continuous coverage of village popu-
    lation, 43, 46
  and establishment of rapport, 43, 48-
    51, 52, 54-55, 56-57, 60, 68
  physical and administrative support facili-
    ties for, 43, 44-47
  and provision of services, 38-39, 43, 46,
    48, 51-53, 61, 123, 165-166
  recruitment of staff for, 43, 48
  six fundamentals of, 43-44, 126
  systematic supervision of, 43, 46, 48
Field procedures, 4, 55-76. See also Data;
    Laboratory procedures
Finland, M., 113
Fitzhardinge, P. M., 132
Flores, M., 7, 34, 37, 51, 68, 70, 104, 111,
    217
Fogón, 15, 16
Food and Agriculture Organization
    (FAO), 214, 298
Food crops, 17, 18-20, 22
Foods, supplemental. See also Diet;
    Weaning
  and growth and development, 217-227,

Foods, supplemental (*continued*) 253, 311, 318, 322, 324–326
  intake of, by breast-fed infants, 202–207
  nutritive value of, for breast-fed children, 211–217, 302–303
Fox, J. P., 84, 86, 228, 256
Friedman, E. A., 113
Fudenberg, H. H., 127, 129

Gangarosa, E. J., 246, 273
García, B., 6, 202
Garn, S. M., 192
Gelfand, H. M., 131, 228, 236
Gestational age (GAGE). *See also* Fetal growth
  and birth weight, 132–136, 137–151, 152–166, 169–201, 321
  data on, collection of, 121, 356–361
  defined, 98, 122
  and growth and development in infancy and childhood, 132–136, 169–201
  infant mortality and, 155–158
  maternal factors and, 137–151
  and serum immunoglobulins, 129–132
  survival during infancy and early childhood and, 152–166
Giardia lamblia, 111, 235, 236, 239, 240, 241, 242, 248–249, 251–252, 265–266, 280, 306, 309, 314
Gibbons, R. J., 252
Gibson, J. R., 164
Giroud, A., 150
Gitlin, D., 129
Goldman, A. S., 209–212, 227
Goldstein, H., 132
Gómez, F. R., 257
Gopalan, C., 209
Gopalan, G., 217, 303
Gorbach, S. L., 229, 237
Gordon, J. E., 4, 43, 163, 164, 227, 233, 244, 246, 247, 254, 270, 272, 273, 291, 303
Gordon, M., 98, 111, 114
Greenhill, J. D., 113
Greenwald, P., 150
Greulich, W. W., 191
Growth. *See also* Fetal growth
  and birth weight, 132–136, 155, 169–201
  breast-feeding, weaning, and, 222–227
  comparison with industrialized countries, 179, 183
  curves, 179, 196–201
  and development in infancy and early childhood, 167–210, 222–227, 304–318, 331–324
  and disease, 258, 277–292

and gestational age, 132–136, 167–201
and infection, 112–113, 252–253
and malnutrition, 293–303, 304–305
and maternal variables, 111, 200–201, 226–227
multivariate analysis of, 89–90, 304–318
supplemental foods and, 214–222
of twins, 192–196

Guaro, 50
Guatemala, 7, 21, 34, 323, 326, 328, 329, 330
  Central Government of, 6, 25, 51–52, 57
  City, 7, 20, 21, 44, 46
  Department of, 20, 21
  Ministry of Health of, 51
Güipil, 23, 204, 205
Guzmán, M. A., 169, 170

Habicht, J. P., 170
Hall, C. E., 228
Hanshaw, J. B., 84
Hansman, C., 172, 295
Hardy, J. B., 132, 166
Harris, A., 84
Harvard School of Public Health, 4, 172
Health Center, village, 6, 7, 36–38, 45, 46, 48, 50, 51–52, 72, 74
Height. *See* Anthropometry, physical
Hematology, 84
Hemoglobin values, 294–294, 302
Herpesviruses, 84, 131, 133, 261, 263
Hollister, A. C., 244, 292
Housing, 7, 9, 10–12, 15, 21, 56, 60–61, 98, 324
Howie, R. N., 124
Hurtado, J. J., 126
Hydropexia, 56
Hygiene and sanitary practices, 6, 12–17, 33, 56, 112, 150–151, 252–253, 317, 323–327, 329

Illness. *See* Disease; Infection; Intestine, infection and colonization of
Immunization, 51, 52, 163, 165–166, 253, 257, 303, 324–326, 329
Immunoglobulins, 84, 265
  file, 88
  secretory, levels and significance of, 84, 209, 212, 227, 252
  serum, levels and significance of, 111–112, 127–132, 145–147, 160–161, 265, 267, 270
Impetigo, 259, 270, 277
INCAP. *See* Institute of Nutrition of Central America and Panama
Indians, 6, 17, 21–25, 27, 33, 48, 50, 51,

Indians (*continued*)
  57, 58, 59, 95, 169, 321, 323, 324,
  326, 330
Infanticide, absence of, 56
Infants (first year of life)
  anemia in, 293–295, 302
  anthropometry of, 346–361
  diet of, 202–227
  growth and development of, 169–201
  and intestinal colonization and infection,
    228–253
  malnutrition in, 293–303
  mortality of, 55–56, 164–166, 302–303
  survival of, 152–166, 302–303
Infection. *See also* Disease; Nutrition-
    infection interaction
  and anemia, 293
  and birth weight, 127–132, 143–144,
    147, 265
  code for, 337–341
  and colonization of the intestine, 228–
    253
  and growth and development in infancy
    and early childhood, 101, 179, 196,
    304–318, 321–323, 325–326, 328,
    329
  prevalence of
    among mothers, 229
    among newborns, 127–132, 145–147,
      229–230
    among pregnant women, 111–115,
      145–147, 150
  relation between nutrition and, 3–4, 98,
    113, 143, 150–151, 277–286, 293
  symptoms of, 341
  treatment for, 341
Injuries, 71–75, 258–259, 270, 337–341
Institute of Nutrition of Central America
    and Panama (INCAP), 6–7, 16, 36–
    37, 44–45, 46, 51, 61, 169, 170, 242,
    259, 293, 295, 298, 303
  dietary recommendations of, 68, 69, 71,
    107, 108, 109, 211, 217
  Nutrition-Infection Study of, 7, 36–37,
    45, 51, 274
Institutional Guide to HEW Policy of Pro-
    tection of Human Subjects, 54
Inter-American Highway, 6, 7
International Committee for Standardi-
    zation in Hematology, 294
International Investigation of Childhood
    Mortality, 164
Intertrigo, 259
Interventions, alternatives and considera-
    tions of possible, 38–39, 90–91, 150–
    151, 166, 201, 227, 252–253, 291–
    292, 302–303, 318, 321–331

Intestine, infection and colonization of.
    See also Diarrheal disease
  data on, collection of, 75–76
  defined, 228
  rates and significance of, 111, 228–253,
    258
  sources of, 117–120, 228–253
Iron, intake of
  by children, 71, 211–214, 293–295
  by pregnant women, 69, 106–111

Jackson, E. C., 150
Jackson, R. L., 170
Johnson, K. M., 237
Johnston, F. E., 179
Joplin, C., 85
Jurado-García, E., 95

Katz, S. H., 295
Kelly, G., 170
Kennedy, W. P., 124
Kennell, J. H., 120
Kinch, R. A. H., 150
Klaus, M. H., 120, 165
Kloene, W., 237
Kronmal, R. A., 85, 86, 202, 305
Kwashiorkor (K), 56, 161, 257, 259,
    298–302
  marasmic (M–K), 298–300

Laboratory procedures, 44, 45, 46, 47, 50,
    52, 62, 76, 78–85. *See also* Field
    procedures
Lactating women
  diet of, 109–111
  pregnancy among, 208
Ladinos, 21–25, 27, 57, 58, 59, 208, 326,
    328, 330
Laga, E. M., 129
Land
  cultivation of, 7, 17–21, 24, 31, 56, 110,
    327–328, 329
  ownership of, 12, 18–19, 21, 22, 25, 34,
    56, 60–61, 324, 327, 330
Latrines, 12, 16, 33, 52, 60–61
Lechtig, A., 84, 113, 126, 127, 132, 143,
    265
Lennette, E. H., 78, 81
Levinson, F. J., 303
Lim, K. A., 81
Lin, C. C., 132
Literacy, 33, 56
Live births. *See also* Newborns
  defined, 98, 122
  number of, 58, 59, 99, 122
Livestock, 12, 18, 20, 22, 56, 60–61, 99,
    327

Love, E. J., 150
Low birth weight. *See* Birth weight
Lubchenco, L. O., 132, 135
Luna-Jaspe, G. H., 55

McGregor, I. A., 265
McKeown, T., 164
Maize. *See also* Tortillas
  cultivation of, 17, 18, 19, 20, 30, 300
  consumption of, 34, 207, 286
  nutritive value of, 106-111, 217, 295
  preparation of, 30, 68, 205
Malcolm, L. A., 196
Malnutrition. *See also* Nutrition-infection
    interaction
  and anemia, 293-295
  classification of, 257-258
  data on, collection of, 55-56
  and fertility, 99
  and fetal growth, 137-151
  and growth and development in infancy
      and early childhood, 101, 150-151,
      293, 295-296, 318, 321-323
  and infectious disease, 3, 55, 161-166,
      251, 277-292, 293-303
  protein-calorie (PCM)
    case fatalities in, 161-163
    epidemic of, 302
    incidence of, 257, 258-259, 270, 293,
        298-302
    and physical growth, 293
    role in infectious disease of, 161-164,
        258, 299-300
    severe forms of, 298-302
    treatment of, 51, 270
  and survival, 158, 163-166
Mancini, G., 84
Marasmus, 161, 257, 258, 298-302
Marriage, 29-30, 95, 151
Martinez, C., 70, 209, 226
Mata, L. J., 37, 46, 48, 52, 78, 79, 80, 83,
    84, 86, 90, 102, 111, 112, 113, 117,
    118, 127, 132, 143, 147, 169, 170,
    179, 209, 212, 214, 229, 233, 236,
    237, 238, 242, 244, 246, 247, 250-
    251, 265, 270, 272, 273, 281, 291
Maternal environment (matroenviron-
    ment), concept and significance of,
    95-120, 137-151, 157-166, 200-
    201, 226-227, 229, 302, 314-318,
    321-323, 324-325, 329. *See also*
    Mothers
Maternal health, defined, 137. *See also*
    Fetal growth; Maternal environment;
    Mothers
Maternal-infant interaction, 98, 118-120,
    165, 203, 207, 227, 314

Maternal variables. *See* Maternal environ-
    ment
Mean corpuscular hemoglobin concentra-
    tion (MCHC), 294-295
Measles
  case fatality in, 55-56, 161-163, 272
  duration and severity of, 270-272, 289
  epidemics of, 34-35
  epidemiologic behavior of, 273-274
  nutrition and impact on, 279-282,
      286-291, 301-302
  rates of, 262, 263
  treatment of, 53, 272
  vaccine for, 52, 163
Mejía, W., 226
Melnick, J. L., 80
Melvin, D. M., 238
Men
  birth and death rates of, 34-39, 55-57
  daily activities and role of, 22, 25-26,
      27, 29, 30, 31
Menchú, M. T., 68, 71
Méndez, J., 169
Mendizábal, C. A., 273
Meredith, H. V., 172
MGDP (mean gross domestic product),
    decline of, 20-23
Microbiology, 80-83
Midwifes, role of
  in birth process, 115-118, 122-123, 142
  in study, 48-49, 61, 99, 115, 121, 123,
      127
Milanesi, M. C., 165
Minifundios, 17
Ministriles, 25, 48, 50, 54
Monif, G. R. G., 131, 132
Monto, A. S., 237, 256
Moore, A. E., 80
Morbidity. *See also* Disease
  code, 71, 72-74
  file, 89
  maternal, and fetal growth, 145-147
  rates, 258, 260-263
  among village women, 98, 113-115
Mortality, 34-37
  causes of, 159-163
  in early childhood, 158, 304
  infant, 155-158
    comparison with industrialized nations,
        164-166
Mothers, 95-98. *See also* Fetal growth;
    Maternal environment; Pregnant
    women
  and birth process, 115-118
  diet of, 103, 104-111
  infection among, 111-115, 145-147,
      229

Mothers (*continued*)
  interaction between infants and, 98,
    118-120
  morbidity among, 113-115, 145-147
  obstetric history of, 98, 99-101
  physical anthropometry of, 101-104,
    137-151
  socioeconomic level of, 98-99, 103, 138,
    145-146, 149-151
Multivariate analyses, 89-90, 304-318
Mycobacterium, 80

Narasinga-Rao, B. S., 214
National Academy of Sciences, 68
National Center for Health Statistics
  (NCHS), 164
National Institutes of Health (NIH), 54,
  83
National Research Council (NRC), Food
  and Nutrition Board of, 68
Naturales, 24
Nelson, D. P., 83
Neva, F. A., 80
Newborns
  anthropometry of, 121-127
    as function of maternal variables,
    137-151
  birth weights of, 137-151
  enrollment and observation of, 58, 59-
    60, 61, 62-64
  file on, 88
  gestational age of, 137-151
  growth and development of, 95-98,
    137-151, 183-192, 305, 318
  infection in, 117-120, 127-133
  and intestinal colonization and infection,
    228-253
  survival of, 95-98, 137-151, 152-166
Niacin, intake of
  by children, 71, 211-214, 217-218, 295
  by pregnant women, 69, 106-111, 144
Niswander, J. D., 135
Niswander, K. R., 98, 111, 114
Nixtamal, 30, 295
Nutrient intake. *See* Diet
Nutrition education, significance of, 217,
  227, 291, 298, 300, 326, 329
Nutrition-infection interaction, 3-4, 38-
  39, 161-166, 220, 227-292, 293-
  303, 318, 321-323, 325
Nutrition-Infection Study, 7, 37, 45, 51,
  274

Oberndorfer, L., 226
Obstetrical experience, 61-62, 98, 99-101,
  113, 115-118, 122-123, 141-142

Occupations, 31-32
Olson, L. C., 237
Oratorio, 12, 15
Ota, W., 237
Otzoy, S., 12
Ounsted, M., 132

Palmer, D. F., 84
Pan American Health Organization
  (PAHO), 44, 86, 164, 293
Parasites, 80, 83, 89, 111, 132, 238-242
Parity
  defined, 98
  and fetal growth, 141-142
  and growth of children, 305, 310, 313,
    316
Parks, W. P., 237
Parrilla-Ríos, C. M., 292
Participation, 48-50, 51, 54-55, 58-60.
  See also Rapport, establishment of,
    between staff and villagers
Pathogens, early invasion by, 235-236
Patroness's Day, celebration of, 27, 50
PCM (protein-calorie malnutrition). *See*
  Malnutrition
Petate, 33
Phillips, D. S., 195
Piñatas, 50
Plank, S. J., 165
Pneumonia. *See* Respiratory disease
Polioviruses, 81, 112, 133, 248, 254
Politics, village involvement in, 25-26, 44,
  48, 50, 54
Population
  data on, collection of, 54-57
  estimates, 55
  file, 88
  growth, 24, 24-39, 321, 323, 324,
    327-328
  target, 57-60
Pradilla, A., 292
Pregnancy. *See* Mothers; Pregnant women
Pregnant women. *See also* Mothers;
    Obstetrical experience
  diet and feeding practices of, 34, 67-68,
    103, 104-111, 143-144, 150-151
  enrollment and observation of, 58-59,
    61-62, 98
  and fetal growth, 137-151
  illness in, 145-147, 150, 340
  physical anthropometry of, 64, 101-103
Premature delivery, low birth weight and.
  See Birth weight
Preterm infant, defined, 122. *See also*
  Gestational age
Primipara, defined, 98

Priorities, recognition of, 326–330
Protein, intake of
   by children, 34, 70–71, 211–214, 217–
      220
   and physical growth of infants and chil-
      dren, 214–226
   by pregnant women, 34, 69, 106–111,
      144
   deficiencies in, 257, 295, 303
Protein-calorie malnutrition. *See* Mal-
   nutrition
Puerperal fever, absence of, 113
Puffer, R. R., 164, 165
Pulique, 30
Pyle, S. I., 191

Quetzal, 21

Rao, K. S. J., 209
Rapport, establishment of, between staff
   and villagers, 43, 46, 48–51, 52, 54–
   55, 56–57, 60, 68
Regression analyses, step-wise (SWRAs),
   149–151
   with parameters of fitted growth curve,
      200–201
   for physical growth, 305–307, 311, 315
Reh, E., 7, 34, 37, 51, 111
Religious activities, 12, 27, 29, 30, 50
Remington, J. S., 84
Respiratory disease
   case fatality in, 161–164, 272
   data on, collection of, 56, 159
   duration and severity of, 270, 289–290
   epidemics of, 34–35
   and growth, 306, 309, 310–313, 318
   and nutrition, impact on, 277, 279, 280,
      286, 301–302
   rates of, 114, 131, 159–164, 259–265
   treatment of, 272
Riboflavin, intake of
   by children, 71, 209, 211–214, 220, 293
   by pregnant women, 69, 106–111, 144
Ritchie, L. S., 83
Rohmann, C. G., 192
Rosa, F. W., 132, 143
Rosales, L., 27
Rosebury, T., 117, 229
Rosen, L., 84
Rowe, D. S., 112, 265
Royal Victoria Hospital, The (Quebec,
   Canada), 165
Rubella, 84, 112, 263, 270, 277

Sabin, A. B., 236
Sacatepéquez, Department of, 7, 20, 21,
   25

Salmonella, 78–79, 83, 111, 233
   antibodies to, investigation of, 84
   duration of, 251
   intestinal infection by, rates of, 247
Salomon, J. B., 289
Sanitation, 6, 12–17, 33, 52, 56, 60–61,
   99, 112, 150–151, 209, 227, 252–
   253, 277, 291, 317, 323–327, 329
Sanjur, D. M., 226
Santa María Cauqué
   climate of, 7, 16–17, 24
   economy of, 17–23, 24, 30–32, 35, 56,
      60–61, 110, 323, 324, 326–330
   government of, 25, 48, 50, 54
   history of, 6
   housing in, 7, 9, 10–12, 15, 56, 60–61,
      98, 324
   location of, 7–8
   sanitation in, 6, 12–17, ⌐, 56, 60–61,
      99, 112, 150–151, 209, 227, 252–
      253, 291, 317, 323–327, 329
Santa María Cauqué, people of
   birth and death rates of, 34–37, 55–57
   clothing of, 23, 25, 56, 60
   diet of, 6, 20, 21, 34
   education of, 32, 33, 56, 60–61
   ethnicity of, 21–25, 56
   hygiene and sanitary practices of, 6, 12–
      17, 33, 56, 60–61, 112, 150–151,
      252–253, 317, 323–327, 329
   population growth among, 34–39, 55–
      57, 324
   social and cultural characteristics of, 18,
      25–32, 50, 56, 60–61, 98
Santiago Sacatepéquez, 55, 57, 99
Schaedler, R. E., 80
Schistosoma, 242
Schmidt, N. J., 78, 81
Scrimshaw, N. S., 4, 7, 16, 37, 51, 206,
   227, 272, 274, 277, 289, 291
SECI. *See* Socioeconomic Index
Serological procedures, 84
Serrano, C. V., 164, 165
Services, provision of, 38–39, 43, 45, 46,
   48, 51–53, 61, 123, 165–166
Sever, J. L., 111, 114
Sex differences
   and anthropometric differences, 124–
      126, 138, 147, 149, 150
   by birth, 56–57, 122
   and deaths, 160
   and disease, 263, 270
   and growth and development in infancy
      and early childhood, 174, 179, 191–
      192, 305
   and kwashiorkor, 299
   and weaning, 205, 208

Shattuck, G. C., 34, 257
Shiga dysentery
  epidemics of, 246, 272–273
  treatment of, 272
Shigella, 78–79, 83, 84, 233, 280
  boydii, 244, 247, 250, 306, 309, 314
  chronicity and duration of, 248–251
  dysenteriae, 244, 245, 246, 247, 250,
    273, 306, 309, 314
  flexneri, 244, 245, 247, 250, 306, 309,
    314, 315, 316, 318
  infection rates of, 265–266
  prevalence of, 111, 118, 236, 242–247,
    265
  sonnei, 244, 250, 305, 306, 309, 314,
    315
Singletons. *See also* Newborns
  anthropometry of, 124–127
  number of, 59, 117, 122
Size
  body, importance of, 167
  maternal and infant, correlation be-
    tween, 138–141
Skin disorders, noninfectious, 258, 259
Smith, C. W., 209–212, 227
Smith, D., 189
Smith, G. H., 20, 21
Social characteristics, 25–32
Socioeconomic Index (SECI)
  computation of, 57, 60–61
  and maternal variables, 98–99, 103, 138,
    145–146, 149–151, 201, 305, 317
  and newborn variables, 138, 145–146,
    149–151
Socioeconomic status, maternal, 98–99
  and fetal growth, 145
  and PCM, 302
Solien-González, N. L., 27
Spanish, 6, 24, 32, 33, 323
Staff
  list, 333–334
  rapport between villagers and, 43, 46,
    48, 51, 52, 61
  recruitment of, 43, 48
  services performed by (*see* Services)
  supervision of, 46
Staphylococcus aureus, 235
Statistical Package for the Social Sciences
  (SPSS), 44–45, 87, 311
Steven, E. M., 132
Stewart, R. J. C., 150
Stiehm, E. R., 127, 129
Stillbirth
  defined, 98, 122
  number, 37, 59, 99, 100, 113, 122, 124
Streptococci, 229–230, 231, 232
Streptococcus pneumoniae, 280

Stuart, H. C., 172
Sukhatme, P. V., 303
Supervision of field operations, sys-
    tematic, 43, 46, 48
Support facilities, physical and adminis-
    trative, for field operations, 43, 44–
    47
Survival, during infancy and early child-
    hood. *See also* Mortality
  birth weight and, 123, 152–166
  disease and, 159–166
  gestational age and, 152–166
  malnutrition and, 163–166
  maternal factors and, 150–151
Suspensions, 80
Susser, M., 132, 143

Tanner, J. M., 150, 196
Tapesco, 33
Taylor, C. E., 4, 132
Temascales, 12–13, 15, 16, 33, 118, 203
Term infant (T), defined, 122. *See also*
  Gestational age
Thiamin, intake of
  by children, 71, 211–214
  by pregnant women, 106–111
Thomson, A. M., 150
Tortillas. *See also* Maize
  consumption of, 30, 106, 206, 207,
    285–286
  nutritive value of, 69, 106–111, 295
  preparation of, 30, 64, 295
Towbin, A., 159
Toxoplasma, 112, 131, 133
  gondii, 84, 132
Treponema pallidum, 84, 112, 132
Trichinella, 242
Trichuris, 111, 240, 242, 306, 309, 314
Tuj. *See* Temascales
Turshen, M., 132, 143
Twins
  anthropometry of, 124–127
  deaths among, 149–160
  growth and development of, 192–196
  infectious disease in, 231–232, 254–256,
    286–289
  number of, 59, 117, 122
Tyrrell, D. A. J., 256

Ullman, B. M., 256
University of Kansas School of Medicine,
  84
University of Washington, 84, 87
  computer analysis of data at, 44–45, 86,
    91
Urrutia, J. J., 79, 85, 167, 209, 233, 254,
  270, 273

US Department of Agriculture, 84
US Department of Health, Education, and Welfare (HEW), 54, 126, 164
Usher, R., 165

Vaccines. *See* Immunization
Valverde, V., 217, 303
Van Zijl, W. J., 244
Varicella, 270, 277, 289
Veillonellae, 230, 231, 232
Viruses, 80-83, 84, 132, 248
Vitamin A (retinol)
  deficiences of, 293, 295
  intake of, 68
    by children, 70-71, 211-212, 217, 220
    by pregnant women, 69, 106-111
Viteri, F. E., 293, 295

Waterlow, J. C., 298, 303
Weaning. *See also* Breast milk, nutritional and immune properties of; Foods, supplemental
  age, 205, 217, 305, 310, 312-315, 317-318
  breast-feeding, growth, and, 222-227, 253, 302-303, 305, 310, 312-315, 317-318, 322, 325, 329
  process, 205-209, 329
  and survival, 165
Weatley, W. B., 83
Wegman, M. E., 164
Weight. *See* Anthropometry, physical; Birth weight
Weiss, W., 150
Weld, J. T., 78, 83
Weller, T. H., 80
Wenner, H. A., 84
Whooping cough
  case fatality in, 55, 161-163, 272
  data on, collection of, 55-56
  duration and severity of, 270-272, 289, 290
  epidemics of, 34-35, 38, 52, 161
  epidemiologic behavior of, 274-275
  and nutrition, impact on, 281-283, 286-291
  rates of, 262, 263
  treatment of, 53
  vaccine for, 52, 163
Wiener, G., 132
Williams, R. C., 252
Women
  birth and death rates of, 34-39, 55-57
  daily activities and role of, 17, 25, 27, 29, 30-31
World Health Organization (WHO), 126, 214, 294, 298

World Medical Association, 54
Wyatt, R. G., 84, 209, 212, 227, 233

Yerushalmy, J., 135
Younger, J. S., 80

Zitcer, E. M., 80